Protocols for Neural Cell Culture

©1997 Humana Press Inc.
999 Riverview Drive, Suite 208
Totowa, New Jersey 07512

For additional copies, pricing for bulk purchases, and /or information about Humana titles, contact Humana at the above address or at any of the following numbers: Tel: 201-256-1699; Fax: 201-256-8341; E-mail: humana@interramp.com

This publication is printed on acid-free paper. ⊗
ANSI Z39.48-1984 (American National Standards Institute
Permanence of Paper for Printed Library Materials

Cover illustration: Figure 4C in Chapter 2, "Microexplant Cultures of the Cerebellum," by Bernard Rogister and Gustave Moonen.

Cover design by Patricia F. Cleary.

Printed in the United States of America. 10 9 8 7 6 5 4 3 2 1

Library of Congress Cataloging-in-Publication Data

Protocols for Neural Cell Culture / edited by Sergey Fedoroff and Arleen Richardson—2nd ed.
    p.   cm.
   Includes bibliographical references and index.
   ISBN 0-89603-454-2 (alk. paper)
   1. Nerve tissue—Cultures and culture media—Laboratory manuals. 2. Neurons—Growth—Laboratory manuals. I. Fedoroff, Sergey. II. Richardson, Arleen.
   [DNLM: 1. Nerve Tissue—cytology—laboratory manuals. 2. Tissue Culture—methods—laboratory manuals. 3. Neurons—cytology—laboratory manuals.WL 25 P967]
   QP356.25.P765 1992
   611'.0188—dc20
   DNLM/DLC
   for Library of Congress   92-1532
                                               CIP

Protocols for Neural Cell Culture

Protocols for Neural Cell Culture

Second Edition

edited by

Sergey Fedoroff and *Arleen Richardson*

Department of Anatomy and Cell Biology, University of Saskatchewan, Saskatoon, Saskatchewan, Canada

Humana Press   **Totowa, New Jersey**

Cover illustration: Figure 4C in Chapter 2, "Microexplant Cultures of the Cerebellum," by Bernard Rogister and Gustave Moonen.

Cover design by Patricia F. Cleary.

Printed in the United States of America. 10 9 8 7 6 5 4 3 2 1

Library of Congress Cataloging-in-Publication Data

Protocols for Neural Cell Culture / edited by Sergey Fedoroff and Arleen Richardson—2nd ed.
    p. cm.
    Includes bibliographical references and index.
    ISBN 0-89603-454-2 (alk. paper)
    1. Nerve tissue—Cultures and culture media—Laboratory manuals. 2. Neurons—Growth—Laboratory manuals. I. Fedoroff, Sergey. II. Richardson, Arleen.
    [DNLM: 1. Nerve Tissue—cytology—laboratory manuals. 2. Tissue Culture—methods—laboratory manuals. 3. Neurons—cytology—laboratory manuals.WL 25 P967]
    QP356.25.P765 1992
    611'.0188—dc20
    DNLM/DLC
    for Library of Congress   92-1532
                                                                           CIP

Preface

In recent years tissue culture has become one of the major methodologies of biomedical research. It has applications in clinical diagnosis, toxicology, and industrial biotechnology. In the future, its usefulness will undoubtedly expand into gene and cell therapies.

Every worker in tissue culture has favorite methods for doing things. The procedures in this book by no means represent the only ways of achieving desired results. However, certain principles prevail. Only proven protocols that are used routinely in well-established laboratories have been selected for the present volume. Most of the protocols have been used successfully for many years in teaching tissue culture at the University of Saskatchewan. Four chapters deal with culturing neurons from the central and peripheral nervous systems and include a protocol for the study of myelination by oligodendrocytes and Schwann cells. Three chapters cover procedures for isolating and growing glia cells, including astrocytes, oligodendrocytes, and microglia from mice, rats, and humans. Protocols for quantification of cells in culture and growth assays, as well as protocols for biological assays for neuroactive agents, are included. Procedures are described for the application of immunocytochemistry to the study of neural cells, the identification of antigens, the preparation of cultures for electron microscopic analysis, and the care and use of dissecting instruments.

To assist users of this volume, we have presented protocols as they are used in the laboratories of origin, even though this has resulted in some duplication and differences in details of similar procedures from chapter to chapter. We believe that good sterile techniques are much more important as preventive measures against contamination than the routine use of antibiotics; therefore, we have avoided inclusion of antibiotics as part of the culture media. We have included general discussion, where appropriate, based on experience gained in our tissue culture laboratory during more than forty years of research and teaching.

This volume is designed to be kept close at hand as a ready reference and a guide to laboratory procedures. It is based on tissue culture manuals used for a number of years at international courses on tissue culture at the University of Saskatchewan, made possible by the generous support of the Canadian Council of Animal Care and the Medical Research Council of Canada.

Sergey Fedoroff
Arleen Richardson

Preface to the Second Edition

The second edition of *Protocols for Neural Cell Culture* adheres to the principles enunciated in the first edition, but the content has been extensively revised and expanded. Two new chapters have been added to reflect the increased interest in the development and differentiation of the nervous system and in the reconstruction of its circuitry in tissue culture. One chapter deals with slice cultures in which the organization of the nervous system is preserved. When slice cultures are combined with explant cultures, afferent and efferent projections can be reconstructed. The other chapter deals with aggregating neural cell cultures, in which "minibrains" can form. Theses are small, uniformly sized spheres of nervous tissue, usually having nerve cells in the center and astrocytes, oligodendrocytes, and microglia in the periphery. Such cultures can be used to study neutral cell interactions in an organized milieu and for qualitative as well as quantitative studies at biochemical and molecular levels.

A new development is the isolation and propagation of progenitor cells that can be stimulated to differentiate into either neurons or various types of glial cells. Two chapters deal with the isolation of neopallial cells and the stimulation of their development into astroglia, microglia, or oligodendroglia. Such cultures can easily be scaled-up and made highly enriched in one cell type.

Highly enriched "pure" cultures of one cell type are often required for the study of a particular cell type or for coculturing with other cell types in order to discern neural cell interactions. We have added a new chapter that reviews a number of procedures for elimination of unwanted (contaminating) neutral or nonneural cells. We have included a chapter on procedures for transfection of cells in culture with nontoxic mutant herpes simplex virus because of the rapid advances in gene therapy as applied to the nervous system, and because nontoxic mutant herpes simplex virus can be used as a vector for transfer of genes to nondividing neurons.

The practical tips gathered together in a new chapter should be useful to those operating a tissue culture laboratory. They will be especially helpful to beginners in the field and serve as reminders to every experienced tissue culturist. As with the first edition, this manual is intended to be a useful, practical companion in the neural cell culture laboratory, and in its improved and expanded version, should be an even more valuable resource.

Sergey Fedoroff
Arleen Richardson

Introduction

The brain, spinal cord, and peripheral ganglia are the epitome of heterogeneous tissues. They contain unique neuronal and glial cells as well as vascular and connective tissue and other miscellaneous cell elements. Glial cells comprise astroglial, oligodendroglial, and microglial cell subsets in the central nervous system or Schwann cells in the peripheral nervous system. Each glial cell subset can be further subdivided based on *in situ* location and phenotypic expression. The categorization of neuronal cell subsets is based on *in situ* criteria, such as anatomical location, developmental age, electrophysiological properties, and molecular expression repertoire. There are perhaps thousands of different neuronal subsets, each with their own particular array of properties and intercellular associations. Any particular property expressed by a neural cell will be controlled to a large extent by molecular signals within the immediate environment. Since environmental signals often change during the life of a cell, the expressed cellular characteristics may also change. The incredible cellular complexity of nervous tissue presents unique problems to the neuroscientist attempting to understand how individual neural cells or cell communities contribute to the proper functioning of the nervous system. Despite the complexities, a driving force in neuroscience research is the belief that a detailed understanding of neural cells will lead to the development of rationales for treating the unacceptable number of developmental abnormalities, pathologies, and traumatic injuries imposed on the human nervous system.

The in vitro approach to the study of the nervous system attempts to reduce cellular complexity and to characterize extrinsic influences. When neural tissue or tissue derivatives are transferred to a culture vessel, the tissue loses to various extents:

1. Contributions to its humoral environment from the remaining organ and organism;
2. Its physiochemical connections with other neuronal, glial, peripheral, and target cells; and
3. The anchorage that enabled it to maintain three-dimensional structure within the tissue.

In vitro, the culture medium and gas phase provide a new humoral environment and artificial growth surfaces provide reanchorage. Although there can be no completely compensatory contribution to the loss of specific intercellular interactions, cultures can be set up to retain or re-establish connections similar to the original tissue.

The culture medium and substratum can be defined to decided extents. However, medium and substratum will become less defined after the cellular elements are introduced, since neural cells will remove certain components and contribute others. A common way to delay and minimize cellular modifications of the in vitro environment is to provide the medium and substratum in large excess relative to the number of neural cells.

The two major experimental advantages of using neural cultures to characterize the nervous system are:

1. Reduced cellular complexity; and
2. Ability to manipulate the cellular environment.

The major disadvantage, promulgated for all in vitro studies, is the uncertainty of physiologically relevant phenotypic expression. However, there is overwhelming evidence that neural cells often express the same properties in vivo and in vitro. Some few examples include astroglial cell production of vimentin and glial fibrillary acidic protein, oligodendroglial and Schwann cell elaboration of myelin, neuronal postmitosis, neuronal expression of action potentials, neurofilaments, growth cone formation, and axonal growth. Neuroscientists generally agree that most, if not all, in vitro phenotypic expressions of neural cells are responses to the extrinsic regulation imposed by the specific culture environment and that, as such, they represent potential properties of the cells in vivo.

The advantages of reducing neural tissue complexity and manipulation of the cellular environment in vitro have permitted scientists to predict and regulate the behavior of specific neural cells in vivo. The purification, characterization, and cloning of neurotrophic factors (NTFs) depended almost entirely on the use of in vitro techniques. NTFs enhance the survival and growth of specific sets of cultured neuronal cells. By administering NTFs or anti-NTF antibodies *in situ*, investigators have demonstrated that specific neurons require NTFs for their survival, maturation, and maintenance.

In practical terms, the following considerations are important in using neural cultures:

1. Source of neural tissue: animal species, animal age, anatomical site of tissue;
2. Type of culture: organ, slice, explant (fragment), disaggregate, reaggregate, cell line;

3. Extrinsic environment: basal medium, medium supplements, substratum, gas phase, temperature.

SOURCE OF NEURAL TISSUE

Nearly all studies have used neural tissues from developing invertebrates, chickens, and rodents. Such organisms were chosen because of the convenience of maintaining colonies of them, the ability to predict the developmental age of their nervous systems, and the specific similarities of their nervous systems with the less accessible human one. Just about every organ and tissue from these animals at almost every age have been used at one time or another for in vitro studies. Particularly popular tissues include the chick embryo sympathetic, parasympathetic, and sensory ganglia, rodent sensory ganglia, and specific chick and rodent spinal cord and brain components. Detailed characterizations of these neural tissues and their component cells make the above systems ideal for continued study.

TYPE OF CULTURE

Organ, slice and explant (fragment) cultures have been favorite preparations for electrophysiological investigations because they retain the greatest degree of original histotypic organization and can be initiated from a same tissue from both developing and adult animals. Disaggregated or reaggregated cells and cell lines have been preferred by those investigators requiring replicate cultures, cell accessibility, and cell subset purification.

EXTRINSIC ENVIRONMENT

Most neural cultures are maintained at body temperature and in a 100% air or 5% carbon dioxide/95% air gas phase. However, the basal medium, substratum (if there is one), and supplements vary considerably, depending on what aspect of the culture is being studied. Usually, except for some invertebrate cells that can be grown in simple salt media, neural cells require specific ions, amino acids, vitamins, cofactors, hormones, mitogens (for proliferating cells), and other growth- and maintenance-promoting substances. Generally, these requirements are fulfilled by supplying the cells with a basal nutrient medium containing fetal bovine, horse, or human serum and crude tissue extracts. Chemically defined media have been developed that allow a more rigorous definition of the chemical requirements of neural cells and permit neuroscientists to manipulate the chemical environment to favor the growth of selected cell subsets. The overall aim of this manual is to give the reader an introductory understanding of the most important aspects of neural cell cultures and to provide enough basic information to allow the reader to set up and use neural cell cultures competently.

Marston Manthorpe

FURTHER READING

Banker, G. and Goslin, K. (eds.) (1991), *Culturing Nerve Cells*. MIT Press, Cambridge, MA.

Bottenstein, J. E. and Sato, G. (eds.) (1985), *Cell Culture in the Neurosciences*. Plenum, New York.

Boulton, A. A., Baker, G. B., and Walz, W. (eds.) (1992), *Practical Cell Culture Techniques*. Humana, Totowa, NJ.

Bunge, R. P. (1975), Changing uses of nerve tissue culture 1950–1975, in *The Nervous System. Vol. 1, The Basic Neurosciences*. (Tower, D. B., ed.) Raven, New York, pp. 31–42.

Crain, S. M. (1976), *Neurophysiological Studies in Tissue Culture*. Raven, New York.

Fedoroff, S. and Hertz, L. (eds.) (1977), *Cell, Tissue, and Organ Cultures in Neurobiology*. Academic, New York.

Fedoroff, S. and Vernadakis, A. (1986), *Astrocytes* Vols. 1–3. Academic, New York.

Fischbach, G. D. and Nelson, P. G. (1977), Cell culture in neurobiology, in *The Nervous System. Vol. 1, Cellular Biology of Neurons, Part 2*. (Kandel, E. R., ed.) American Physiol. Soc. Bethesda, MD, pp. 719–774.

Giacobini, E., Vernadakis, A., and Shahar, A. (eds.) (1980), *Tissue Culture in Neurobiology*. Raven, New York.

Harvey, A. L. (1984), *The Pharmacology of Nerve and Muscle in Tissue Culture*. Liss, New York.

Lendahl, U. and McKay, R. D. G. (1990), The use of cell lines in neurobiology. *TINS* **13,** 132–137.

Lumsden, C. E. (1968), Nervous tissue in culture, in *The Structure and Function of Nervous Tissue*. Vol. 1 (Bourne, G. H., ed.) Academic, New York, pp. 67–140.

Murray, M. R. (1965), Nervous tissue *in vitro*, in *Cells and Tissues in Culture*. Vol. 2 (Willmer, E. N., ed.) Academic, New York, pp. 373–455.

Nelson, P. G. (1975), Nerve and muscle cell in culture. *Physiol. Rev.* **55,** 1–61.

Nelson, P. G. and Leiberman, M. (1981), *Excitable Cells in Tissue Culture*. Plenum, New York.

Norenberg, M. D., Hertz, L., and Schousboe, A. (eds.) (1988), *The Biochemical Pathology of Astrocytes*. Liss, New York.

Pfeiffer, S. E. (ed.) (1982), *Neuroscience Approached Through Cell Culture*. Vol. 1. CRC, Boca Raton, FL.

Pfeiffer, S. E. (ed.) (1982), *Neuroscience Approached Through Cell Culture*. Vol. 2. CRC, Boca Raton, FL.

Ransom, B. R. and Kettenmann, H. (eds.) (1991), Glial cell lineage. *Glia* **4,** 121–243.

Sato, G. (ed.) (1973), *Tissue Culture of the Nervous System*. Plenum, New York.

Schubert, I. (ed.) (1984), *Developmental Biology of Cultured Nerve, Muscle and Glia*. Wiley, New York.

Seil, F. J. (1979), Cerebellum in tissue culture. *Rev. Neurosci.* **4,** 105–177.

Shahar, A., de Vellis, J., Vernadakis, A. and Haber, B. (eds.) (1989), *A Dissection and Tissue Culture Manual of the Nervous System*. Liss, New York.

Varon, S. (1975), Neurons and glia in neural cultures. *Exp. Neurol.* **48,** 93–134.

Contents

Chapter Nineteen
Tips in Tissue Culture   **253**
Sergey Fedoroff and Arleen Richardson

Chapter Twenty
Use of Dissecting Instruments in Tissue Culture   **263**
Arleen Richardson

Contributors

Jack P. Antel • *Department of Neurology and Neurosurgery, Montreal Neurological Institute, Montreal, PQ, Canada*

Colin J. Barnstable • *Department of Ophthalmology and Visual Science, Yale University School of Medicine, New Haven, CT*

Jürgen Bolz • *Cerveau et Vision, INSERM, Bron, France*

Richard P. Bunge • *Miami Project, University of Miami School of Medicine, Miami, FL*

Robert B. Campenot • *Department of Anatomy and Cell Biology, University of Alberta, Edmonton, AB, Canada*

Valerie Castellani • *Cerveau et Vision, INSERM, Bron, France*

Ruth Cole • *Neurobiochemistry Group, University of California at Los Angeles, CA*

Jean de Vellis • *Beurobiochemistry Group, University of California at Los Angeles, CA*

Richard M. Devon • *College of Dentistry, University of Saskatchewan, Saskatoon, SK, Canada*

Angela P. Dyer • *Department of Microbiology, University of British Columbia, Vancouver, BC, Canada*

Sergey Fedoroff • *Department of Anatomy and Cell Biology, University of Saskatchewan, Saskatoon, SK, Canada*

Paul Honneger • *Institut de Physiologie, Faculté de Médecine, Universite de Lausanne, Switzerland*

Mary I. Johnson • *Division of Child Neurology, Department of Pediatrics, University of Arizona Health Science Center, Tucson, AZ*

Bernhard H. J. Juurlink • *Department of Anatomy and Cell Biology, College of Medicine, University of Saskatchewan, Saskatoon, SK, Canada*

Marston Manthorpe • *Vical, San Diego, CA*

Florianne Monnet-Tschudi • *Institut de Physiologie, Faculté de Médecine, Universite de Lausanne, Switzerland*

Gustave Moonen • *Science de Physiologie Humaine et de Physiopathologie, Institut Léon Fredericq, University of Liege, Belgium*

Arleen Richardson • *Department of Anatomy and Cell Biology, College of Medicine, University of Saskatchewan, Saskatoon, SK, Canada*

Bernard Rogister • *Science de Physiologie Humaine et de Physiopathologie, Institut*

Léon Fredericq, University of Liege, Belgium

Shawn K. Thorburne • *Department of Anatomy and Cell Biology, College of Medicine, University of Saskatchewan, Saskatoon, SK, Canada*

Frank Tufaro • *Department of Microbiology, University of British Columbia, Vancouver, BC, Canada*

Voon Wee Yong • *Department of Neurology and Neurosurgery, Montreal Neurological Institute, Montreal, PQ, Canada*

Chapter One

Outgrowth Assays and Cortical Slice Cultures

Valérie Castellani and Jürgen Bolz

1. OUTGROWTH ASSAY

A simple outgrowth assay is described that allows the quantification of the growth behavior of specific axon populations on known and unknown substrates. Small explants prepared from various regions of the brain are placed on substrate-coated coverslips in Petriperm dishes with culture medium. This permits the observation of axonal growth patterns (axon elongation and branch formation) continuously over time. In addition, by blocking molecules that might control the growth and guidance of axons (e.g., with antibodies or lectins), this assay is well-suited to examine factors that promote or inhibit axonal growth and/or induce or prevent the formation of axon collaterals (Gotz et al., 1992; Henke-Fahle et al., 1996).

1.1. Preparation of Substrata

1. Materials:
    Laminin-polylysine solution (300 μL).
    Phosphate buffer, calcium- and magnesium-free (25 mL).
    Culture medium (3 mL).
    Forceps, fine.
    Petri dishes (100-mm) (2).
    Petri dish, sterile, glass (100-mm) (1).

Protocols for Neural Cell Culture, 2nd Ed. • Eds.: S. Fedoroff and A. Richardson • Humana Press, Inc., Totowa, NJ

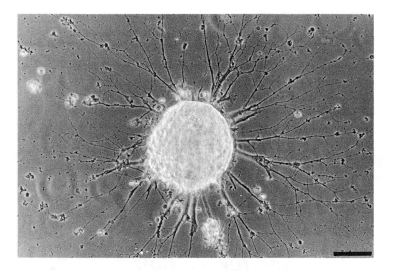

Fig. 1. Phase contrast micrograph of fiber outgrowth from a cortical explant on postnatal cortical membranes. The explant was prepared at E16 and fixed after 3 d in culture. Scale bar 100 μm.

> Petriperm dishes (2).
> Coverslips, 11 × 22 mm (4).
> Membrane solution (100 μL).
> Sterile pipet tips.

2. Preparation of a laminin/polylysine substrate: The extracellular matrix protein laminin has proven to be a good substrate for axonal growth; however, different types of axon populations respond differently to the growth-promoting properties of laminin. Polylysine is "sticky;" it enhances the attachment of the explants, which is necessary for fiber extension, but it also might reduce axonal growth. Therefore, different combinations of laminin-polylysine, as well as laminin alone, should be tested.

    a. Sterilize forceps using the hot bead sterilizer. When the temperature reaches 250°C, insert dry and clean instruments for at least 5–10 s, depending on their size. When sterile, put the forceps into a sterile <u>glass</u> Petri dish and keep the ends covered with the lid.

    b. With fine forceps, place two cleaned and sterile coverslips on the bottom of a 100-mm Petri dish. Pipet 100 μL of the laminin-polylysine solution on each coverslip. Prepare two "sandwiches" by covering each coverslip with a second one.

    c. Cover the Petri dish and incubate the sandwiches for at least 30 min at 37° in a humid atmosphere of 5% CO_2, 95% air.

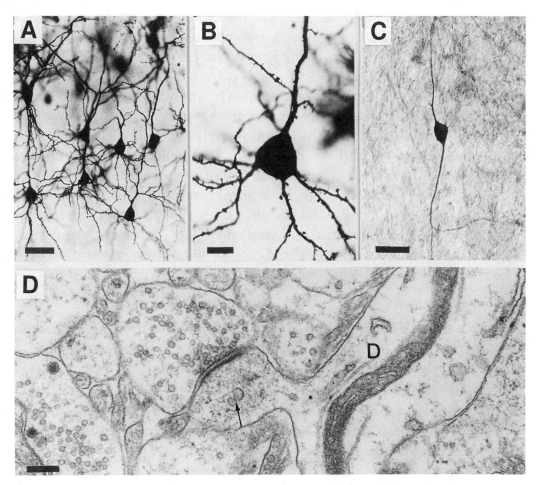

Fig. 2. Organotypic organization of cortical slice cultures. **(A,B)** Golgi stained pyramidal cells; **(C)** GABA immunoreactive nonpyramidal cell; **(D)** electron micrograph showing a synapse on a dendritic spine. The slices were prepared from 6 d old rats and kept for 2 wk in culture. The scale bar is 200 μm in (A) 50 μm in (B) and (C), and 0.2 μm in (D).

    3. Preparation of membrane carpets: Different components of cortical cell membrane preparations promote or inhibit the growth of cortical and thalamic axons, and some of these molecules act differentially on these two axon populations. Moreover, cortical cell membranes prepared at different developmental stages revealed that their expression can be developmentally regulated. The preparation of cell membranes (in which molecules from the extracellular matrix copurify) is described in the appendix.

      a. Open one of the two sandwiches with a forceps and rinse each coverslip with phosphate-buffered saline (PBS), twice with 1 mL on the side coated with laminin-polylysine solution, and once with 1 mL on the other side.

b. Place one coverslip on the bottom of another 100-mm Petri dish, coated side up. Pipet 100 μL of the membrane solution on this coverslip. Again make a sandwich by placing the second coverslip **coated side down** on the first one.

c. Place the two Petri dishes (one with laminin-polylysine sandwich and one sandwich with membrane solution) for 2 h in the incubator.

d. After incubation, open the laminin-polylysine sandwich and rinse the two coverslips with PBS, as in 3a above. Place both coverslips, **coated side up**, in a Petriperm dish and add 750 μL of culture medium.

e. Open the sandwich with membrane preparation. Let the membrane solution drip briefly, but do not rinse. Place both coverslips, **coated side up**, in a Petriperm dish and add 750 μL culture medium. Store the two Petriperm dishes in the incubator until the explantation of the cortical tissue.

1.2. Cortical Explants

Dissection of the fetuses involves removing the brain, trimming it down to isolate the cerebral cortex, and cutting the block of cortex twice at orthogonal orientations with the McIlvain tissue chopper (Mickle Laboratory Engineering, Mill Works, UK). This produces many tissue cubes of roughly the same size.

1. Dissecting out fetuses: **Note: The following procedure is performed outside of the laminar flow-hood; extra caution should be exercised to prevent contamination.**

   a. Materials:
      Scissors, large (1).
      Scissors, medium (1).
      Forceps, large (1).
      Forceps, small (1).
      Petri dish, glass (100-mm).
      Pregnant rat with E16–E18 fetuses.
      70% ethanol.
      Cork board and pins (8).
      Gauze squares, 2 × 2 in. (4).

   b. Euthanize the pregnant rat by carbon dioxide inhalation followed by cervical dislocation.

   c. Pin the rat down on a cork board, ventral side up. Prepare the ventral surface of the rat by soaking with 70% ethanol.

   d. Using the large sterile scissors and large forceps, cut laterally across the lower abdomen just above the vaginal orifice. Cut through the skin, but not the underlying muscle. Then cut up the left side and laterally across the chest. Move the skin to the side and pin. Again soak the exposed area with 70% ethanol.

e. Using the medium sterile scissors and small forceps, make an incision, as before, through the muscle layer, taking care not to pierce the intestines. Grasp one horn of the uterus, dissect it out of the abdominal cavity, and transfer the intact uterus to the 100-mm glass Petri dish. Quickly transfer this glass Petri dish to the laminar flow hood.

Note: All subsequent procedures are performed in the laminar flow-hood.

2. Removal of fetuses from uterus
   a. Materials:
      Scissors, small (1).
      Forceps, small (1).
      Petri dish (35 mm) (1).
      Petri dish, sterile, glass (100 mm) (1).
   b. Sterilize instruments using the hot bead sterilizer. When the temperature reaches 250°C, insert dry and clean instruments for at least 5–10 s, depending on their size. When sterile, put the instruments into a sterile glass Petri dish and keep the ends covered with the lid.
   c. Using the small scissors and forceps, cut through the length of the uterus and separate the fetuses from their placentas and accompanying amniotic membrane. Transfer the fetuses to a 35-mm Petri dish.

3. Preparation of cortical explants
   a. Materials:
      Gey's balanced salt solution/glucose (GBSS/glucose) (30 mL).
      Culture medium (15 mL).
      Petri dish (100 mm) (1).
      Petri dish (1).
      Scissors, small (1).
      Forceps, Dumont (2).
      Scalpel blade.
      Spatula, large (1).
      Spatula, small (1).
      Ice bucket and ice.
   b. Sterilize instruments using the hot bead sterilizer. When the temperature reaches 250°C, insert dry and clean instruments for at least 5–10 s, depending on their size. When sterile, put the instruments into a sterile glass Petri dish and keep the ends covered with the lid.

c. Place the GBSS/glucose in an ice bath. Pipet 6 drops (1 mL each) of this solution about equally spaced in a 100-mm Petri dish.

d. Decapitate three embryos with small scissors and put each head in one drop of GBSS/glucose.

e. Under a dissecting microscope, remove the skin and skull together with two fine forceps. Take out the whole brain with a small spatula and put it in a second drop of GBSS/glucose. Cut between the two hemispheres. Place one hemisphere pia side down and hold the tissue with forceps placed in the striatum. With a scalpel, make a small cut at the anterior and posterior pole of the hemisphere and then unfold the hemisphere with a second forceps. Make two lateral cuts to obtain a rectangular block of (neo)cortex. Transfer each block to a third drop of GBSS/glucose.

f. Transfer all blocks of cortex to the disk on the tissue chopper, cut at 200 μm, rotate the disk by 90°, and cut again at 200 μm.

g. Collect the cortex cubes with a large spatula and place them in a 35 mm dish about half-filled with culture medium. Incubate the tissue for 1–2 h at 37°C in a humidified atmosphere of 5% CO_2, 95% air. This allows the diffusion of proteolytic enzymes released by damaged cells.

h. Under the dissecting microscope, explant the cortex cubes with a pipet in 15 μL medium on the coated cover slips in the Petriperm dishes. Repeat this until there are enough explants on the four coverslips (two coated with laminin-polylysine, two coated with membrane solution), but allow a reasonable distance between the explants. To keep the volume of the medium (750 μL) constant, remove 15 μL from the medium each time you transfer explants on one of the coverslips (the explants do not adhere to the substrate if there is too much fluid).

i. Wait 10 min, then carefully transfer the Petriperm dishes into the incubator. Note that most explants have not yet adhered to the substrate, so do not shake or tilt the dishes. Incubate for 30 min at 37°C in a humidified atmosphere of 5% CO_2, 95% air. Most explants should then have adhered to their substrate.

j. Remove the explants from the incubator and **slowly** add 1250 μL of culture medium to each dish. Return to the incubator.

Note: Examine fiber outgrowth after 2–4 d in vitro. To confirm the neuronal origin of the fibers, explants can be stained with antibodies directed against neuronal markers, e.g., MAP5 (Sigma, St. Louis, MO), SMI31 (Sternberger Monoclonals Inc., Baltimore, MD) and glial markers, e.g., GFAP (Bioscience Products AG, Emmenbrücke, Switzerland), vimentin (Sigma).

2. CORTICAL SLICE CULTURES

In cortical slice cultures, the intrinsic organization is organotypically preserved and the morphological and neurochemical maturation and differentiation of cortical neurons continues in this culture system. By culturing cortical slices next to explants from regions of the brain that are interconnected with the cortex in vivo, it is possible to reconstruct afferent and efferent projections under in vitro condition (for review, *see* Bolz et al., 1993). Different techniques have been used to sustain slices in vitro long enough for neurons to establish connections with cocultured targets. In a procedure initially described by Gähwiler (1981), slices are embedded in a plasma clot on glass coverslips and cultured in a roller tube, to alternate exposure of the tissue to air and medium. Alternatively, the slices are plated on collagen-coated membranes and kept stationary in an incubator, with the level of the medium just below the surface of the explants (Stoppini et al., 1991). The slices placed on collagen-coated membranes show little spontaneous fiber outgrowth, and axons invade cocultured explants only when the slices are in direct contact or when migrating cells form bridges between the two cultures. Here we describe the roller culture technique. Slices cultured according to this method flatten to 1–3 cell layers after a few days in vitro (which greatly facilitates electrophysiological recordings), while retaining their histotypic organization. In addition, the plasma clot has proven to be a good substrate for axonal outgrowth and also appears to stabilize diffusible chemoattractant molecules.

2.1. Materials

GBSS/glucose (30 mL).
GBSS (2 mL).
Chicken plasma (20 µL).
Thrombin solution (20 µL).
Medium (3.0 mL).
Petri dishes (100-mm) (2).
Petri dish, sterile, glass (100 mm).
Coverslips (11 × 22 mm) (4).
Plastic tubes, Nunc, flat (110 × 16 mm).
Scissors, large (1).
Scissors, small (1).
Forceps, fine (2).
Scalpel blade.
Spatula, large (1).
Spatulas, small (2).
Ice bucket and ice.

Roller drum.

Tissue chopper (McIlvain).

2.2. Preparation of Cortical Slices

1. Preparation for dissection:
   a. Sterilize instruments using the hot bead sterilizer. When the temperature reaches 250°C, insert dry and clean instruments for at least 5–10 s, depending on their size. When sterile, put the instruments into a sterile glass Petri dish and keep the ends covered with the lid.
   b. Place the GBSS/glucose in an ice bath. Pipet 4 drops (1 mL each) of this solution about equally spaced in a 100-mm Petri dish.
2. Dissection:
   a. Anesthetize a young postnatal rat by Metofane™ inhalation, then decapitate the animal with large scissors. Using forceps, hold the head on the bottom of the Petri dish. With small scissors, cut the skin along the midline and unfold the skin with two forceps. Then cut the skull along the midline and remove the whole brain with a large spatula and place it in a drop of GBSS/glucose in the Petri dish.
   b. Cut the two hemispheres apart with a scalpel blade and place them pia side down in a drop of GBSS/glucose. Under a dissecting microscope, hold the tissue with forceps placed in the striatum. With a scalpel, make a small cut at the anterior and posterior pole of the hemisphere and then unfold the hemisphere with a second forceps. Make two lateral cuts to obtain a rectangular block of (neo)cortex. Transfer each block to a third drop of GBSS/glucose. Remove the pia carefully with two forceps.
3. Cortical slices:
   a. Add 5 mL cold GBSS/glucose to a 100-mm Petri dish.
   b. Place a block of cortex with pia side down on the tissue chopper, remove fluid with a pipet, and cut 300-μm thick slices.
   c. Transfer the slices with a large spatula into a new 100-mm Petri dish containing cold GBSS and glucose. Under a dissecting microscope, carefully separate the slices with a small spatula.
   d. Store the slices at 4°C for 30–45 min. This allows the diffusion of enzymatic factors released by damaged cells.

2.3. Preparation of the Plasma Clot

1. Place four glass coverslips in a 100 mm petri dish; pipet 20 μL chicken plasma solution in the center of each coverslip. Transfer a slice into the plasma drop (see Section 3.6.).

2. Pipet 20 μm thrombin solution next to the plasma clot and gently hold the coverslip with forceps on the bottom of the Petri dish (see Section 3.7.). Then carefully mix the two drops with a small spatula and spread the mixture over the entire surface of the coverslip. Keep the slices 30–45 min in the Petri dish to allow coagulation of the plasma.
3. Place the coverslip in a Nunc plastic tube and add 750 μL of culture medium (*see* Section 3.1., item 2.)
4. Transfer the tubes in a roller-drum incubator (10 revolutions/h) at 37°C. in dry air.

2.4. Maintenance of the Cultures

1. Change the medium every 2–5 d, depending on the size and metabolic activity of the slices, as indicated by a change in color of the medium from orange to yellow.
2. After 2–3 d in vitro, to prevent excessive growth of glia and other neuronal cells, 7.5 μL of mitotic inhibitor solution is added to each culture tube for 24 h.

3. APPENDIX

3.1. Medium

1. Medium for outgrowth assay: 100 mL Eagle's basal medium (Gibco 41100025), 50 mL Hanks' balanced salt solution, 50 mL Horse serum.
   a. Mix Eagle's basal medium and Hanks' balanced salt solution.
   b. Add 0.8 g (4 mg/mL) methylcellulose (Sigma M-7027). Agitate at 4°C for 2 h or until dissolved.
   c. Inactivate the horse serum at 56°C, for 30 min.
   d. Add 0.1 mM glutamine and 6.5 mg/mL glucose.
   e. Add antibiotics (streptomycin 10 mg/mL; penicillin, 10,000 U/mL); antifungics (amphotericin B 2.5 mg/mL); and the horse serum.
   f. Sterilize by filtration through a 0.2 μm filter.
2. Medium for cortical slices: Same medium as for outgrowth assay, but without the methylcellulose. Annis et al. (1990) described a serum-free medium for organotypic slice cultures.
3. Gey's balanced salt solution/glucose
   a. Gey's balanced salt solution (Gibco-BRL 14260-020).
   b. Add 6.5 mg/mL glucose.
   c. Sterilize by filtration through a 0.2-μm filter.

3.2. Laminin and Polylysine

1. 1 mg/mL Laminin (Sigma L-2020, Gibco-BRL 23017-015).
   a. Sterilize with a 0.2 μm filter (nonpyrogenic, hydrophilic).

      b. Aliquot and store at −20°C.
2. Poly-L-Lysine hydrobromide (Sigma P1399).
      a. Dilute to 1 mg/mL with high quality distilled water.
      b. Sterilize by filtration through a 0.2-μm filter.
      c. Aliquot into 10-μL amounts and store at −20°C.
3. Laminin-polylysine solution: Add 3 μL of laminin and 3 μL of polylysine stock solution to 300 μL of Gey's balanced salt solution (GBSS).

3.3. Homogenization Buffer (H-Buffer)

Tris-HCl, pH 7.4	10 mM
$CaCl_2$	1.5 mM
Spermidine (Sigma-4139)	1 mM
Aprotinine (Sigma A-1153)	25 μg/mL
Leupeptine (Sigma L-2884)	25 μg/mL
Pepstatine (Sigma P-4265)	5 μg/mL
2,3-dehydro-2-deoxy-N-acetyl-neuraminic acid (Sigma D-4019)	15 μg/mL

3.4. Membrane Preparation

1. Dissect the postnatal cortex (P0–P7) in Gey's balanced salt solution (GBSS) supplemented with glucose (6.5 mg/mL) and remove the pia.
2. Pool blocks of cortex in an ice-cold homogenization buffer (H-buffer).
3. Homogenize the cortex first with a 1 mL pipet tip and then with a 27-gage injection canula.
4. Centrifuge for 10 min at 50,000g with a Beckman ultracentrifuge (rotor TLS 55) in a sucrose step gradient (upper phase 150 μL of 5% glucose; lower phase 350 μL of 50% sucrose).
5. Wash the interband containing the membrane fraction twice in calcium and magnesium-free phosphate-buffered saline (PBS) which also contains the inhibitors leupeptine, pepstatine, aprotinine and 2,3-dehydro-2-deoxy-N-acetylneuraminic acid (same concentration as in the H-buffer) at 14,000 rpm (approx 12,000g) in an Eppendorf Biofuge.
6. After resuspension in calcium- and magnesium-free PBS without the inhibitors, the concentration of the purified membranes is determined by its optical density at 220 nm with a spectrophotometer. For this prepare a blank of 2940 μL 2% SDS and 210 μL PBS. For the sample, add 70 μL PBS to the tube with membranes, mix, and remove 70 μL of the membrane solution. Adjust the concentration of the membrane suspension, so that an aliquot diluted 1:15 in 2% SDS has an optical density of 0.1.
7. You can store the membranes frozen in a solution of 50% calcium- and magnesium-free PBS and 50% glycerol solution. In this case, adjust the optical density to about 0.2 and make aliquots of 200 μL. Before use, add 1 mL

calcium- and magnesium-free PBS, recentrifuge, and resuspend in 300 μL PBS. Adjust the optical density to 0.1.

3.5. Mitotic Inhibitor Solution

1. Dissolve 2.46 mg 5-fluoro-2-deoxyuridine (Sigma F-0503) in 10 mL distilled water.
2. Dissolve 2.8 mg cytosine-D-arabinofuranoside (Sigma C-6645) in 10 mL distilled water.
3. Dissolve 2.4 mg uridine (Sigma U-3750) in 10 mL distilled water.
4. Mix 5-fluoro-2-deoxyuridine, uridine, and cytosine-D-arabinofuranoside 1:1:1. Sterilize by filtration using a 0.2-μm filter.
5. Store at −20°C in 200 μL aliquots.

3.6. Plasma

Chicken plasma (Sigma P-3266) is reconstituted with 1 mL sterile distilled water. Sterilize by filtration using a 0.2 μm filter. Five hundred microliter aliquots are stored frozen at −20°C.

3.7. Thrombin

1. Reconstitute thrombin (10,000 U; Sigma T-4648) with 8 mL distilled water.
2. Centrifuge for 30 min at 2500 rpm.
3. Sterilize by filtration using a 0.2 μm filter.
4. Store 30 μL aliquots frozen at −20°C.
5. Before use, add 1 aliquot of 30 μL to 1 mL GBSS.

FURTHER READING

Annis, C. M., Edmond, J., and Robertson, R. T. (1990), A chemically-defined medium for organotypic slice cultures. *J. Neurosci. Methods* **32,** 63–70.

Annis, C. M., O'Dowd, D. K., and Robertson, R. T. (1994), Activity-dependent regulation of dendritic spine density on cortical pyramidal neurons in organotypic slice cultures. *J. Neurobiol.* **25,** 1483–1493.

Annis, C. M., Robertson, R. T., and O'Dowd, D. K. (1993), Aspects of early postnatal development of cortical neurons that proceed independently of normally present extrinsic influences. *J. Neurobiol.* **24,** 1460–1480.

Bolz, J., Götz, M., Hübener, M., and Novak, N. (1993), Reconstructing cortical connections in a dish. *Trends Neurosci.* **16,** 310–316.

Bolz, J., Novak, N., Götz, M., and Bonhoeffer, T. (1990), Formation of target-specific neuronal projections in organotypic slice cultures from rat visual cortex. *Nature* **346,** 359–362.

Bolz, J., Novak, N., and Staiger, V. (1992), Formation of specific afferent connections in organotypic slice cultures from rat visual cortex co-cultured with lateral geniculate nucleus. *J. Neurosci.* **12,** 3054–3070.

Caeser, M., Bonhoeffer, T., and Bolz, J. (1989), Cellular organization and development of slice cultures from rat visual cortex. *Exp. Brain Res.* **77,** 234–244.

Distler, P. G. and Robertson, R. T. (1993), Formation of synapses between basal forebrain afferents and cerebral cortex neurons: an electron microscopic study in organotypic slice cultures. *J. Neurocytol.* **22,** 627–643.

Gähwiler, B. H. (1981), Organotypic monolayer cultures of nervous tissue. *J. Neurosci. Methods* **4,** 329–342.

Götz, M. and Bolz, J. (1989), Development of vasoactive intestinal polypeptide (VIP)-containing neurons in organotypic slice cultures from rat visual cortex. *Neurosci. Lett.* **107,** 6–11.

Götz, M. and Bolz, J. (1992), Preservation and formation of cortical layers in slice cultures. *J. Neurobiol.* **23,** 783–802.

Götz, M. and Bolz, J. (1994), Differentiation of transmitter phenotypes in rat cerebral cortex. *Eur. J. Neurosci.* **6,** 18–32.

Götz, M., Novak, N., Bastmeyer, M., and Bolz, J. (1992), Membrane bound molecules in rat cerebral cortex regulate thalamic innervation. *Development* **116,** 507–519.

Henke-Fahle, S., Mann, F., Götz, M., Wild, K., and Bolz, J. (1996), Dual action of a carbohydrate epitope on afferent and efferent axons in cortical development. *J. Neurosci.* **16,** 4195–4206.

Hübener, M., Götz, M., Klostermann, S., and Bolz, J. (1995), Guidance of thalamocortical axons by growth-promoting molecules in developing rat cerebral cortex. *Eur. J. Neurosci.* **7,** 1963–1972.

Molnár, Z. and Blakemore, C. (1991), Lack of regional specificity for connections formed between thalamus and cortex in coculture. *Nature* **351,** 475–477.

Novak, N. and Bolz, J. (1993), Formation of specific efferent connections in organotypic slice cultures from rat visual cortex co-cultured with lateral geniculate nucleus and superior colliculus. *Eur. J. Neurosci.* **5,** 15–24.

Roberts, J. S., O'Rourke, N. A., and McConnell, S. K. (1993), Cell migration in cultured cerebral cortical slices. *Dev. Biol.* **155,** 396–408.

Stoppini, L., Buchs, P.-A., and Muller, D. (1991), A simple method for organotypic cultures of nervous tissue. *J. Neurosci. Methods* **37,** 173–182.

Wolburg, H. and Bolz, J. (1991), Ultrastructural organization of slice cultures from rat visual cortex. *J. Neurocytol.* **20,** 552–563.

Yamamoto N., Kurotani, T., and Toyama, K. (1989), Neural connections between the lateral geniculate nucleus and visual cortex in vitro. *Science* **245,** 192–194.

Yamamoto, N., Yamada, K., Kurotani, T., and Toyama K. (1992), Laminar specificity of extrinsic cortical connections studied in coculture preparations. *Neuron* **9,** 217–228.

Chapter Two

Microexplant Cultures of the Cerebellum

Bernard Rogister and Gustave Moonen

1. INTRODUCTION

This chapter is devoted to a simple method for culturing developing rat cerebellum. The method can also be used for rat hippocampus embryonic age 18 (E18), cerebral cortex (E18), and even spinal cord, but at an earlier stage of development (E14). This method was initially designed to obtain long-term survival of cerebellar macroneurons, Purkinje cells, and deep nuclear macroneurons (Moonen et al., 1982; Neale et al., 1982). Indeed, in cultures in which a single cell suspension is seeded, virtually all the neurons die between 5 and 10 d, whereas significant survival is obtained if small aggregates of cells (microexplants) rather than single cells are seeded. The term "microexplant" was used to stress the difference from the classic cerebellar explants that consist of a thin cerebellar slice, which are much more "organized" tissue samples.

Microexplant cultures have also been adapted to serum-free conditions for short-term experiments of <1 wk duration (Section 3.1.). These preparations have been used for the study of survival factors for cerebellar neurons (Grau-Wagemans et al., 1984), protease release by neural cells, proliferation of astroglia cells, neuronal migration on different substrates, and modulation of neuritic behavior (Fischer et al., 1986).

1. PREPARATION OF CEREBELLUM

1.1. Materials

Newborn rats, 0–2 d of age.
Petri dishes, sterile, glass (100 mm) (2).
Petri dishes, sterile, plastic (100 mm) (2).

Protocols for Neural Cell Culture, 2nd Ed. • Eds.: S. Fedoroff and A. Richardson • Humana Press, Inc., Totowa, NJ

95% Ethanol.

70% Ethanol.

Hanks' balanced salt solution (Hanks' BSS) (50 mL).

Forceps, large (1).

Forceps, medium, curved (1).

Scissors, large (1).

Scissors, small (1).

Forceps, fine, curved (1).

Forceps, fine (10 cm) (1).

Scissors, pointed, curved (10 cm) (1).

Petri dish (35 mm) (1).

Minimum essential medium (MEM) with glucose and insulin, MEMgI (10 mL).

1.2. Procedure for Gross Dissection (Figs. 1 and 2)

1. Preparation for gross dissection:
   a. Sterilization of instruments: Sterilize instruments by immersing them in 70% alcohol and drying them in air inside the laminar flow hood or by inserting them in a hot bead sterilizer for 5–10 s at 250°C. When sterile, put the instruments into a sterile glass Petri dish and keep the ends covered with the lid.
   b. Pipet 15 mL Hanks' BSS into one 100-mm glass Petri dish and one 100-mm plastic Petri dish. Replace covers.
   c. Pipet 1 mL MEMgI medium into a 35-mm Petri dish.
2. After sacrificing the newborn rat pups by carbon dioxide or Metofane™ inhalation, pick up and completely immerse a newborn rat into 95% ethanol. Hold the newborn rat over the empty 100-mm plastic Petri dish and decapitate using the large scissors. Repeat for each newborn rat.
3. While holding the head with curved forceps, use the small scissors to cut the skin. Begin at the neck, proceed along the midline, and pull the skin aside (Fig. 1A).
4. Using the scissors, cut the skull (mainly cartilage at this age) by making a Y-shaped cut (the base of the Y begins at the neck). Without damaging the brain, gently pull apart the flaps of the skull (Fig. 1B).
5. Remove the entire brain by using the curved forceps like a spatula cutting all the cranial nerves. Lift the brain out of the brain case and place it in the 100-mm glass Petri dish containing 15 mL Hanks' BSS (Fig. 1C).
6. Excision of the cerebellum (Fig. 2):
   a. Place the Petri dish containing the brain under the dissecting microscope. Using the small scissors, make the following cuts:
      i. A slightly angled cut is made between the cerebellum and the midbrain on one side.

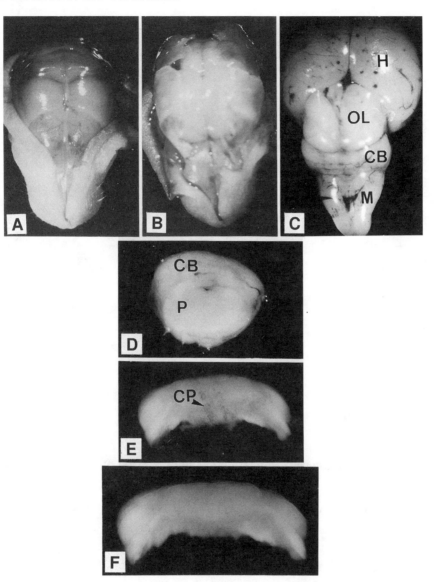

Fig. 1. Dissection of neonatal rat brain. H: Cerebral hemispheres. OL: Optic lobes. CB: Cerebellum. P: Pons. CP: Choroid plexus. M: Medulla (**A**) Removal of skin from neonatal rat. (**B**) Removal of the skull. (**C**) Neonatal rat brain removed from the skull. (**D**) Isolated cerebellum showing the pons. (**E**) Cerebellum with meninges and choroid plexus. (**F**) Isolated cerebellum with meninges and choroid plexus removed.

    ii. A similar slightly angled cut is made on the other side, so that the two cuts meet at the midline and the cerebellum is separated from the more rostral structures.

   iii. A third cut is made between the cerebellum and the medulla separating these two structures.

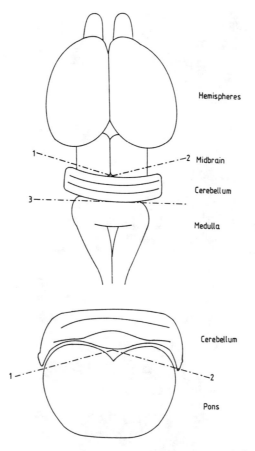

Fig. 2. Schematic representation of the dissection of the cerebellum.

    b. The "slice" containing the cerebellum (dorsal) and the pons (ventral) is now dissected (Fig. 1D). Place the isolated cerebellum into the plastic Petri dish containing Hanks' BSS.

    c. Repeat the excision of cerebellum procedures for each remaining brain.

7. Using the fine forceps, remove the meninges and choroid plexi from each isolated cerebellum (Fig. 1E).

8. Transfer each cerebellum to one 35-mm Petri dish that contains 300–500 μL MEMg (the volume of MEM should be the minimum in order to cover all the cerebella in a corner of the dish).

2. MICROEXPLANT CULTURES

2.1. Materials

Scissors, small (1).
Erlenmeyer flasks (10-mL) (2).

Petri dishes (35-mm) (2).

Centrifuge tubes, sterile (15-mL) (2).

Stoppers, sterile (2).

Aluminum foil pieces, sterile (2).

MEMgI.

Pipet, glass, curved, large aperture.

2.2. Preparation of Microexplants

1. Mince the cerebella in the 35-mm Petri dish into small fragments using the sterile scissors.
2. After mincing the tissue, add MEMgI medium up to 1 mL/cerebellum. (i.e., for 2 cerebella, add up to 2 mL.)
3. Separate the microexplants from smaller clumps, single cells, or debris as follows:
   a. Transfer the minced tissue in medium to the sterile tube. Allow the tissue to sediment for 2–3 min.
   b. Aspirate and discard the supernatant, being careful to retain the microexplants. Resuspend the pellet in fresh medium up to the original volume (1 mL/cerebellum).
   c. Repeat the sedimentation procedure (steps a and b), if necessary.

2.3. Microexplant Suspension Culture

1. Transfer the mixed microexplant suspension to a 10-mL sterile Erlenmeyer flask.
2. Gas the Erlenmeyer flask with a 5% carbon dioxide–95% air mixture and tightly stopper the flask. Cover the stopper with a piece of aluminum foil and place the flask on a gyratory shaker at 90 rpm ($4.5g$) at 37°C for 24 h.

2.4. Microexplant Culture

1. After 24 h remove the Erlenmeyer flask from the shaker.
2. Using the sterile glass, curved, large aperture pipet, transfer the microexplant suspension from the flask. Usually not all the microexplants are recovered. Add one more milliliter of MEMgI to the Erlenmeyer flask in order to recover the remaining microexplants. Transfer the 2 mL to a sterile 15-mL centrifuge tube. Allow the tissue to sediment, discard the supernatant, and resuspend the pellet in 1 mL of MEMgI.
3. Plate the microexplant suspension from one flask into one 35-mm Petri dish coated with either poly-L-ornithine or laminin.
4. Repeat steps 1–3 for each flask prepared.

5. Incubate the microexplant cultures in a humidified 5% carbon dioxide–95% air incubator at 37°C.

6. After 6 h, add 0.5 mL MEMgI to each 35-mm Petri dish.

Note: At 10 d, significant cell death is observed; however, a portion of the neurons will survive and can be maintained for up to several months. Four-week-old cultures are used for electrophysiological studies (Gibbs et al., 1982; MacDonald et al., 1982; Cull-Candy et al., 1987).

2.5. Comments on Substrates

On poly-L-ornithine-coated dishes, neuritic outgrowth is optimal, whereas outward migration of cells including neurons is minimal. On laminin-coated dishes, not only radial neuritic outgrowth is observed, but also outward migration of neurons and glial cells (Figs. 3 and 4). (*See* Selak et al., 1985 for further details.)

3. APPENDIX

3.1. Medium

1. Eagle's Minimum Essential Medium (MEM) (Gibco-BRL 410-2500) formulation (Eagle, 1959):

Components	mg/L
Inorganic salts:	
$CaCl_2$ (anhyd.)	200.00
KCl	400.00
$MgSO_4$ (anhyd.)	97.67
NaCl	6800.00
$NaH_2PO_4 \cdot H_2O$	140.00
Other components:	
D-Glucose	1000.00
Phenol red	10.00
Amino acids:	
L-Arginine $\cdot$ HCl	126.00
L-Cystine $\cdot$ 2HCl	31.29
L-Glutamine	292.00
L-Histidine HCl $\cdot$ H_2O	42.00
L-Isoleucine	52.00
L-Leucine	52.00
L-Lysine HCl	72.50
L-Methionine	15.00

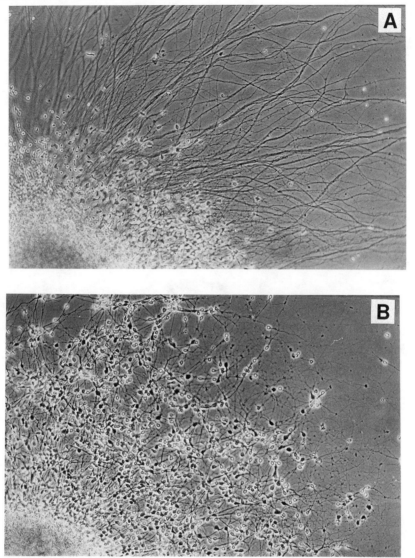

Fig. 3. Newborn rat cerebellum microexplants cultured for 4 d in MEMgI medium on (**A**) poly-L-ornithine-coated substratum and (**B**) laminin-coated substratum. In (B), a more extensive outward migration of cerebellar granule cells is observed. Phase contrast picture.

L-Phenylalanine	32.00
L-Threonine	48.00
L-Tryptophan	10.00
L-Tyrosine (disodium salt)	52.10
L-Valine	46.00
Vitamins:	
D-Ca pantothenate	1.00
Choline chloride	1.00

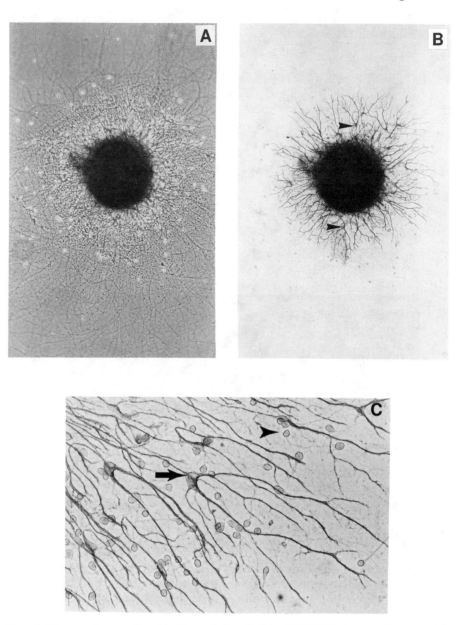

Fig. 4. Cerebellum microexplant cultured for 3 d in MEMgI on a poly-L-ornithine-coated substratum and observed after immunohistochemical demonstration of the glial fibrillary acidic protein. **(A)** Low-power phase contrast microphotograph allowing demonstration of the massive outward neuritic growth. **(B)** Low-power bright field microphotograph showing that the GFAP positive radial glial cell remain close to the microexplant (large arrow). **(C)** High-power phase contrast microphotograph of an area of (A) that is close to the microexplant. Phase contrast was used for this picture to demonstrate the GFAP-positive radial glial cells (large arrow) as well as the GFAP negative granule neurons (small arrow). As can be seen, neurons remain in the vicinity of the glial process.

Folic acid	1.00
i-Inositol	2.00
Nicotinamide	1.00
Pyridoxal HCl	1.00
Riboflavin	0.10
Thiamine HCl	1.00

2. For short-term cultures, MEM is supplemented with glucose at a final concentration of 6 g/L and bovine insulin at a final concentration of 5 µg/mL (MEMgI). The insulin is added just prior to use at low pH.

3. For long-term cultures, serum is added to the medium. MEM is supplemented with glucose at a final concentration of 6 g/L, 10% heat-inactivated (56°C, 30 min) horse serum (v/v), and 10% fetal bovine serum (FBS) (v/v). Both serum are obtained from Gibco-BRL.

4. The following method may be used to avoid overgrowth of cultures by nonneuronal cells when cultures are grown in the presence of serum:

   a. Culture cells in MEM supplemented with glucose at a final concentration of 6 g/L, 10% heat-inactivated (56°C, 30 min) horse serum (v/v), and 10% FBS (v/v).

   b. After 4 d in culture, the culture can be treated for 48 h with the following medium: 15 µg/mL 5'-fluoro-2'-deoxyuridine (FdR) and 35 µg/mL uridine in MEM supplemented with 10% heat-inactivated horse serum.

   c. After 48 h of treatment with the antimetabolite, the cells are cultured in MEM supplemented with 10% heat-inactivated horse serum.

3.2. Poly-L-Ornithine and Laminin-Coated Plates

1. Preparation of solutions:

   a. Poly-L-ornithine hydrobromide mol wt 30,000–70,000 (Sigma, St. Louis, MO, catalog #P3655) should be stored desiccated at –20°C.

      i. Add 0.1 g poly-L-ornithine to 100 mL pH 8.4 boric acid buffer to form a stock solution of 1.0 mg/mL.

      ii. Sterilize by filtration through a 0.2-µm filter.

      iii. Store at 4°C for up to 2 mo.

      iv. For use, dilute 10 mL poly-L-ornithine stock solution to a final volume of 100 mL with sterile distilled water to get a working solution of 0.1 mg/mL.

   b. Preparation of boric acid buffer:

      i. Make up an excess amount of 0.15*M* boric acid buffer: 1.59 g boric acid + 0.75 g NaOH/125 mL distilled water.

      ii. Adjust pH to 8.4 by adding HCl and testing aliquots. **Do not** put the pH electrode in the buffer.

    c. Mouse laminin (EY Laboratories, Inc., San Mateo, CA, cat. #2404 or Gibco-BRL cat. #6260 LA):

        i. Stock solutions should be reconstituted to about 1 mg/mL in sterile phosphate buffered saline (PBS), pH 8.0.

       ii. For use, dilute laminin to a concentration of 1 μg/mL by the addition of sterile PBS.

  2. Coating of plates with poly-L-ornithine and laminin:

    a. Coating plates with poly-L-ornithine:

        i. Make up stock solution of poly-L-ornithine at 1.0 mg/mL.

       ii. Dilute 10-fold with sterile distilled water to get a working solution of 0.1 mg/mL.

      iii. Add 1 mL poly-L-ornithine solution to 35-mm tissue culture dish. Make sure the entire surface of the dish is covered.

      iv. Allow to dry at room temperature in a laminar flow hood for 1–24 h.

       v. At least 30 min before planting the cells, wash each dish twice with 2.0 mL sterile distilled water. Replace the last water wash with 1 mL medium.

      vi. Incubate 30 min in a 5% carbon dioxide–95% air incubator at 37°C. When ready to seed cells, remove the medium from the Poly-L-ornithine-coated dish; add cells and fresh medium.

    b. Coating plates with laminin:

        i. Dilute laminin in sterile water, serum-free medium, or PBS to a working concentration of 10 μg/mL.

       ii. Apply laminin to the growth surface at a concentration of 10 μg/cm^2 or at a concentration of 10 μg/mL.

      iii. Allow to stand for 2–24 h at 37°C.

      iv. Remove from incubator and either seal in plastic bags and freeze at –20°C or remove excess laminin solution and add medium in preparation for culture.

       v. Do not allow plates to dry out.

FURTHER READING

Cull-Candy, S. G. and Usowicz, M. M. (1987), Multiple-conductance channels activated by excitatory amino acids in cerebellar neurons. *Nature* **325,** 525–528.

Eagle, H. (1959), Amino acid metabolism in mammalian cell cultures. *Science* **130,** 432–437.

Fischer, G., Kunemund, V., and Schachner, M. (1986), Neurite outgrowth patterns in cerebellar microexplant cultures are affected by antibodies to the cell surface glycoprotein L1. *J. Neurosci.* **6,** 605–612.

Gibbs, W., Neale, E. A., and Moonen, G. (1982), Kainic acid sensitivity of mammalian Purkinje cells in monolayer cultures. *Dev. Br. Res.* **4,** 103–108.

Grau-Wagemans, M.-P., Selak, I., Lefebvre, P. P., and Moonen, G. (1984), Cerebellar macroneurons in serum-free cultures. Evidence for intrinsic neuronotrophic and neuronotoxic activities. *Dev. Br. Res.* **15,** 11–19.

MacDonald, R. L., Moonen, G., Neale, E. A., and Nelson, P. G. (1982), Cerebellar macroneurons in microexplant cell culture. Postsynaptic amino acid pharmacology. *Dev. Br. Res.* **5,** 75–88.

Moonen, G., Neale, E. A., MacDonald, R. L., Gibbs, W., and Nelson, P. G. (1982), Cerebellar macroneurons in microexplant cell culture. Methodology, basic electrophysiology, and morphology after horseradish peroxidase injection. *Dev. Br. Res.* **5,** 59–73.

Neale, E. A., Moonen, G., MacDonald, R. L., and Nelson, P. G. (1982), Cerebellar macroneurons in microexplant cell cultures: ultrastructural morphology. *Neuroscience* **7,** 1879–1890.

Selak, I., Foidart, J. H., and Moonen, G. (1985), Laminin promotes cerebellar granule cells migration *in vitro* and is synthesized by cultured astrocytes. *Dev. Neurosci.* **7,** 278–285.

Chapter Three

Aggregating Neural Cell Cultures

Paul Honegger and Florianne Monnet-Tschudi

1. INTRODUCTION

Aggregating brain cell cultures are primary, three-dimensional cell cultures consisting of even-sized, spherical structures that are maintained in suspension by constant gyratory agitation. Because the avidity of freshly dissociated fetal cells to attach to their counterparts, cell aggregates form spontaneously and rapidly under appropriate culture conditions. The reaggregated cells are able to migrate within the formed structures, and to interact with each other by direct cell-cell contact, as well as through exchange of nutritional and signaling factors. This tissue-specific environment enables aggregating neural cells to differentiate, and to develop specialized structures (e.g., synapses, myelinated axons) resembling those of brain tissue *in situ*. Aggregating cell cultures are therefore classified as organotypic cultures (Doyle et al., 1994).

The basic methodology of rotation-mediated aggregating brain cell culture was introduced by Moscona (1961) and subsequently applied to cells of the central nervous system (CNS) for morphological and biochemical investigations (e.g., De Long and Sidman, 1970; Seeds, 1971). The original culture procedure was subsequently modified by using a mechanical sieving technique for tissue dissociation, instead of the enzymatic procedure (Honegger and Richelson, 1976), and by developing an appropriate chemically defined culture medium (Honegger et al., 1979). These modifications greatly simplified the procedure for the culture preparation and provided a means to grow large numbers of highly reproducible replicate cultures for multidisciplinary studies. Furthermore, the availability of a chemically defined

Protocols for Neural Cell Culture, 2nd Ed. • Eds.: S. Fedoroff and A. Richardson • Humana Press, Inc., Totowa, NJ

medium greatly facilitated the study of the role of hormones and endogenous messengers in the brain. (For protocols that use enzymatic tissue dissociation for aggregating neural cell cultures, *see* Choi et al., 1993).

2. PREPARATION OF AGGREGATING NEURAL CELL CULTURES

It is important to start with immature brain tissue of an appropriate, well-defined developmental stage. The optimal gestational period for culture preparation depends on both the species and the brain region. The protocols presented here use fetal rat brain tissues because of the relative ease in obtaining well-timed and large numbers of fetuses from this species. The cellular composition and developmental potential of the cultures are influenced greatly by the properties of the starting brain tissue (Honegger and Richelson, 1976). Using rat tissue for culture preparation, the spinal cord should be taken not later than at gestational d 14; whole brain not later than gestational d 15; and the telencephalon not later than gestational d 16. The use of mice has some advantage, because of the ever-increasing number of mutant and transgenic mice available. There is no fundamental difference between mouse and rat cells in the preparation and handling of aggregate cultures, nor in their developmental characteristics.

The rats are usually mated overnight and then separated the next morning. The day of separation is counted here as d 0. As a rule of thumb, with an average of 12 fetuses/animal, it would take about 7 timed-pregnant rats to prepare 50 replicate cultures of 16-d fetal rat telencephalon cells; or 10 animals for 50 replicate cultures of 15-d fetal rat telencephalon cells. Ideally, 2–3 persons should participate, setting up a large number of replicate cultures: one person can kill the timed-pregnant animals and remove the embryos, the other(s) can do the dissection in a sterile hood with horizontal air flow. During the entire dissection, the biological material is kept in the cold (close to 4°C).

3. PREPARATION FOR DISSECTIONS

3.1. Materials

Puck's salt solution D and gentamicin-sulfate (Puck's D-GS). (*See* Section 11.3., items 1 and 2.)
Tube, plastic, sterile (50-mL) (1).
Ice bucket and ice.
Petri dish, plastic (60 mm) (2).

3.2. Preparation

1. Add 40 mL of Puck's D-GS to a 50-mL plastic tube (for the storage of the dissected tissue).
2. Add 25 mL of Puck's D-GS to 50-mL plastic tubes (one tube for each pregnant animal, for the reception and transfer of the fetuses); place the tubes in ice.

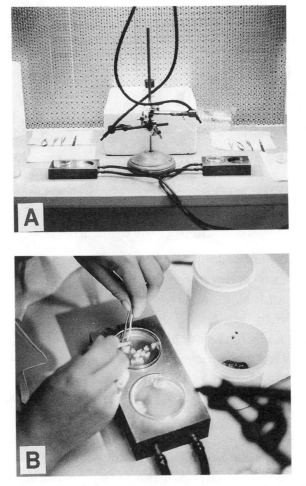

Fig. 1. Dissection of fetal neural tissue. (**A**) Setup of the sterile hood for dissection (for two persons). The dissecting blocks are perfused with an ice-cold liquid and illuminated by a lamp with fiber optics. The dissection instruments lay on sterile pads. A styrofoam box filled with ice is used to store the tubes and Puck's D-GS. (**B**) Close-up of a dissecting step: extraction of the fetal brain.

3. Set up the sterile hood for the dissection (Fig. 1A).
4. Add 8 mL of Puck's D-GS to two 60-mm plastic Petri dishes and place them on the dissecting block (or on ice, if no dissecting block is available).
5. Set up the lab for the decapitation and for the excision of the whole uterus containing the fetuses.

4. REMOVAL OF RAT FETUSES

Prior to the removal of fetuses from the pregnant rat, assemble all required instruments and solutions in the laminar flow hood.

4.1. Materials

Scissors, large (1).
Scissors, small, pointed (1).
Forceps, large (1).
Forceps, small, curved (1).
Gauze squares (2 × 2-in.) (4).
95% Ethanol denatured with 2% ketone.
Absorbent toweling.
Plastic 50-mL tube containing 25 mL ice-cold Puck's D-GS.

4.2. Dissecting Out Fetuses

Note: The following procedure is performed outside of the laminar flow hood; extra caution should be exercised to prevent contamination.

1. Sterilize instruments using the hot bead sterilizer. When the temperature reaches 250°C, insert dry and clean instruments for at least 5–10 s, depending on their size. Instruments may also be sterilized by autoclaving prior to needing them or by immersing them in 70% ethanol for 5–10 min and drying them inside the laminar flow hood.
2. Sacrifice the pregnant rat by decapitation. (Make sure to avoid all unnecessary stress to the animal and to follow the ethical guidelines).
3. Lay the decapitated animal on its back on an absorbent towel and, using the gauze, swab down the abdomen with 95% alcohol.
4. Using the large forceps, grasp the skin about 1 cm above the genitalia. With the large scissors, cut through the skin and fascia, and extend the cut on both sides of the abdomen, until the entire peritoneal cavity lays open.
5. Remove the uterine horns containing the fetuses, using small curved forceps and small pointed scissors, and transfer them to the 50-mL plastic tube containing 25 mL of ice-cold Puck's D-GS.
   Note: All subsequent procedures are performed in the laminar flow hood.

5. DISSECTION OF FETAL BRAIN TISSUE

5.1. Materials

Scissors, curved Vannas (1).
Forceps, fine curved (1).
Forceps, Extrafine, Dumont no. 5 (1).
Scalpel holder and #11 blade.
Petri dishes, plastic (60 mm), fitting on a dissecting block or on ice.
Ice bucket and ice.
Puck's D-GS (1–2 bottles of 500 mL). (*See* Section 11.3., items 1 and 2.)
Plastic 50-mL tube filled with 40 mL of Puck's D-GS.

5.2. Dissection of Fetal Brain Tissue

1. Sterilize instruments using the hot bead sterilizer. When the temperature reaches 250°C, insert dry and clean instruments for at least 5–10 s, depending on their size. Instruments may also be sterilized by autoclaving prior to needing them or by immersing them in 70% ethanol for 5–10 min and drying them inside the laminar flow hood.

2. Transfer the uterine horns to one of the Petri dishes placed on the cold dissecting block.
   Note: Make sure that during the entire dissection procedure, the biological material is always immersed in cold Puck's D-GS.

3. Open the uterine horns with the Vannas scissors and, using small forceps, transfer the fetuses to a new Petri dish.

4. Using the Vannas scissors and small forceps, separate the fetuses from their amniotic sacs and placentae and transfer them to a new Petri dish.

5. Transfer one fetus to a new Petri dish containing Puck's D-GS and dissect the brain.
   a. Hold the head of the fetus fixed in a lateral position with the aid of the Dumont forceps (Fig. 1B).
   b. Make an extended lateral incision at the base of the brain using the Vannas scissors by cutting skin and cartilage from the region of the brain stem to the most frontal point.
   c. Extract the entire brain by lifting it through this opening using the blunt side of the closed Vannas scissors. Keep the brain and discard the rest of the fetus.

6. Repeat step 5 for the rest of the fetuses from the same animal.

7. Using the scalpel, dissect the region(s) to be selected for preparation of cultures.

8. Transfer the dissected brain tissue to the 50-mL plastic tube filled with 40 mL of Puck's D-GS.
   Note: During dissection, replace the supernatant of this tube several times with fresh cold Puck's D-GS.

9. Repeat steps 3 and 4 of Sections 4.2. and 5.2. for each pregnant rat.
   Note: The duration of the dissection should not exceed 2 h. An experienced person can dissect 40–60 fetuses/h.

6. MECHANICAL DISSOCIATION OF FETAL BRAIN TISSUE

To dissociate the dissected and collected brain tissue, a sieving procedure according to Rose (1965), Schrier (1973), and Varon and Raiborn (1969) is used in a slightly modified form (Honegger and Richelson, 1976).

6.1. Materials

Nylon mesh bags, 200 μm pore size, fitted around a glass funnel (1 or 2).

Nylon mesh bag, 115 μm pore size, fitted around a glass funnel and attached with tape. (*See* Section 11.2, item 3.)

Glass rods (0.6 cm diameter, 20 cm long), with blunt, fire-polished ends (1 or 2).

Plastic centrifuge tubes, 50 mL conical (two per batch).

Cold Puck's D-GS.

Nigrosin or Trypan blue for cell viability tests.

Hemocytometer (or electronic cell counter).

Chemically defined medium. (*See* Section 11.1.)

Plastic culture flask of appropriate size to hold the total culture volume.

Ice buckets filled with ice (2).

6.2. Preparation

1. Set up the laminar flow hood for the dissociation procedure.
2. If necessary, divide the pooled brain tissue into batches of not more than 50 whole brains (or 100 brain parts) per batch.
3. Rinse each batch of tissue three times with about 40 mL of cold Puck's D-GS.
4. Add 25 mL of cold Puck's D-GS to the 50-mL plastic tubes (1/batch) and place them in ice, together with the empty 50-mL tubes (1/batch).

6.3. Dissociation Protocol

1. Take the 200 μm mesh bag (with a glass funnel fitted in the inside) and place it in a 50-mL plastic centrifuge tube containing 25 mL of Puck's D-GS. Keep on ice.
2. Pour the pooled brain tissue of one batch into the bag. Rinse the funnel, if necessary, with 2 mL of Puck's D-GS.
3. Remove the funnel, close the bag, and hold its upper ends against the outer side of the tube wall, *making sure that the tissue remains immersed.*
4. Using the glass rod, gently stroke downward, from the outside of the bag, to squeeze the tissue through the mesh into the surrounding solution.
5. After this first dissociation step, take the second nylon bag (115 μm mesh), attached with tape to a short glass funnel, and place it on top of an empty 50-mL conical plastic tube.
6. Using a 5-mL serological plastic pipet, transfer the cell/tissue suspension to the nylon bag and let the suspension pass through the filter by gravity flow into the 50-mL tube. Toward the end of the filtration, add Puck's D-GS up to a final volume of 50 mL.

Note: If there is a second batch, repeat steps 1–6.

7. Centrifuge the resulting filtrate (300g, 15 min at 4°C, with slow acceleration and deceleration).

8. After centrifugation, place the tube(s) on ice.
   a. Discard the supernatant using a pipet.
   b. Add 2.5 mL of fresh cold Puck's D-GS and resuspend the pellet by trituration (5–6 strokes up and down using a 5-mL plastic pipet, but *avoid foaming*).
   c. Bring the volume of this suspension to 50 mL with cold Puck's D-GS and take an aliquot (0.1 mL) for cell counting.

9. Centrifuge the cell suspension(s) (300g, 15 min at 4°C, as above).

10. Count the cells (from step 8c).
    a. Determine the total cell number in each batch. An aliquot of 0.1 mL cell suspension is mixed with 50 mL of Puck's D-GS (dilution 1:500), and the total cell number determined by the use of either a hemocytometer or an electronic cell counter.
    b. Viability: It may be useful (particularly for beginners) to examine also cell viability (determination of the percentage of cells that exclude a test dye, such as nigrosin or trypan blue). Usually, this test shows a viability of about 50%.

11. At the end of the second centrifugation, discard the supernatant and resuspend the pellet by trituration (as described for step 8b).

12. Fill the plastic culture flask with the appropriate amount of cold culture medium to obtain a final cell density of 7.5×10^6 viable cells/mL. Add the cell suspension to the medium and mix well.
    Note: The final cell density should be increased if tissue of a more advanced developmental stage is used for dissociation.

7. INITIATION AND MAINTENANCE OF AGGREGATING NEURAL CELL CULTURES

Culture initiation is the most critical step in the entire procedure, since, in order to obtain truly replicate cultures, it is crucial that all steps in the procedure are rigorously adhered to (*see* Table 1). This is particularly important for the phase of cell reaggregation under gyratory agitation, since a balance between attracting and shearing forces has to be established. For the importance of uniformity, *see* Section 11.2., item 2.

Cell aggregation starts immediately after the cell suspension has been placed in the incubator. However, during the period of warming up, the pH of the culture medium will rise above physiological values. In order to keep this critical period, as short as possible, two persons should work together during culture initiation, one who pipets the aliquots of the cell suspension, and one who transfers the flasks to the incubator.

Table 1
Outline of the Preparation of Aggregating Neural Cell Cultures

Day 0	Day 1	Day 2
Fetal CNS tissue, pooled and rinsed	Orbital shaker: 73 rpm (morning)	Transfer of aggregates to 50-mL Erlenmeyer addition of 4 mL medium
Mechanical dissociation in Puck's D-GS	74 rpm (evening)	
Passage through 200 μm nylon mesh		
Filtration through 115 μm nylon mesh		Orbital shaker: 77 rpm
Centrifugation (300g, 15 min, 4°C)		
Resuspension of pellet (trituration)		
Cell count		
Centrifugation (300g, 15 min, 4°C)		
Resuspension of pellet (trituration)		
in cold serum-free medium		
Final cell density: 7.5×10^6 cells/mL		
Incubation (CO_2 incubator, 37°C)		
Aliquots (4 mL) in 25-mL Erlenmeyer		
Orbital shaker: 68 rpm (at start)		
70 rpm (evening)		

7.1. Materials

Gyratory shaker, 25 mm shaking diameter. (*See* Section 11.2., item 1.)
Erlenmeyer flasks, 25 mL. (*See* Section 11.2., item 2.)
Erlenmeyer flasks, 50 mL. (*See* Section 11.2., item 2.)
Gas permeable plastic caps for Erlenmeyer flasks (Bellco Biotechnology, Vineland, NJ).

7.2. Protocol for Culture Initiation and Maintenance

1. Prepare the required number of 25-mL Erlenmeyer flasks (Schott Duran, modified, as described in Section 11.2.) and loosen the gas-permeable plastic caps.
2. Transfer 4 mL aliquots of the final cell suspension to the 25-mL Erlenmeyer flasks.
3. Place the flasks onto the platform of a rotating gyratory shaker in the CO_2 incubator (Fig. 2) at 37°C, with a CO_2 atmosphere in accordance with the bicarbonate concentration in the medium (e.g., 10% CO_2 and 90% humidified air, with medium containing 3.7 g bicarbonate/L). The initial frequency of agitation is *68 rpm*.
4. In the evening of the day of culture preparation (d 0), increase the agitation frequency to *70 rpm*.
5. The next day, increase agitation to *73 rpm* (in the morning) and then to *74 rpm* (in the evening).

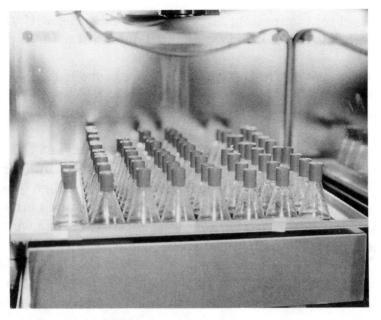

Fig. 2. View inside an incubator containing a gyratory shaker. The culture flasks (here 50-mL Erlenmeyer flasks with gas-permeable caps) are kept in ranges of 10 (max. load 100 flasks). Attached to the shaker platform is a thermometer to show the local temperature (kept between 36.5 and 37°C).

6. At d 2, transfer cultures to 50-mL Erlenmeyer flasks equipped with gas-permeable plastic caps. Pour the content of each flask carefully along the glass wall of a new flask and repeat exactly the same movement by adding an additional 4 mL of fresh prewarmed medium, with which the original flask was rinsed. Ideally, *no aggregates should remain attached on the wall of the new culture vessel*.

Note: Again, this procedure will cause a rise in the pH of the medium (as at culture initiation, *see above*). Therefore, care should be taken to keep this operation as short as possible (not exceeding 30 min/series). Allow to equilibrate for 1–2 h before a further series is transferred.

7. After completion of the transfer, increase the frequency of agitation to *77 rpm*, and thereafter every day by *1 rpm*, until the maximal rotation speed *(80 rpm)* is attained at d 5.
8. At d 5, the culture medium is replenished for the first time.
   a. Warm the required amount of fresh culture medium in a water bath.
   b. Take the culture flasks in groups of five, put them on a slanted support, and allow the aggregates to settle.
   c. With a 5-mL pipet, remove 5 mL of medium, and add an equal volume of fresh medium.

Note: To avoid contamination, always use a fresh pipet with fresh medium.

9. The medium is replenished every third day until d 14, and every other day thereafter.

10. At d 20, because of the greatly increased metabolic rate of the cultures, the content of each flask has to be divided into two separate cultures ("splitting"). At the same time, medium containing albumin-bound lipids (*see* Section 11.1., step 9e) will be added.

    a. Use a 2-mL plastic pipet to split the cultures. Tilt the flask containing the aggregates, quickly resuspend the aggregates by short aspiration and brisk expulsion of the supernatant medium, and then quickly take a 2-mL aliquot and transfer it to a fresh flask containing 4 mL of medium.

    b. Transfer a second 2-mL aliquot in exactly the same way.

    c. Replace the missing volume in the original flask with 4 mL of fresh medium.

    Note: The new culture flasks containing 4 mL of fresh medium have to be equilibrated in the incubator for at least 1 h before splitting.

11. A second split may be necessary at d 30.

8. BRAIN CELL AGGREGATES ENRICHED WITH EITHER NEURONS OR GLIAL CELLS

It may sometimes be necessary to compare the regular aggregate cultures with aggregate cultures enriched with either neurons or glial cells. The preparation of aggregates from cells purified and grown initially in monolayer culture was found to be tedious, and the resulting cultures difficult to grow (Guentert-Lauber et al., 1985). Therefore, a pharmacological approach was taken (Honegger and Werffeli, 1988; Corthésy-Theulaz et al., 1990), to eliminate either the neurons by a single treatment with cholera toxin or the glial cells by an early treatment with cytosine arabinoside.

8.1. Preparation of Glial Cell-Enriched Aggregate Cultures

Aggregate cultures are treated at d 7 (i.e., 24 h prior to the regular medium change) with a single dose of cholera toxin (100 nM). During the following 2 wk, the neurons progressively disappear from the aggregates, giving rise to glial cell-enriched aggregate cultures.

Note: The commercially available cholera toxin (*Vibrio cholerae* type Inaba 569B from Gibco-BRL or Calbiochem) usually contains NaN_3, which is cytotoxic (Calbiochem offers now an azide-free preparation for tissue culture). To remove the azide, cholera toxin is dialyzed against 0.9% NaCl, buffered with HEPES (0.5 mM, pH 7.4), and subsequently sterilized by filtration (0.2 μm). It has to be kept in mind that cholera toxin is a very labile compound; thus, solutions of cholera toxin should not be frozen and thawed repeatedly.

8.2. Preparation of Neuron-Enriched Aggregate Cultures

Aggregate cultures of 15-d fetal rat telencephalon are treated twice (at d 2 and d 4) with cytosine arabinoside (Ara-C, Sigma no. C-1768; 0.4 μM final concentration in culture). In such cultures, the majority of glial cells proliferate during the first week. Therefore, cultures treated with Ara-C contain mostly neurons and only few glial cells. However, the virtual absence of glial cells greatly affects neuronal maturation. Therefore, to enhance neuronal maturation in cultures devoid of glial cells, depolarizing concentrations of KCl (30 mM final concentration in culture) have to be added to the culture medium from d 7 onward (Riederer et al., 1992). KCl is added to the medium from an iso-osmolar stock solution (174 mM KCl).

Note: The most rigorous glial cell depletion is obtained by a combined treatment at d 2 with both Ara-C (0.4 μM) and epidermal growth factor (EGF, receptor grade, Collaborative Biomedical, Bedford, MA, 5 ng/mL). The treatment with Ara-C is repeated at d 4, this time without EGF. Subsequently, the cultures require high potassium medium for neuronal maturation. Perhaps, in the future, selected neurotrophic factors could be used. On the other hand, cultures derived from somewhat more mature tissue (e.g., from 16-d rat telencephalon), exhibit less intense mitotic activity and seem to contain a small population of postmitotic glial cells (predominantly astrocytes) that are not affected by Ara-C. These cultures do not require elevated KCl concentrations for neuronal maturation.

9. ANALYSIS OF AGGREGATING NEURAL CELL CULTURES

Initially, aggregating cell cultures were used exclusively for light microscopic morphological studies (e.g., Moscona, 1961; Delong and Sidman, 1970). The application of biochemical criteria was introduced by Seeds (1971), and thereafter has been considerably extended and combined with the techniques of molecular biology. Furthermore, morphological studies at the electron microscopic level, and cytochemical evaluations have been introduced.

For the different analytical approaches, aggregates are washed with phosphate-buffered saline (PBS) (*see* Section 11.3., item 3). For morphological analyses, the PBS is prewarmed; for biochemical and molecular biological techniques, the PBS is used ice-cold. In stationary suspensions, the sedimentation of aggregates by gravity is sufficiently rapid; only very early cultures (in vitro d 1–2) require gentle centrifugation (75g, 1 min) for washing.

9.1. Morphological Analyses

Aggregating neural cell cultures, in contrast to substrate cell cultures, do not permit direct microscopic observation; they require an approach similar to that used for tissue fragments. However, all basic light microscopic and electron microscopic techniques can be applied.

1. Fixation and embedding: Specific fixation and embedding procedures are used for immunocytochemistry, histochemistry, and electron microscopy. For immunocytochemistry, the best preservation of antigenicity is obtained by omitting tissue fixation. Therefore, cryostat sections are routinely used. In certain cases, immunostaining can be obtained on paraffin sections after a classical deparaffination, but only a few antigens resist the high temperature during embedding.

   a. For cryostat sections (10 µm), the PBS-washed aggregates are transferred to a gelatin capsule (Feton International, Brussels, no. 00) by using a 1-mL plastic pipet. The supernatant is then removed with a Pasteur pipet and the aggregates are covered with cryoform (Cryomatrix; Shandon Scientific, Runcorn, Cheshire, England). The capsule is immediately immersed in isopentane cooled in liquid nitrogen. The temperature of the isopentane is critical for good tissue preservation. It is optimal when the first white spots of solid isopentane appear at the bottom of the container. Frozen capsules are transferred to a plastic tube kept in dry ice to prevent accidental fracturing. They are stored at –80°C. The day before cutting on the cryostat, the frozen capsules are transferred to –20°C.

   b. For paraffin sections, the aggregates are fixed either in 4% paraformaldehyde (for immunocytochemistry) or in Carnoy solution (for histochemistry and regular light microscopy). For paraformaldehyde fixation, the PBS-washed aggregates are immersed in PBS containing 4% paraformaldehyde for 1 h at 4°C. For Carnoy fixation, the aggregates are transferred to glass tubes. The supernatants are discarded and freshly prepared Carnoy solution (*see* Section 11.3., item 4) is added for 1 h at room temperature. The Carnoy solution is changed once, after 15 min of fixation. The aggregates are then dehydrated by sequential passage to 100% ethanol (2 × 15 min), ethanol/toluol (15 min), and toluol (15 min).

   The fixed aggregates are transferred to gelatin capsules (Feton, 000) and placed on a prewarmed support in an oven kept at 60°C. The aggregates are covered with melted paraplast using a prewarmed 1-mL disposable plastic pipet. Thirty minutes later, the paraffin is removed and replaced by a fresh bath. After two more baths of 30 min each, the support with the capsules is taken out of the oven. Once room temperature is attained, the gelatin capsules are removed and the paraffin cylinders are embedded in paraffin blocs.

   c. For electron microscopy, the PBS-washed aggregates are fixed for 1 h at room temperature, in PBS containing 1.5% glutaraldehyde and 0.5% paraformaldehyde. Thereafter, they are rinsed in PBS for 1 h and then transferred to 1.5-mL Eppendorf tubes. The aggregates are postfixed for 1 h in 2% osmium tetroxide and dehydrated in ethanol (successively in 30, 70, 90%, and 100%, for 10 min at each concentration), and finally in propylene oxide for 5 min. The aggregates are then embedded in TAAB 812™, either in bean capsules (8 mm) or in gelatin capsules (Feton, 0). Between each step of the dehydration and embedding protocol, the aggregates are sedimented by centrifugation (500g, 5 min).

2. Immunocytochemistry: For cryostat sections, the pre-equilibrated (–20°C) block is attached to the cryostat support with cryoform, and the gelatin capsule is removed with the use of a razor blade. Ten micrometer cryostat sections are transferred to glass slides coated twice with undiluted polylysine (slide adhesion solution, Sigma P-8920) and kept at room temperature. The sections are fixed in acetone (10 min at room temperature) and then kept overnight at 4°C until staining. For best results, staining is always done on freshly cut sections.

    a. Immunofluorescence staining: For immunofluorescence staining, the sections are rehydrated in PBS for 10 min, the unspecific sites blocked with serum (normal rabbit serum DAKO no. X-0902 if monoclonal antibodies are used; normal swine serum DAKO no. X-0901 with polyclonal antibodies; both diluted 1:25 in PBS), and then exposed to the primary antiserum (overnight at 4°C in a moisture chamber). Thereafter, they are washed three times for 20 min in PBS and then exposed (30 min) to the fluorescent secondary antibody (DAKO, 1:50 in PBS), filtered just before use through Gelman Acrodisc PF no. 4187, 0.8 μm/0.2 μm. Then the sections are washed again in PBS (20 min), and mounted in a semipermanent medium according to Lennette (1978). The polymerization of the medium requires 1–2 h at 4°C. The sections are stored at 4°C.

    b. Peroxidase staining: For peroxidase staining, the sections are first treated for 30 min with methanol containing 0.3% H_2O_2, then with 95% ethanol, and finally dried in the air. The dried sections are encircled with a delimiting pen (DAKO no. S-2002). After rehydration with PBS, the same procedure is used as described above for the immunofluorescence. Biotinylated immunoglobulins and avidin-biotin bound to peroxidase are obtained from Vector Laboratories. After avidin-biotin (30 min), sections are sequentially rinsed, first in PBS (15 min), followed by Tris-HCl, pH 7.6 (5 min); Tris-HCl containing 0.2% nickel sulfate (10 min); 0.05% diaminobenzidine/0.2% nickel sulfate (10 min); and finally by 0.05% diaminobenzidine/0.003% H_2O_2/0.2% nickel sulfate (5 min). This nickel enhancement procedure is according to Adams (1981). After two washes in Tris-HCl, the sections are counterstained with 0.5 % toluidine blue (30 s), differentiated, dehydrated, and mounted in Pertex (Histolab, Göteborg, Sweden).

3. Histochemistry: Histochemical staining is used for the detection of microglial cells in rat brain cell aggregate cultures (Monnet-Tschudi et al., 1995). Microglial cells express a surface glycoprotein recognized specifically by the isolectin B4 isolated from *Griffonia simplicifolia*. This staining technique was first described by Streit and Kreutzberg (1987) and Ashwell (1990). In brief, the 5 μm paraffin sections are deparaffinized and rehydrated, then blocked with H_2O_2 (0.3% in methanol) followed by ethanol 100 and 96%. The dried sections are encircled with a delimiting pen (DAKO) and rehydrated in Tris saline (see Section 11.3., item 5). They are incubated overnight at 4°C in isolectin B4 from *Griffonia simplicifolia* conjugated with peroxidase (Sigma L-5391; 12.5 mg dissolved in 1 mL Tris saline containing 1% Triton X-100). For the peroxidase staining with nickel enhancement, the same procedure is used as described above for immunocytochemistry.

4. Autoradiography: For autoradiography, both cryostat sections and paraffin sections can be used. The dried sections are dipped in Ilford L4 emulsion and exposed for 4 wk. They are developed in phenizol (Ilford no. 34 Do 57; dilution 1:4 in H_2O), dried, and finally counterstained with toluidine blue as described in Section 9.1., step 2.

9.2. Biochemical Analyses

Because of the high reproducibility of aggregate cultures and the possibility to prepare numerous replicate cultures that contain relatively large amounts of material, this culture system is particularly suitable for multidisciplinary studies. Biochemical analyses are most convenient for quantitative routine assays. For example, by measuring the activities of neuronal and glial marker enzymes (point 1), developmental events and changes in the cellular composition can be easily monitored. Metabolic labeling studies are available to monitor cell proliferation (point 2), synthesis of proteins and neurotransmitters (Honegger and Richelson, 1979), or changes in metabolic activity (point 3). Furthermore, the expression of specific proteins can be studied at both the transcriptional and the protein level, following standard protocols (point 4). For more detailed studies, subcellular extraction protocols can be applied, e.g., for the quantitative extraction of synaptosomes or myelin (point 5). In most cases it is sufficient to use three parallel cultures for quantitative analysis. Often, only a fraction of one flask is necessary for a series of assays. It is also possible to perform sequential assays with aggregates from the same flask, e.g., for sampling at different time points. There seem to be no obvious limits to the use of aggregating neural cell cultures. Examples of some tested applications are given below.

1. Enzymatic activities, total protein, and DNA content: The aggregates are washed twice in 5 mL of ice-cold PBS and homogenized in 2×250 μL of 2 mM potassium phosphate containing 1 mM EDTA, pH 6.8, using conical glass-glass homogenizers (Bellco). The homogenates are briefly sonicated (2×2 s pulses of 30 W using a microtip), divided into aliquots for the different assays, and stored at –80°C for analysis. The activities of cell type-specific enzymes, such as choline acetyltransferase, glutamic acid decarboxylase, tyrosine hydroxylase (all neuron-specific), glutamine synthetase (representing astrocytes), and 2',3'-cyclic nucleotide 3'-phosphohydrolase (typically oligodendroglial), are determined using either radiometric or colorimetric assays (Seeds, 1971; Wilson et al., 1972; Honegger and Richelson, 1976; Honegger and Schilter, 1992). Specific enzymatic activities are expressed as a function of either the protein or the DNA content.

   Total protein is determined either by the Folin phenol method (method of Lowry et al., modified by Wilson et al., 1972) or by the Coomassie blue dye binding method of Bradford (1976), using the Bio-Rad dye reagent (no. 500-0006) according to the protocol of the supplier. The DNA content is measured by a fluorimetric assay (Downs and Wilfinger, 1983).

2. Mitotic activity: DNA synthesis is determined by measuring the incorporation of [^{14}C]thymidine into a macromolecular fraction (Lenoir and Honegger, 1983). The cultures are incubated for 4 h in regular medium containing [^{14}C-methyl]thymidine (0.5 μCi/flask, specific activity 61 mCi/mmol). Aggregates are then washed three times with ice-cold PBS, homogenized in 0.4 mL of 0.05% (v/v) Triton X-100, using conical glass-glass homogenizers (Bellco), and sonicated briefly. Aliquots (20 and 40 μL) of the homogenate are placed on separate glass fiber filter disks (Whatman GF/A 2.5 cm) and dried under an infrared heat lamp. The filters are then transferred to supports on a filtration manifold and washed once with 5 mL of 10% (w/v) trichloroacetic acid (TCA) and three times with 5 mL of 5% TCA. Thereafter, they are rinsed in 200 mL of ethanol/ether (1:1) and subsequently in 200 mL of ether. The filters are then transferred to glass scintillation vials, air dried, and incubated overnight with 0.5 mL of NCS tissue solubilizer (Amersham). After neutralization of the digest with 17 μL of glacial acetic acid, 10 mL of scintillation cocktail (Optifluor, Packard) is added for counting.

3. Uptake of 2-deoxyglucose: The uptake of [^{3}H]2-deoxy-D-glucose is measured according to Yu et al. (1993). Aliquots of aggregates are transferred to 15-mL conical plastic tubes, washed once with 4 mL of culture medium, taken up in 4 mL of fresh medium, and transferred to 25-mL culture flasks. After 1 h of equilibration in the CO_2 incubator (culture conditions as usual), 50 μL (3.2 μCi) of 2-deoxy-D-[1-^{3}H]glucose (specific activity 17 Ci/mmol) is added to the medium and the incubation continued for 30 min. The incubation is termi-

nated by the addition of 4 mL of ice-cold PBS. The aggregates are immediately transferred to conical glass homogenizers (Bellco) and washed three times with 5 mL of ice-cold PBS. They are then homogenized in 2×200 μL of 2 mM potassium phosphate buffer, pH 6.8. The homogenates are sonicated, and aliquots are then taken for protein assay and liquid scintillation counting. For the latter, 0.3 mL aliquots of the homogenates are mixed with equal volumes of lysis solution (10 mM NaOH containing 0.1% Triton X-100), transferred to scintillation vials, and counted after addition of 7.5 mL Pico-Aqua scintillation cocktail (Packard). **Note:** Small samples of aggregates (e.g., one-eighth of the content of one flask) are incubated in a final volume of 0.8 mL using 12-well plates (Costar no. 3512). In this case, the uptake is initiated with 10 μL aliquots of 2-deoxy-D-[1-^{3}H]glucose and terminated by the addition of 2 mL of ice-cold PBS.

4. Protein expression:

    a. Total cellular RNA: Total cellular RNA can be extracted from the cultures by using standard protocols, e.g., according to Chomczynski and Sacchi (1987). From the aggregates of each flask, 100–200 μg of total RNA can be obtained, depending on the developmental stage of the cultures. Isolated total RNA (or mRNA obtained by further purification) will serve for specific applications, such as Northern blot analysis, polymerase chain reaction, and cDNA cloning (Corthésy-Theulaz et al., 1990; Bardoscia et al., 1992; Taylor et al., 1994; Appel et al., 1995).

    b. Relative rate of protein synthesis: The relative rate of protein synthesis can be examined by metabolic labeling using [^{35}S]-methionine as a radioactive tracer in serum-free medium lacking unlabeled methionine (Corthésy-Theulaz et al., 1990). The labeled cultures are washed in ice-cold PBS containing 5 μg/mL cycloheximide and solubilized in 0.4% deoxycholic acid, 1% Nonidet P-40, 60 mM EDTA, and 10 mM Tris-HCl, pH 7.4, containing protease inhibitors (10 μg/mL each of leupeptin [Sigma no. L-0649], antipain [Sigma no. A-6191], and pepstatin [Sigma no. P-4265]); 5 μg/mL of E-64 (Sigma no. E-3132); and 1 mM aminoethylbenzene-sulfonylfluoride (Sigma no. A-5938). The nonsolubilized material is eliminated by centrifugation (2 min, 8000g). The resulting supernatant is used for further purification steps, including immunoprecipitation, and for final analyses. Inhibition of protein synthesis at the transcriptional and translational levels can be achieved according to Pan and Price (1984), using actinomycin D (0.1 μM final concentration) and cycloheximide (1 μM final concentration), respectively.

    c. Western blot analysis: For Western blot analysis (Riederer et al., 1992; Monnet-Tschudi et al., 1995), PBS-washed aggregates are homogenized in 2 mM phosphate buffer, pH 6.8, in the presence of protease inhibitors

(10 µg/mL each of leupeptin, antipain, and pepstatin); 5 µg/mL of E-64; and 1 mM aminoethylbenzene-sulfonylfluoride, as described above. Proteins (10–50 µg/slot) are separated by sodium dodecyl sulfate-poly-acrylamide gel electrophoresis (SDS-PAGE). The gels are taken for the electrophoretic transfer of proteins to nitrocellulose sheets (BA-S 85; Schleicher and Schuell). Specific proteins are probed by incubation overnight with specific antibodies. Blots are revealed either by the peroxidase-conjugated antibody technique, using peroxidase-conjugated rabbit antimouse IgG (DAKO no. P-0260) for monoclonal antibodies, or goat antirabbit IgG (Nordic, GAR/IgGH+L/PO) for the polyclonal antibodies, both diluted 1:10^3, and either the chromogen chloro-1-naphthol or the chemiluminescence kit of Boehringer Mannheim. The nitrocellulose sheets are exposed to hyperfilm MP (Amersham), which is then developed in a Curix 60 (Agfa) developing apparatus.

    d. ELISA and RIA: For the quantitation of specific proteins by ELISA or by radioimmunoassay (RIA), total culture homogenates can be used, e.g., to measure myelin basic protein content by RIA (Kerlero de Rosbo et al., 1990).

5. Subcellular fractions: Pooled aggregates from a minimum of five flasks, taken at an advanced developmental stage, can be used for the quantitative extraction of myelin (Matthieu et al., 1979) or for the preparation of synaptosomal fractions (Monnet-Tschudi et al., 1995).

10. CHARACTERISTICS OF SERUM-FREE AGGREGATING NEURAL CELL CULTURES

Aggregating cell cultures can be grown in up to 150 replicate cultures per batch, each flask containing more than 1000 individual aggregates. It is important to obtain even-sized aggregates with a final diameter of 300–400 µm. At the outset, the dissociated cells appear to reaggregate in a random fashion, but in the formed aggregates, the cells reorganize in a tissue-specific way (Fig. 3). Thus, the neurons tend to be localized more towards the center of the aggregate, and oligodendrocytes and astrocytes are more concentrated toward the periphery. A small population of microglial cells is found scattered throughout the aggregates. No fibroblasts and no macrophages can be found in these cultures.

During the first 2 wk in vitro, most of the glial cells proliferate. Thereafter, little mitotic activity is observed. The differentiation of neurons and glial cells progresses for several weeks. Myelination of axons starts in the third week, and attains a maximum after 4 wk of culture. The neuronal maturation and synapse formation may persist for 2 mo or more. With the progression of maturation, the metabolic rate increases dramatically and the neurons exhibit spontaneous electrical activity.

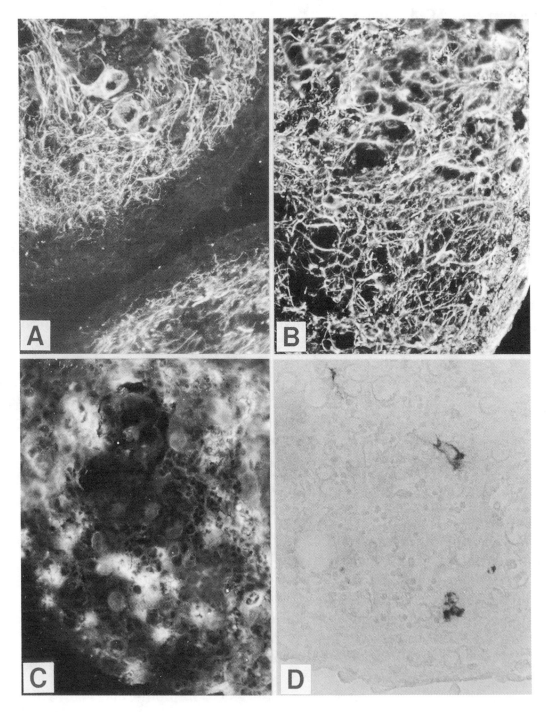

Fig. 3. Examples of morphological analyses of aggregating cell cultures of fetal rat telencephalon. **(A)** Immunostaining for neurofilament protein (NF-M); **(B)** immunostaining for glial fibrillary acidic protein (GFAP); **(C)** immunostaining for myelin basic protein (MBP); **(D)** histochemical staining for microglial cells using isolection B4 from Griffonia simplicifolia. (A–C) Cryostat sections of aggregates grown for 35 d in chemically defined medium. (D) Paraffin section of 15-d aggregate fixed in Carnoy solution. Magnification: 400×.

11. APPENDIX

11.1. Chemically Defined Culture Medium

Because aggregating neural cell cultures form tissue-like structures, many endogenous factors necessary for cell survival, development, and maintenance are provided by cell-cell interactions within the aggregates. It is probably for this reason that they were among the first neural cell cultures to grow in a serum-free, chemically defined medium (Honegger et al., 1979). The original defined medium has been modified only slightly through the years, and should be considered as a minimal growth medium. An increasing number of growth and maturation factors, which can be added to the chemically defined media described here, are able to enhance the development of neurons and glial cells. The protocol for the preparation of 10 L of serum-free culture medium is as follows:

1. Purchase Dulbecco's modified Eagle's medium (DMEM) powder mix for 10 L (Gibco cat. no. 52100-039), containing high glucose (4.5 g/L) and L-glutamine, but no bicarbonate and no pyruvate.
2. Fill a glass jar (Pyrex) with 8 L of ultrapure water and dissolve the powder under gentle continued stirring (use large magnetic stirring bar).
3. Add the following supplements:

Choline chloride (Sigma C-7527)	1.35 g
L-Carnitine (Fluka, Buchs, Switzerland, 22018)	20 mg
Lipoic acid (Sigma T-5625)	2 mg
Vitamin B12 (Fluka 95190)	13.6 mg

4. Add 1 mL of each of the following 10^4-fold concentrated stock solutions of trace elements (stored frozen at $-20°C$):

$CdSO_4 \cdot 8H_2O$ (Merck, Darmstadt, 2028)	50 μM
$CuSO_4 \cdot 5H_2O$ (Merck 2790)	100 μM
$MnCl_2 \cdot 4H_2O$ (Merck 5927)	50 μM
Na_2SeO_3 (Serva, Heidelberg, 30210)	150 μM
$NaSiO_3 \cdot 5H_2O$ (Fluka 71746)	2.5 mM
$(NH_4)_6Mo_7O_{24} \cdot 4H_2O$ (Sigma M-0878)	5 μM
$NiSO_4 \cdot 6H_2O$ (Merck 6727)	2.5 μM
$SnCl_2 \cdot 2H_2O$ (Merck 7815)	2.5 μM
$ZnSO_4 \cdot 7H_2O$ (Merck 8883)	50 μM

5. Adjust the pH of the medium close to the final pH with NaOH ($1N$)
6. Add sodium bicarbonate according to the CO_2 atmosphere used in the incubator (e.g., 3.7 g/L, if cultures are kept at 10% CO_2), and immediately gas with 10% CO_2 in air until the pH is adjusted to 7.4.

7. Adjust the osmolarity of the medium to 340 ± 2 mOsm by adding the required volume of water.

8. Sterilize the medium by filtration using MediaKap-10 hollow fiber filters (Microgon, 0.2 μm) and a peristaltic pump. Store the medium in 500-mL bottles (Pyrex) with gas-tight closures, at 4°C in the dark.

9. Just before use, complete the medium with the following additions:
   a. BME vitamins (Gibco-BRL no. 21040-035) from a 100-fold concentrated stock solution.
   b. Vitamin A alcohol and vitamin E (trace concentrations; *see* Note below).
   c. Transferrin (Sigma T-2252; 1 mg/L final concentration).
      Triiodothyronine (Na$^+$ salt, Sigma T-2752; 30 nM final concentration).
      Insulin (Sigma I-5500; 5 mg/L final concentration).
      Hydrocortisone-21-phosphate (Sigma H-4251; 20 nM final concentration).
      Gentamicin sulfate (Sigma no. G-1264; 25 mg/L final concentration) as antibiotic.
   d. In addition, for cultures up to 20 d in vitro; add linoleic acid (Na$^+$ salt, Sigma no. L-8134, 3 mg/L final concentration).
   e. For cultures older than 20 d in vitro; substitute linoleic acid by albumin-bound lipids (Albumax II, Gibco-BRL no. 11021-011; final concentration 0.1% w/v); all other medium components are the same as above.

   Note: The stock solutions of transferrin, linoleic acid, triiodothyronine, insulin, and hydrocortisone-21-phosphate are prepared as 10^3-fold concentrated aqueous solutions and stored at –20°C. The gentamicin sulfate stock solution, 500-fold concentrated, is also stored at –20°C. The Albumax II stock solution (stored at 4°C) is prepared 100-fold concentrated (10% w/v), its pH adjusted to 7.4 with 0.2N NaOH, using phenol red (15 mg/L final concentration, from a 50-fold concentrated sterile stock solution) as indicator.

   Preparation of the stock solution for vitamins A and E: 114 mg vitamin A alcohol (Fluka no. 95144) is dissolved in 200 μL of absolute alcohol and mixed with 2.0 mL of α-tocopherol (Sigma T-3251), stored at –20°C. Of this mixture, 50 μL is transferred to 10 mL of medium, sonicated, and added to one bottle (500 mL) of medium by sterile filtration (Gelman Acrodisc PF no. 4187, 0.8 μm/0.2 μm).

11.2. Materials

1. Gyratory shaker: Besides the standard equipment of a tissue culture laboratory, aggregating cell cultures require a gyratory shaker that fits inside a CO_2 incubator. Care should be taken to purchase a heavy duty-type gyratory

shaker built to function at 100% humidity. It should be driven by magnetic induction rather than by a driving belt, and it should not create too much heat in the incubator. The incubator, on the other hand, should be able to tolerate the heat produced by the shaker.

2. Culture flasks: Uniform Erlenmeyer-type culture flasks are required for aggregating cell cultures. It is difficult to find a large batch of uniform so-called DeLong flasks on the market (between batches there are enormous variations in the geometry of the flasks). Therefore, it is best to purchase a large batch of standard Erlenmeyer flasks directly from the factory (for example, Schott Duran 25- and 50-mL Erlenmeyer flasks), if possible with unfinished necks, and to have the necks modified (short straight neck, outside diameter 18 mm) suitable for a gas-permeable plastic cap (Bellco). To adjust for an optimal vortex, it is best to keep the shaking protocol (*see* Section 7.), and to vary, if necessary, the volume of the culture medium in the flask.

3. Nylon mesh filter sacs: The nylon mesh (nybolt, nylon monofilament, 200/ 360 and 11P-115, Swiss Silk Bolting Cloth, Zurich) can be purchased in large sheets. Suppliers for this material in Canada and the United States: B. & S. H. Thompson, Quebec, and TETKO, Elmsford, NY. The filter sacs can be produced from double sheets by cutting with a suitable soldering iron (40 W for 200-μm mesh and 30 W for 115-μm mesh), so that the sacs are cut and sealed at once.

   The filter sacs and appropriate funnels are prepared in the following sizes:
   a. The 200 μm mesh sacs are 3.5 cm large and 14 cm long; the appropriate funnels have a 12 cm long stem and outside diameters of 2.5 cm (top) and 1.6 cm (bottom).
   b. The 115 μm mesh sacs are 5.0 cm large and 5.5 cm long; the appropriate funnels have a 4 cm long stem and outside diameters of 4.5 cm (top) and 2.5 cm (bottom).

11.3. Solutions

1. Puck's salt solution D (Puck's D) according to Wilson et al., 1972:

NaCl	8 g/L
KCl	400 mg/L
$Na_2HPO_4 \cdot 7H_2O$	45 mg/L
KH_2PO_4	30 mg/L
D-glucose	1 g/L
Sucrose, pH 7.4, 340 mOsm	20 g/L

   Store at 4°C.

2. Puck's salt solution D containing gentamicin-sulfate (Puck's D-GS). Just *before use*, add to Puck's D 25 mg/L gentamicin-sulfate (Sigma G-1264). Adjust the pH to 7.4 with 0.2N NaOH (approx 0.5 mL/500 mL Puck's D).

3. PBS:

NaCl	6.43 g/L
KCl	395 mg/L
$Na_2HPO_4 \cdot 7H_2O$	540 mg/L
D-Glucose	4.5 g/L
Sucrose	24 g/L
$MgCl_2 \cdot 6H_2O$	160 mg/L
$CaCl_2$	200 mg/L
Gentamicin-sulfate (Sigma G-1264)	325 mg/L

pH 7.3, 340 mOsm. Store at 4°C.

Note: Neutralize the solution before adding the Mg^{2+}- and Ca^{2+}-salts.

4. Carnoy solution: Ethanol (100%): chloroform:glacial acetic acid, 30:15:5. Protect solution from light.

5. Tris saline for histochemistry:

Trizma-base	1.94 g/L
Trizma-HCl	13.22 g/L
NaCl	9 g/L

Dissolve in H_2O, final pH 7.4.

11.4. Washing the Glassware

The detergents for washing the culture glassware should be devoid of organic additives. We recommend using a product line like Neodisher® (Chem. Fabrik Dr. Weigert, Hamburg). The culture glassware should never dry before it is clean. Used glassware is stored immersed in a basic detergent solution (e.g., neodisher LM-10; 5% v/v). After washing with special detergent (e.g., neodisher FT), the glassware is rinsed with cold tap water and then with a citric acid solution (e.g., neodisher Z) to remove traces of detergent. Thereafter, the glassware is rinsed several times with deionized water, and finally with ultrapure water. After drying in an oven, the glassware is sterilized.

11.5. Sterilization Procedures

The culture flasks with gas-permeable plastic caps in place are sterilized in an autoclave (120°C) with pulsed vapor. After a first sterilization, they are wrapped in a layer of aluminum foil and sterilized once more. The nylon filter bags, each with their glass funnel inside, are loosely wrapped in aluminum foil and autoclaved in a vapor-permeable box at 120°C. Cotton-plugged glass pipets are sterilized in an oven (4 h at 180°C). For the sterilization of dissecting instruments, see Sections 4.2. and 5.2.

11.6. Useful Antibodies for Immunocytochemical Studies in Neural Cell Aggregates

Antigen recognized	Designation*	Dilution	Source
Glial fibrillary acidic protein	GFAP (m)	1:800	BioMako/Sigma no. 6077
Vimentin	Vim (m)	1:10	Dako no. M-0725
Glutamine synthetase	GS (p)	1:50	Juurlink et al. (1981)
Glial hyaluronate protein	GHAP (m)	1:40	Bignami and Ashner (1992)
Ganglioside GD3	GD3 (m)	1:10	Dr. Pallmann AG, München
Galactocerebroside	GalC (m)	1:50	Boehringer no. 1351 621
Myelin basic protein	MBP (m)	1:500	Boehringer no. 1118 099
Myelin oligodendrocyte glycoprotein	MOG (m)	1:50	Linington et al. (1984)
Neurofilament 200 kDa	NF H (m)	1:100	Boehringer no. 814 342
Neurofilament 160 kDa	NF M (m)	1:200	Boehringer no. 814 334
Neurofilament 60 kDa	NF L (m)	1:10	Riederer et al. (1993)
Microtubule associated protein 2	MAP2 (m)	1:10	Huber and Matus (1984)
Microtubule associated protein 5	MAP5 (m)	1:10	Riederer et al. (1986)
Synaptophysin	SYN (m)	1:10	Boehringer no. 902 314

*m and p indicate monoclonal and polyclonal antibodies

FURTHER READING

Adams, J. (1981), Heavy metal intensification of DAB-based HRP reaction product. *J. Histochem. Cytochem.* **29,** 775.

Appel, K., Honegger, P., and Gebicke-Haerter, P. (1995), Expression of interleukin-3 and tumor necrosis factor-β mRNA in cultured microglia. *J. Neuroimmunol.* **60,** 83–91.

Ashwell, K. (1990), The distribution of microglia and cell death in the developing mouse cerebellum. *Dev. Brain Res.* **55,** 219–230.

Bardoscia, M. T., Amstad, P., and Honegger, P. (1992), Expression of the proto-oncogene c-fos in three-dimensional fetal brain cell cultures and the lack of correlation with maturation-inducing stimuli. *Mol. Brain Res.* **12,** 23–30.

Bignami, A. and Aschner, R. (1992), Some observations on the localization of hyaluronic acid in adult, newborn and embryonal rat brain. *Int. J. Dev. Neurosci.* **10,** 45–57.

Bradford, M. M. (1976), A rapid and sensitive method for the quantitation of microgram quantities of protein utilising the principle of protein dye binding. *Analyt. Biochem.* **72,** 248–254.

Choi, H. K., Won, L., and Heller, A. (1993), Dopaminergic neurons grown in three-dimensional reaggregate culture for periods of up to one year. *J. Neurosci. Meth.* **46,** 233–244.

Chomczynski, P. and Sacchi, N. (1987), Single-step method of RNA isolation by acid guanidinium thiocyanate-phenol-chloroform extraction. *Analyt. Biochem.* **162,** 156–159.

Corthésy-Theulaz, I., Mérillat, A.-M., Honegger, P., and Rossier, B.C. (1990), Na$^+$-K$^+$-ATPase gene expression during in vitro development of rat fetal forebrain. *Am. J. Physiol.* **258** (*Cell Physiol.* **27**), C1062–C1069.

DeLong, G. R. and Sidman, R. L. (1970), Alignment defect of reaggregating cells in cultures of developing brains of reeler mutant mice. *Dev. Biol.* **22,** 584–599.

Downs, T. R. and Wilfinger, W. W. (1983), Fluorimetric quantification of DNA in cells and tissues. *Analyt. Biochem.* **131,**538–547.

Doyle, A., Griffiths, J. B., and Newell, D. G. (Principal Editors) (1994), *Cell and Tissue Culture: Laboratory Procedures.* Wiley, Chichester.

Guentert-Lauber, B., Monnet-Tschudi, F., Omlin, F. X., Favrod, P., and Honegger, P. (1985), Serum-free aggregate cultures of rat CNS glial cells: biochemical, immunocytochemical and morphological characterization. *Dev. Neurosci.* **7,** 33–44.

Honegger, P., Lenoir, D., and Favrod, P. (1979), Growth and differentiation of aggregating fetal brain cells in a serum-free defined medium. *Nature* **282,** 305–308.

Honegger, P. and Richelson, E. (1976), Biochemical differentiation of mechanically dissociated mammalian brain in aggregating cell culture. *Brain Res.* **109,**335–354.

Honegger, P. and Richelson E. (1977), Biochemical differentiation of aggregating cell cultures of different fetal rat brain regions. *Brain Res.* **133,**329–339.

Honegger, P. and Richelson, E. (1979), Neurotransmitter synthesis, storage and release by aggregating cell cultures of rat brain. *Brain Res.* **162,**89–101.

Honegger, P. and Schilter, B. (1992), Serum-free aggregate cultures of fetal rat brain and liver cells: methodology and some practical applications in neurotoxicology, in *The Brain in Bits and Pieces. In vitro Techniques in Neurobiology, Neuropharmacology and Neurotoxicology,* Zbinden, G., ed., MTC Verlag, Zollikon, Switzerland, pp. 51–79.

Honegger, P. and Werffeli, P. (1988), Use of aggregating cell cultures for toxicological studies. *Experientia* **44,** 817–823.

Huber, G. and Matus, A. (1984), Differences in the cellular distribution of two microtubule-associated proteins, MAP1 and MAP2, in rat brain. *J. Neurosci.* **4,** 151–160.

Juurlink, B. H., Schousboe, A., Jorgensen, O. S., and Hertz, L. (1981), Induction by hydrocortisone of glutamine synthetase in mouse primary astrocytes. *J. Neurochem.* **36,** 136–142.

Kerlero de Rosbo, N., Honegger, P., Lassmann, H., and Matthieu, J.-M. (1990), Demyelination induced in aggregating brain cell cultures by a monoclonal antibody against myelin/oligodendrocyte glycoprotein. *J. Neurochem.* **55,** 583–587.

Lennette, D. A. (1978) An improved mounting medium for immunofluorescence microscopy. *Am. J. Clin. Pathol.* **69,** 647,648.

Lenoir, D. and Honegger, P. (1983), Insulin-like growth factor I (IGF I) stimulates DNA synthesis in fetal rat brain cell cultures. *Dev. Brain Res.* **7,** 205–213.

Linington, C., Webb, M., and Woodhams, P. L. (1984), A novel myelin-associated glycoprotein defined by a mouse monoclonal antibody. *J. Neuroimmunol.* **6**, 387–396.

Matthieu, J.-M., Honegger, P., Favrod, P., Gautier, E., and Dolivo, M. (1979), Biochemical characterization of a myelin fraction isolated from rat brain aggregating cell cultures. *J. Neurochem.* **32**, 869–881.

Monnet-Tschudi, F., Zurich, M.-G., Pithon, E., van Melle, G., and Honegger, P. (1995), Microglial responsiveness as a sensitive marker for trimethyltin (TMT) neurotoxicity. *Brain Res.* **690**, 8–14.

Moscona A. A. (1961), Rotation-mediated histogenetic aggregation of dissociated cells: a quantifiable approach to cell interactions in vitro. *Exp. Cell Res.* **22**, 455–475.

Pan, L. C. and Price, P. A. (1984), The effect of transcriptional inhibitors on the bone gamma-carboxyglutamic acid protein response to 1,25-dihydroxyvitamin D3 in osteosarcoma cells. *J. Biol. Chem.* **259**, 5844–5847.

Riederer, B., Cohen, R., and Matus, A. (1986), MAP5: a novel microtubule-associated protein under strong developmental regulation. *J. Neurocytol.* **15**, 763–775.

Riederer, B. M., Monnet-Tschudi, F., and Honegger, P. (1992), Development and maintenance of the neuronal cytoskeleton in aggregated cell cultures of fetal rat telencephalon and influence of elevated K⁺ concentrations. *J. Neurochem.* **58**, 649–658.

Riederer, B. M., Porchet, R., Marugg, R. A., and Binder, L. I. (1993), Solubility of cytoskeletal protein in immunohistochemistry and the influence of fixation. *J. Histochem. Cytochem.* **41**, 609–616.

Rose, S. P. R. (1965), Preparation of enriched fractions from cerebral cortex containing isolated, metabolically active neuronal cells. *Nature (London)* **206**, 621,622.

Schrier, B. K. (1973), Surface culture of fetal mammalian brain cells: effect of subculture on morphology and choline acetyltransferase. *J. Neurobiol.* **4**, 117–124.

Seeds N. W. (1971), Biochemical differentiation in reaggregating brain cell culture. *Proc. Natl. Acad. Sci. USA* **68**, 1858–1861.

Streit, W. J. and Kreutzberg, G. W. (1987), Lectin binding by resting and reactive microglia. *J. Neurocytol.* **16**, 249–260.

Taylor, V., Miescher, G. C., Pfarr, S., Honegger, P., Breitschopf, H., Lassmann, H., and Steck, A. J. (1994), Expression and developmental regulation of Ehk-1, a neuronal Elk-like receptor tyrosine kinase in brain. *Neuroscience* **63**, 163–178.

Varon, S. and Raiborn, C. W., Jr. (1969), Dissociation, fractionation, and culture of embryonic brain cells. *Brain Res.* **12**, 180–199.

Wilson, S. H., Schrier, B. K., Farber, J.-L., Thompson, E. J., Rosenberg, R. N., Blume A. J., and Nierenberg, M. W. (1972), Markers for gene expression in cultured cells from the nervous system. *J. Biol. Chem.* **247**, 3159–3169.

Yu, N., Martin, J.-L., Stella, N., and Magistretti, P. (1993), Arachidonic acid stimulates glucose uptake in cerebral cortical astrocytes. *Proc. Natl. Acad. Sci. USA* **90**, 4042–4046.

Chapter Four

Primary Cell Cultures
of Peripheral and Central Neurons and Glia

Mary I. Johnson and Richard P. Bunge

1. INTRODUCTION

Tissue culture allows the separate establishment of neurons and glia under a variety of conditions of substrate and media. By subsequent recombination of relatively pure cell populations, specific questions of neuronal development and neuronal–glia interactions may be studied. In vivo, axons of dorsal root ganglion (DRG) neurons course through both the central nervous system (CNS) and peripheral nerve trunks, and induce myelination by both central (oligodendrocytes) and peripheral (Schwann cells) neuroglia. In culture, either PNS or CNS glial cells can be added to the networks of nonneuronal cell-free disaggregated DRG neurons. When provided with suitable medium, the glia expand in number and myelination occurs in several weeks. Similarly, cultures of sympathetic neurons have been utilized to study factors influencing neurotransmitter and dendritic development as well as axonal growth, particularly the form and function of growth cones. Studies of substrate requirements and molecular interactions underlying neurite extension have utilized explants of both central and peripheral neurons.

2. PREPARATION OF RAT EMBRYOS

2.1. Materials

Pregnant rat (timed pregnancy of desired embryonic age).
Cork board with pins (8).
Ethanol (80%).

Protocols for Neural Cell Culture, 2nd Ed. • Eds.: S. Fedoroff and A. Richardson • Humana Press, Inc., Totowa, NJ

Ethanol (95%).
Alcohol burner and matches.
Septisol solution.
Shaver.
Petri dishes, plastic or glass (100 mm) (2).
Sterile tube containing 15 mL L-15 medium.
Scissors (6–8 in.) (3).
Forceps (6–8 in.) (3).
Gauze squares, 4 × 4 in. (4).

2.2. Sterilization of Instruments

Sterilize forceps and scissors by immersing them in 80% alcohol (minimum of 20 min) and drying them in air inside the laminar flow hood. When sterile, put the instruments into a sterile glass Petri dish and keep the ends covered with the lid.

2.3. Removal of Uterus

1. The pregnant rat is sacrificed by overdosing with Metofane™ before immobilizing on a cork board ventral side up.
2. Preparation of adult pregnant rat:
   a. Shave abdomen (animal clippers or razor).
   b. Squeeze septisol solution onto the abdomen of the rat and scrub with gauze. Repeat once.
   c. Wash the shaved area with 80% ethanol, cover the abdomen with gauze, and drench gauze with 80% ethanol.
3. With sterile scissors and forceps (set #1), make a lateral cut across the lower abdomen just anterior to the vaginal orifice. Cut through just the skin of the rat and not through the underlying muscle. Continue the incision up the left side of the animal and laterally across the chest of the rat.
4. Retract the skin to the left side and pin it to the board.
5. With new sterile scissors and forceps (set #2), cut through the muscle layer, making the same type of incision as before, except extend the cut up the animal.
6. With new sterile scissors and forceps (set #3), free each horn of the uterus and remove it to a Petri dish containing L-15 medium.

Note: All subsequent procedures are performed in the laminar flow hood.

3. PREPARATION OF DRG

3.1. Materials

E15 rat embryos.
L-15 medium, 25 mL.

Petri dishes, plastic (100 mm) (2).
Forceps (3–4 in.) (2).
Scissors, fine (2).
Spring scissors.
#5 Jeweler's forceps (2).
Petri dish, 100 mm, containing two 35-mm plastic Petri dish bottoms.
Dissecting microscope.
Petri dish, 100 mm.
Ethanol (80%).

3.2. Preparation for Removal of Rat Embryos

1. Sterilization of instruments: Sterilize forceps and scissors by immersing them in 80% alcohol (20 min) and drying them in air inside the laminar flow hood. When sterile, put the instruments into a sterile Petri dish and keep the ends covered with the lid.
2. Preparation:
   a. Pipet 15 mL of L-15 medium into a 100-mm plastic Petri dish.
   b. Pipet 1 mL of L-15 medium into a 100-mm plastic Petri dish.
   c. Pipet 2 mL of L-15 medium into each of two 35-mm plastic Petri dish bottoms contained in a glass 100-mm Petri dish.

3.3. Removal of Rat Embryos from the Uterus and Dissection

1. With sterile fine scissors and forceps, make a cut throughout the length of the uterus.
2. Remove each embryo with the disk-shaped placenta and transfer (with or without amniotic membranes) to a 100-mm plastic Petri dish containing 15 mL of L-15 medium.
3. Dissection of embryo:
   a. Remove membranes if they are still intact.
   b. Before proceeding with the dissection, check the maturity of the embryo. The digits on fore- and hindlimbs should be well defined. The eye also is developed (and open) at this point. E15 embryos are at a good age to ensure that DRGs are pulled out with the cord. The vertebral bodies are soft enough to cut through and the body as a whole is fragile and should be handled with care. DRGs mature in a rostral to caudal direction. The rootlets (connecting the ganglia to the cord) for a lumbar ganglia are quite short, making it more difficult to remove the ganglia; cervical ganglia are probably the easiest to dissect out.
   c. Remove the head at the cervical flexure.

d. Remove viscera by cutting with fine sterile scissors on each side of the body from tail to head just anterior to the vertebral column.
e. Lay the remaining tissue on the dorsal surface so that the ventral surface is uppermost.
f. Repeat steps a–e for each embryo.

3.4. Removal of Spinal Cord

Note: The following is performed under the dissecting microscope. Use the 100-mm Petri dish with 1 mL of L-15 medium. Use a fine spring scissors and a #5 forceps.

1. Clean the ventral surface of the embryo of any remaining viscera, such as the aorta.
2. Make a ventral cut, in a rostral (from where the head was removed) to caudal direction, through the vertebral bodies to expose the cord throughout its length. Alternatively, the vertebral pedicles can be cut on each side, and the strip of vertebral bodies removed *en bloc*.
3. Using the medulla as a "handle," pull straight up (toward the microscope) on the cord, freeing it from the vertebral canal. Try to minimize side-to-side movement of the cord in order to ensure that DRGs will remain attached to the cord.
4. Place dissected cord in one of the two 35-mm Petri dishes filled with L-15 medium.
5. Rinse the cord at least once with L-15 medium to free it of debris and blood. Transfer the washed cord to the second 35-mm Petri dish filled with L-15 medium.
6. Repeat steps 1–5 for each spinal cord.

3.5. Removal of Ganglia

1. Using two fine forceps (#5), pinch off ganglia from the spinal cord and at the same time try to minimize the amount of meninges that may come off with the ganglia.

Note: The particular advantage in using the 15-d rat embryos is that the ganglia come out of the vertebral column with the cord and can be easily plucked off the cord. With practice, one can obtain approx 40 ganglia/embryo. If the litter has 15 embryos, it is therefore possible to obtain 600 ganglia (in approx 3 h). With a yield of about 5000 cells/ganglion, this can give 3×10^6 neurons.

2. Repeat above step for all spinal cords.

Note: If possible (or necessary), discard ganglia that have too much of the meninges attached.

4. PREPARATION OF PURE DRG NEURON CULTURES

4.1. Materials

Plastic Petri dish, 35 mm, containing ganglia.
Trypsin solution, 0.25% in Hanks' calcium/magnesium-free basic salt solution
(4 mL).
Maintenance medium (*see* Section 12.1., 3b) (25 mL).
Polypropylene centrifuge tube, sterile (15 mL).
Petri dishes, plastic, collagen coated (35 mm) (3).
Sterile Pasteur pipet (tip constricted to 0.5 mm).

4.2. Trypsin Digestion

1. After all the ganglia are collected (up to a maximum of 150 ganglia/dish), amass the ganglia in the center by swirling the Petri dish. Carefully pipet off the L-15 medium.
2. Add 2 mL 0.25% trypsin solution to the Petri dish. Incubate at 37°C for 40 min.
3. After 40 min, remove the Petri dish from the incubator and add a few drops of maintenance medium to inactivate the enzyme.

4.3. DRG Neuron Disaggregation and Plating

1. Using a bent tip, cotton-plugged pipet, remove ganglia to a sterile 15-mL centrifuge tube. Wash the dish with an additional few drops of maintenance medium and add this wash to the rest of the ganglia in the tube.
2. Centrifuge the ganglia at 200–300g at room temperature for 5 min.
3. Remove and discard the supernatant without disturbing the pellet. Add 2 mL maintenance medium. Triturate with a small-bore disposable Pasteur pipet until no cell clumps are visible.
4. Centrifuge the cell suspensions at 200–300g at room temperature for 5 min.
5. Remove and discard the supernatant. Add sufficient maintenance medium to obtain a concentration of approx 20 ganglia/3 mL medium.
6. Resuspend cells and plate 3 mL of the medium–ganglia cell suspension into each 35-mm Petri dish. Plate 2–3 dishes.
7. Incubate at 37°C in a 5% carbon dioxide incubator.

5. CULTURES OF DRGs

After the cultures are established as disaggregated cells, they contain a mixture of neurons, fibroblasts, Schwann cells, phagocytes, and various other cell types. The cells that are capable of division (essentially all other cell types except neurons) must be removed. The neurons will survive treatment with antimitotic agents, because almost all of the sensory neuronal population has finished its proliferative phase prior to the time the tissue is taken. The object of the antimitotic medium is to drive proliferation of the dividing cells in the presence of a drug that is lethal for dividing cells. This is accomplished by the following protocol:

Maintenance medium	d 1
Antimitotic medium	d 2–4
Maintenance medium	d 4–6
Antimitotic medium	d 6–8
Maintenance medium	d 8–10
Antimitotic medium	d 10–12
Maintenance medium	d 12 +

This procedure is more effective when using human placental serum than when using fetal bovine serum (FBS). During this period, considerable cell death is observed because the nonneuronal cells die and much cell debris is evident.

6. MYELINATION BY OLIGODENDROCYTES

A variety of glial populations may be used to obtain myelination after seeding onto disaggregated populations of DRG neurons (Wood and Williams, 1984). Cervical spinal cord is dissected from rat embryos on d 15 of gestation (*see* Section 3.4.). The meninges and the dorsal half of the cord are removed, leaving only the two ventral halves connected by the ventral commissure. This tissue is cut into lengths of approx 1 mm and the resulting fragments are disaggregated without enzyme treatment by triturating 12–24 times in maintenance medium. To obtain a moderate glial cell density after plating, the tissue fragments from each cervical ventral cord are disaggregated in 3–4 drops of maintenance medium. After filtration through a nylon filter with 15-µm pores, one drop of this suspension containing $5–10 \times 10^4$ cells is then added to each culture. Three hours after the addition of cord cells, the supernatant medium is drained off and the cultures are refed with maintenance medium.

After the addition of spinal cord cells, the cultures are refed on alternate days for three feedings. Subsequently, cultures to be used for autoradiography are refed with maintenance medium, but all cultures that are to be allowed to myelinate are refed with standard medium (61 mL EMEM, 25 mL human placental serum, 10 mL 9-d chick embryo extract, 3 mL 20% glucose, 0.7 mL 200 m*M* glutamine, and nerve growth factor). The usual concentration of NGF is approx 25 biological U/mL of medium. (A more defined medium may also be used in some instances; *see* Section 12.1., item 3.)

A variety of other methods may be used to isolate oligodendrocytes, including that of McCarthy and de Vellis (1980). More recently, we have obtained functional oligodendrocytes from adult rat by the following method.

Lumbosacral spinal cord is dissected from 4-mo-old female Sprague Dawley rats and stored in cold L-15 medium. The spinal root and meninges are stripped off and the whole cord placed in 0.2% trypsin plus 20 µg/mL DNase in Ca^{2+}-free Hanks' BSS and cut into small pieces. These are incubated 45 min at 35°C. At the end of this incubation, serum is added and the cord fragments recovered by centrifugation. The fragments are triturated through a small-bore pipet in cold L-15 with 10% heat-inactivated serum and the resulting suspension is filtered through a 15-µm pore size nylon filter. This suspension is carefully layered over 2.0 mL of 40% Percoll in a 50:50 mixture of $0.25M$ sucrose in $0.05M$ phosphate buffer, pH 7.4, and L-15 serum and centrifuged at $10,000g$ for 30 min. The myelin layer and a shallow layer of cells just beneath the myelin are discarded. Oligodendrocytes distributed throughout the remaining gradient are harvested, diluted fivefold with L-15 serum, and collected by low-speed centrifugation. Cells resuspended in plating medium (EMEM with 10% serum) are added to cultures containing disaggregated DRGN prepared as previously described (Wood and Williams, 1984), or to empty collagen-coated dishes. Staining with anti-GalCer$^+$ and a rhodamine-conjugated second antibody showed that 30–50% of the viable cells adhering to neurons after 24 h are GalCer$^+$ and 30–50% extend processes. These cells are distinguished from macrophages by:

1. Their brighter fluorescence;
2. Evenly distributed fluorescence (macrophages display a distinct punctate staining pattern); and
3. The presence of slender processes.

We routinely obtain $2–3 \times 10^5$ cells from each lumbosacral cord plated with $10^3–10^4$ cells per culture. Advantages of this procedure include:

1. Easily obtained material;
2. Improved yield of viable cells compared to the mechanical disaggregation method;
3. Enrichment in oligodendrocytes; and
4. Removal of myelin debris and consequent proteolytic activity.

7. MYELINATION BY SCHWANN CELLS

7.1. The Wood Method

The Wood (1976) approach is to establish DRG cultures as explants and to utilize an intermediate level of treatment with antimitotic agents (as compared to that used for neurons). Establishing the neurons as an explant allows them ultimately to be cut out of the culture, the harvest of the surrounding outgrowth of Schwann cells providing the desired pure Schwann cell population. Success here depends on the fibroblasts being more susceptible to antimitotic treatment than are the Schwann cells. Although the treatment does kill many Schwann cells, those that survive subsequently proliferate substantially to repopulate the neuritic outgrowth and are fully functional in that they are capable of going on to myelination. The transplantation procedure expedites the repopulation of the outgrowth because the remaining Schwann cells proliferate vigorously in response to a new neuritic outgrowth.

1. Preparation of Schwann cell progenitors:
   a. Pregnant rat is etherized and the uterine horns removed (*see* Section 2.3.).
   b. Remove E16 embryos from the uterus as previously described in disaggregated neuron preparation (*see* Section 3.3.).
   c. Remove spinal cord and associated DRG by the same method as described for the E15 disaggregated neuron preparation (*see* Section 3.4.). In embryos of this age, however, only cervical and lumbar DRG will remain firmly attached to the cord during its removal.
   d. Once DRGs have been removed from the spinal cord, dissect and remove remaining remnants of the roots in a dish of L-15 containing 10% FBS.
   e. Transfer DRG with a Pasteur pipet that has been wet with L-15 10% FBS to a fresh dish of L-15 10% FBS (serum prevents ganglia from sticking to the pipet surface).
   f. Separate ganglia into groups of three or four. Transfer each of these groups of ganglia with a serum-wet pipet to an Aclar™ dish that has been coated with ammoniated collagen, dried, and wet again with 10 drops of antimitotic medium.
   g. With sterile forceps, arrange ganglia so that they are an equal distance apart from each other and are centrally located within the Aclar dish. Take care not to nick the collagen surface of the dish with forceps, or to poke or squeeze the ganglion in the process of arranging it in the dish.
   h. Once the ganglia are properly arranged in the Aclar dish, remove 4–5 drops of the medium from the dish to prevent ganglia from floating. Do not remove too much of the medium because the tissue will dry out.
   i. These progenitor cultures receive alternating 2-d pulses of maintenance and antimitotic medium for a period of 2 wk to eliminate fibroblasts and are then transplanted.
2. Transplantation procedure:
   a. Materials:
      Sterilized blade holders and razor blades.

Sterilized #5 forceps and #5 Biologie forceps.
35-mm Dishes filled with L-15 10% FBS (2).
Collagen-coated (ammoniated and dried) Aclar dishes.

b. With small pieces of razor blade in blade holders, cut around the central cluster of neurons.

c. With forceps, lift the explant of neurons by the edges (without squeezing the explant) and transfer to a dish of L-15 10% FBS.

d. When all of the explanted neurons have been removed in this manner, carefully strip off the collagen surface from the bottom of the explants, taking care not to poke or squeeze the explant with the forceps. The collagen is readily distinguished from the granular neuronal surface under transillumination in the scope by its shiny appearance.

e. Once all of the collagen has been removed from the explants, transfer explants to a fresh dish of L15 10% FBS and separate into small groupings of explants in the number desired for each dish.

f. Add 10 drops of N2 (defined medium) to each Aclar dish, transfer explants to the dish, arrange proper placement of explants on the dish, and remove a portion of medium to prevent explants from floating (as previously described above).

Note: Transplanted cultures are fed 4–6 drops of N2 medium per Aclar dish every 2 d for a period of 2–3 wk until fully repopulated. Repopulated cultures may then provide Schwann cells for disaggregated neuron cultures.

7.2. The Brockes Method

This procedure has been published in detail by Brockes et al. (1979). We utilized the procedure essentially as published. The approach is to obtain the considerable number of Schwann cells present in the neonatal rat sciatic nerve trunk, at which point in development the nerve contains relatively few fibroblasts. One pulse of antimitotic treatment with cytosine arabinoside is utilized and subsequently, as the cells are passaged, they are treated while in suspension with an antibody (plus complement) to the Thy-1 antigen, which is expressed on fibroblasts but not on Schwann cells. The Schwann cell populations obtained can be expanded and subsequently used for transfer onto DRG neurons, where full functional expression is observed (Porter et al., 1986).

7.3. Obtaining Myelination by Schwann Cells

The objective now is to transfer the pure populations of Schwann cells obtained by either of the two methods described above onto the pure population of DRG neurons. Schwann cells prepared by the Wood method are grown on collagen and must be removed by enzymatic treatment. Schwann cells can also be transferred to certain plastic culture dishes and removed by scraping prior to transferring to the neuronal cultures, if it is desired to avoid a trypsinization step prior to seeding.

Seeding disaggregated neuronal cultures with Schwann cells prepared by the Wood method:

1. Rinse progenitor culture one or two times with Earle's BSS to remove medium.
2. With blade breakers, cut around the ganglion and remove neurons from the dish.
3. Once all neurons have been removed, scrape off collagen plus Schwann cell layer and collect in a test tube.
4. On average, each ganglion yields approx 2×10^5 cells. Add 1 mL 0.05% collagenase solution to every 5–6 layers of collagen to be digested, making sure none of the layers is stuck to the side walls of the tube.
5. Place in desiccator and gas with 150 cm^3 CO_2.
6. Agitate at approx 80 rpm on rotator for 30 min.
7. Centrifuge for 5 min, 1000 rpm.
8. Discard supernatant.
9. Add 0.1% trypsin (10 mg/10 mL Hanks' BSS without calcium and magnesium).
10. Place on rotator (approx 80 rpm) for 30 min.
11. Add an equal volume of myelination medium to quench the reaction.
12. Centrifuge 5 min at 1000 rpm and discard supernatant.
13. Resuspend cells in approx 2 mL (40 drops) myelination medium.
14. Triturate and count the cells in suspension.
15. Seed with approx 1.5×10^4 cells/Aclar dish in a volume of 0.75 mL of maintenance medium/Aclar dish added to 0.25 mL of maintenance medium already in the dish of disaggregated neurons to be seeded.
16. Incubate 18–24 h without disturbing.

8. THE SYSTEM: DISHES AND CONDITIONS OF INCUBATION

8.1. Dishes

In 1970, our laboratory undertook the development of new methods for culturing tissue. The Maximow double-coverslip assembly had been successfully used for a number of years, but was cumbersome in its maintenance and limited the number of cultures available for experimentation. A major need was flexibility in the amount of medium used, allowing the culture of either smaller or larger amounts of tissue, while retaining the capability of observing the cultures at higher magnifications with the compound microscope. We wanted to be able to use a limited feed volume for several reasons:

1. Cultures are sometimes maintained for extended periods and medium components may not be available in large quantities;
2. Cultured nervous tissue may benefit from a degree of self-conditioning of its medium;
3. Some cultures appear to develop more satisfactorily with a shallow overlay of medium because (presumably) of better oxygen exchange with the atmosphere;
4. Expensive drugs or chemicals are most advantageously applied in a small volume; and
5. Smaller "aliquots" of tissue allow more variables per experiment and more cultures per variable.

We therefore developed a small plastic "minidish" with raised edges to contain the culture medium (Bunge and Wood, 1973).

These dishes are molded from inert plastic with a properly machined aluminum punch and die (Aclar 33 C; 5 mil; Allied Chemical Corporation). The punch is heated on a hot plate and the plastic (roughly cut to size) is molded by applying pressure with the cold die. The edges of the small Aclar dishes are then trimmed, cleaned in 70% nitric acid, rinsed first in running tap water and then in distilled water, and finally soaked overnight in double-distilled water. They are then sterilized in 80% ethanol, dried, and coated with collagen. The Aclar dishes are often housed in groups of six in 100×10 mm glass Petri dishes and monitored with an inverted compound microscope. The Aclar dish provides the advantages listed above and has, in addition, the features that its bottom can be cut out after fixation and used as a coverslip to carry the cultures through various staining procedures, and fixation and embedding for electron microscopy can be done directly in the dish and the inert plastic then shelled off the polymerized embedding resin. The flat (2–3 mm thick) disk of polymerized resin allows reviewing of the tissue and marking of specific regions of the culture (even specific myelin segments) for electron microscopic analysis.

Alternately, we use standard plastic culture dishes (35 or 60 mm) or multiwell dishes usually after collagen coating (*see* Section 12.2.). One may also use glass coverslips inside plastic culture dishes or multiwell dishes. These are usually collagen- or laminin-coated before being placed into the housing dishes.

8.2. Incubation Conditions

Instead of CO_2 incubators to house our cultures, we have employed a system of segregating groups of cultures in sealed containers to help prevent spread of mold and fungus infections. Of note is the fact that we use no antibiotics in our feeds, except in some cases during the first days of culture. The cultures are housed in desiccator jars (#3118, 160 mm Pyrex™, Corning Glass Works, Corning, NY) thoroughly cleaned with alcohol, and autoclaved. Sterile water is added to the bottom reservoir to provide a humidified atmosphere. High vacuum grease (Dow Corning Corp., Midland, MI) is used to seal ground glass surfaces (used sparingly to prevent contamination of culture glassware). Depending on the type of medium in use (*see below*), CO_2 is added to maintain pH of approx 7.3. This amount is approx 100 mL for our standard medium and approx 180 mL for the defined medium. The desiccator jars are then placed in an incubator at 37°C.

9. PREPARATION OF RAT SUPERIOR CERVICAL GANGLIA (SCG)

9.1. Embryonic Ganglia

Embryos are removed from pregnant rats as detailed in Sections 2. and 3.3. (1 and 2). Ganglia from gestational d 15–21 can then be used as explants or to generate disaggregated neurons.

1. Isolation of SCG:
   a. Cut into the thorax and through the heart to assure quick exsanguination and reduce bleeding during the dissection.
   b. Using 25-gage needles, pin the embryos supine onto a Petri dish half-filled with hardened wax. Gently hyperextend the head to provide better exposure of the neck.
   c. Remove skin, glands, and muscle, exposing the carotid bifurcation, behind which lies the SCG. All of these steps can be accomplished in embryos using two #5 fine forceps. Care should be taken not to confuse the SCG with the more lateral nodose ganglion. After birth, the nodose ganglion becomes progressively separated form the SCG, making such confusion less likely.
   d. Free the SCG from surrounding tissue before lifting out using both forceps. The younger the embryo, the more fragile the SCG.
   e. Collect the ganglia in L-15 medium (in a 35-mm Petri dish housed within a 100-mm Petri dish).
2. Preparation of SCG cultures:
   a. A well-defined capsule is present on the SCG from E19–E21, and its removal is facilitated by using extrafine forceps (Biologie #5). For SCG from E15–E17, only thin wisps of capsule can be distinguished. Removing the capsule is desirable if nonneuronal cell-free cultures are needed.
   b. Remove the nerve trunks from the decapsulated ganglia and cut them into approx 1-mm chunks using two number 11 blades (Sterisharps, Seam-

less Hospital Products Co., Wallingford, CT) crossed in a scissoring motion. Ganglia from E15 can be cut in half or, more often, are placed into culture intact.

c. Rinse the explants in L-15 to remove tissue debris and transfer them in a small volume of medium to the appropriate culture dish with a fire-polished pipet. To promote explant attachment, the culture dishes should initially contain a small volume of maintenance medium (3–4 drops in a dish 2.2 cm in diameter). After 12–18 h, gently add enough medium to cover the explants to the side of the dish.

9.2. Postnatal Ganglia

The dissection of the SCG from postnatal rats differs only in some details from that described above for the embryonic ganglion. For all ages, ether or CO_2 anesthesia can be used and the dissection done after sterile preparation of the neck.

Preparation of SCG for culturing:

1. Use three sets of sterile instruments for the dissection of skin, glands and muscles, and the SCG, to facilitate the sterile removal of the ganglia.
2. Collect the ganglia in L-15 containing penicillin (100 U/mL) and streptomycin (100 mg/mL), and remove loose connective tissue and blood vessels.
3. The ganglionic capsule can be removed from postnatal rats up to 5–7 d of age. By approx postnatal d 10, it is virtually impossible to remove the true capsule without excessively damaging the ganglion.
4. Free the ganglia of nerve trunks and cut into explants with a maximum diameter of 1 mm. Rinse the explants several times in the antibiotic containing L-15 before transfer to culture dishes. Using these precautions and the inclusion of antibiotics in the medium for several days makes infection a rare problem.

10. PREPARATION OF DISSOCIATED NEURONS

Preparation of dissociated neurons from rats of all ages begins with the preparation of explants as described above. Dissociation procedures then differ according to the age of rat under study.

10.1. Embryonic Neurons

Rinsed explants can be treated by two methods to achieve disaggregation. Mechanical disaggregation as described by Bray (1970) is preferred when exposure of the neurons to enzymes is for some reason undesirable. This procedure has the disadvantage of a lower yield (10–15%) compared to enzyme disaggregation (as high as 90%). Mechanical disaggregation also gives less satisfactory results for the younger embryonic SCGs (E15–E17), since these neurons seem more adherent to one another and, without enzyme treatment, remain in clumps.

1. Mechanical method:
   a. Gently pull apart the SCG explants using two fine forceps.
   b. Transfer to a test tube and agitate with a Vortex mixer. This generates a cell suspension with some remaining fragments.
   c. Filter as described below.
2. Enzyme method: Enzyme dissociation utilizes 0.25% trypsin (TRL-3, No. 3707, Worthington Diagnostics, Freehold, NJ) in L-15 or Hanks' calcium/magnesium-free basic salt solution (filter sterilized). This should be made up fresh or used from a stock solution stored at –80°C.
   a. Incubate the explants with gentle rotation in the trypsin solution at 37°C for 30–45 min.
   b. Rinse three times with L-15 and finally in the medium (maintenance medium is often used) to be used for plating the cells. Serum-containing medium has a naturally occurring trypsin inhibitor. If plating in a chemically defined medium is desirable, further L-15 rinses are recommended, and both trituration and plating should be performed in defined medium with 2.5 mg/mL of bovine serum albumin.
   c. Using an approx 1-mL vol, triturate the chunks against the side of the tissue culture tube with a pipet fire-polished to reduce the bore at the tip to 0.5–1 mm.
   d. After four or five squirts, allow the fragments to settle, remove the cell suspension, and add more medium (0.5–1.0 mL) to the chunks.
   e. Repeat the trituration and combine the two suspensions with any remaining small fragments. This two-step procedure may reduce trauma to the cells released in the first trituration.
   f. Filter the cell suspension (generated by either mechanical or enzyme dissociation) through a nylon mesh (pore size 15 µm, Nitex™ HD3-15, TETKO, Inc., Des Plaines, IL) to remove cell aggregates and other tissue fragments. This step may reduce the yield and may be eliminated if small fragments are not a problem for the experimental design.
   g. Plate filtered suspension onto the prepared culture dishes. To promote uniform plating, the suspension should be agitated frequently, and only four or five dishes seeded between agitations. For optimum attachment and growth, the final layer of collagen should be applied to the dishes and air-dried just shortly (approx 1 h to allow for drying time) before

plating the cells. Under these conditions, the cell suspension can be applied as several drops to the center of the dish. The neurons will be confined by surface tension to the area of the initial drop, facilitating the counting of all cells on the dish at a later date.

10.2. Postnatal Rat SCG Neurons

The disaggregation procedure using trypsin for embryonic rats can be used for the SCGs from young rats up to 3–4 d postnatal with similar results. Dissociated neurons can still be obtained from rats up to 10–12 d of life, but with reduced yields. With trypsin alone, it is virtually impossible to obtain substantial numbers of single neurons from rats over 2–3 wk of age. The best disaggregation and subsequent survival (5–10%) are obtained using the following procedure.

1. Incubate SCG explants in 0.25% collagenase (No. 4194 CLS, Cooper Biochemical, Freehold, NJ) with gentle agitation in a 35-mm Petri dish in a humidified atmosphere (37°C, pH 7.4).
2. After 45–60 min, the explants are quite sticky and clumped. Tease them apart and gently stretch each one out using fine forceps.
3. Remove the old collagenase and add fresh collagenase. Continue incubation for another 45–60 min. If the tissue is incubated for 90–120 min continuously in collagenase without being teased apart, the yield is considerably reduced.
4. Rinse the chunks once in L-15 and incubate (45–60 min) in 0.25% pronase (No. 53702 B Grade, Calbiochem-Behring Corp., La Jolla, CA) in L-15, pH 7.4. Enzyme solutions should be prepared and filter-sterilized shortly before use.

Note: Empirically, it has been found that not all lot numbers of either enzyme give the same results. For pronase in particular, some lots give few, if any, viable neurons. Therefore, check several lots and order a supply of a given lot that gives satisfactory results. The enzymes store well as powders at −20°C.

5. Transfer chunks to a test tube and rinse four times (3 mL each) in L-15 and once in medium. Trituration is carried out as for embryonic neurons. A two- or even three-step procedure with subsequent combining of supernatants is particularly important in avoiding unnecessary trauma to the neurons released during the initial trituration. Usually, very few tissue fragments remain, but they can be allowed to settle, and the supernatant is removed. Filtration through Nitex is omitted. Plating is done as described above for embryonic neurons. Because no inhibitors of these enzymes are available as for trypsin, careful rinsing is particularly important. In addition, a thicker collagen substratum, i.e., 3–4 drops for the air-dried layer on

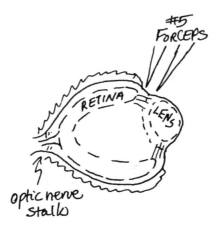

Fig. 1. Diagram of rodent eye. Drawing by N. Kleitman.

2.5-cm dishes, promotes initial attachment of the neurons and avoids break-down of the substrate after a few days of culture.

11. PREPARATION OF RETINAL EXPLANTS

Embryos are removed from pregnant rats as detailed in Sections 2. and 3.3. (1 and 2). Optimal neurite growth is obtained from embryos of gestational d 15, and therefore, dissections for both retina and DRGs (Section 3.) can utilize the same pregnant rat.

11.1. Dissection

1. Separate eyes from extraocular tissue using two #5 forceps. Slip forceps under the eye, gently lifting it in the socket, and pinch off the optic nerve to free the whole eye. Place in Leibovitz's L-15 medium.
2. Using two #5 fine forceps, hold the eye at junction of sclera and lens and gently tear away the lens. The retina and sclera (and so on) are now joined only at the rim of the eye cup and the optic nerve stalk (Fig. 1).
3. Carefully free the retina from the sclera. The retina is thinner and more delicate than the sclera, and will be recognizable by its smooth contour and translucent whitish appearance. Transfer the retina to fresh L-15, being careful to "cradle" retinas when lifting rather than pinching them with the forceps, or the surface tension of the L-15 medium will cause tearing.
4. Bisect or trisect the retina through the optic disk.
5. Place retinal explants on prepared dishes (see note on transferring in step 3 above). Feed with 10% serum in EMEM or DME (NGF not required). Vigor-

ous neurite growth will occur within 24–48 h on air-dried collagen (*see* Section 12.2.) and on living Schwann cells.

12. APPENDIX

12.1. Medium

1. L-15 (Leibovitz) medium (Leibovitz, 1963)

Components	mg/L
Inorganic salts	
$CaCl_2$ (anhyd.)	140.00
KCl	400.00
KH_2PO_4	60.00
$MgCl_2 \cdot 6H_2O$	200.00
$MgSO_4 \cdot 7H_2O$	200.00
NaCl	8000.00
$Na_2HPO_4 \cdot 7H_2O$	359.00
Other components	
D(+)galactose	900.00
Phenol red	10.00
Sodium pyruvate	550.00
Amino acids	
DL-Alanine	450.00
L-Arginine (free base)	500.00
L-Asparagine	250.00
L-Cysteine (free base)	120.00
L-Glutamine	300.00
Glycine	200.00
L-Histidine (free base)	250.00
DL-Isoleucine	250.00
L-Leucine	125.00
L-Lysine (free base)	75.00
DL-Methionine	150.00
DL-Phenylalanine	250.00
L-Serine	200.00
DL-Threonine	600.00
L-Tryptophan	20.00
L-Tyrosine	300.00
DL-Valine	200.00

Vitamins

DL-Ca pantothenate	1.00
Choline chloride	1.00
Folic acid	1.00
i-Inositol	2.00
Niacinamide	1.00
Pyridoxine HCl	1.00
Riboflavin-5'-phosphate, sodium	0.10
Thiamine monophosphate	1.00

2. Eagle's Minimum Essential Medium (EMEM) (Eagle, 1959):

Components	mg/L
Inorganic salts	
$CaCl_2$ (anhyd.)	200.00
KCl	400.00
$MgSO_4 \cdot 7H_2O$	200.00
NaCl	6800.00
$NaHCO_3$	2200.00
$Na_2HPO_4 \cdot H_2O$	140.00
Other components	
D-glucose	1000.00
Phenol red	10.00
Amino acids	
L-Arginine $\cdot$ HCl	126.00
L-Cystine	24.00
L-Glutamine	292.00
L-Histidine HCl $\cdot$ H_2O	42.00
L-Isoleucine	52.00
L-Leucine	52.00
L-Lysine HCl	72.50
L-Methionine	15.00
L-Phenylalanine	32.00
L-Threonine	48.00
L-Tryptophan	10.00
L-Tyrosine	36.00
L-Valine	46.00
Vitamins	
D-Ca pantothenate	1.00
Choline chloride	1.00

Folic acid	1.00
i-Inositol	2.00
Niacinamide	1.00
Pyridoxal HCl	1.00
Riboflavin	0.10
Thiamine HCl	1.00

3. Media for growth and maintenance:
   a. Chemically defined standard medium: The formula for the defined medium we have used is modified from that designated N2 by Bottenstein and Sato (1979). Unlike the initial N2, no HEPES, antibiotics, or bicarbonate is added. In addition, 1.4 mM of L-glutamine and 100 ng/mL of purified 2.5 S NGF are added. Finally, the cultures are grown in a 7% CO_2 atmosphere (vs 5% for standard medium) to maintain the pH at approx 7.4. Since the pH of this medium drifts upward rapidly under ambient air, any handling and feeding of the culture should be done expeditiously. Combine the components in the following order:

i.	Dulbecco's Modified Eagle's Medium (DMEM) (Gibco-BRL [Gaithersburg, MD], #320-1965, with L-glutamine and glucose [4.5 g/L] without sodium pyruvate)	50% (v/v)
ii.	Transferrin* (Chrompure Rat Transferrin, Jackson Immunoresearch Labs, West Grove, PA; store desiccated 0–5°C)	10 mg/L
iii.	Progesterone (Sigma, St. Louis, MO, #P0130)** ethanol (added with progesterone), 214 μM = 0.0012% (v/v)	20 nM
iv.	Putrescine (Sigma #P7505)**	100 mm
v.	Insulin (bovine, crystalline, Sigma #I-5500; store desiccated below −20°C)	5 mg/L
vi.	Na SeO$_3$ (Pfaltz and Bauer, Waterbury, CT, #S97150, LD$_{50}$ = 50 nM/kg)	30 nM

*The original formula called for human transferrin, but because of concern regarding the danger of concentrated human blood products, we have shifted to the use of rat transferrin.
**These components are not needed for the growth of sympathetic neurons.

vii. NGF (2.5S)   100 ng/mL
viii. Ham's F-12 medium (F-12)   50% (v/v)
      (Gibco #320-1765, with L-glutamine)

b. Maintenance medium

Component	mL
EMEM containing 2 mM L-glutamine	90.00
Glucose (200 mg/mL solution)	1.13
Crude nerve growth factor (50 ng/mL)	0.05
Serum	10.00

c. Antimitotic medium: Maintenance medium as above with the following addition to give a final concentration of ($10^{-5}M$) mixture of both fluorodeoxyuridine and uridine (1:1 ratio).

d. Myelination medium for peripheral tissue

Component	mL
EMEM containing 2 mM L-glutamine	85.00
Glucose (200 mg/mL solution)	1.15
Crude nerve growth factor (50 ng/mL)	0.05
Human placental serum	15.00
L-Ascorbic acid (5 mg/mL)	1.00

Note: L-Ascorbic acid is filter-sterilized immediately prior to use. This ingredient has recently been observed to replace embryo extract in meeting the requirements for Schwann cell myelination (Eldridge et al., 1987).

e. "Old reliable" medium: 100 mL of the standard medium includes 61 mL of Eagle's Minimum Essential Medium, 25 mL of human placental serum, 10 mL of 9-d chick embryo extract (50% in BSS), 3 mL of 20% glucose, and 0.7 mL of 200 mM glutamine and NGF. The usual concentration of NGF is approx 25 biological U/mL of medium. This "old" medium is still in frequent use.

f. Comments concerning medium components: Antimitotic agents are generally regarded as having little effect on the nondividing neuronal population. However, recent studies have shown a decrease in the rate of neurite extension from explants when fluorodeoxyuridine is continuously present in the medium. This effect is most dramatic when neurons are derived from early embryonic or older postnatal rats.

Studies with a variety of media formulations have shown the importance of the concentration of certain components. Thus, the concentration of human placental serum or embryo extract can affect the development of choline acetyltransferase activity. Elevated K$^+$ levels are known to increase survival for some neuronal types, but in SCG cultures, it will also affect neurotransmitter synthesis of the neurons (for review, *see* Johnson and Argiro, 1983). Because of this, hemolyzed serum must be used with caution, since the K$^+$ concentrations may be increased.

We have used human placental serum almost exclusively, since it yields consistent results and is available to us from an affiliate hospital. Other sera (horse serum, human adult serum, fetal calf serum) may be used, but from our experience, we recommend that the effects of any serum be well characterized before routine use. In particular, commercially available sera may vary considerably from lot to lot.

12.2. Substrata

We continue to use our own rat tail collagen to provide a stable substratum for myelinating cultures that are carried for many weeks. Many alternate substrata (polylysine or laminin) lose their adhesiveness after several weeks in culture and the cells are lost before the experiment is finished. Commercial collagen preparations should be tested for stability before use in long-term experiments.

1. Collagen preparation: Collagen is prepared by a modification of the method of Bornstein (1958). Because standardization of this procedure has proven critical for obtaining consistent culture results, it is given here in detail. Tails from 6-mo to 1-yr old male rats are used, because those from younger males or female rats give unsatisfactory preparations. Each tail is thoroughly scrubbed with antiseptic soap, rinsed once each in 80% alcohol and tap-distilled water, placed in a filter-paper-lined Petri dish, and frozen for 24 h or longer at –20°C. The tail is sterilized in 95% alcohol for 20 min and dried in a large Petri dish with filter paper. With the tail held at 1–1.5 cm from the small end with a hemostat, the skin is cut completely around the tail using bone-cutting forceps and starting distal to the point where the hemostat is applied. The object now is to fracture the vertebrae of the tail without cutting the tendons that run from the pelvic muscles all along the tail and attach to each vertebrae. If the vertebrae is cracked free and pulled laterally to separate it from the rest of the tail, the attached tendons are pulled out with it and then hang free from the detached vertebral fragment. The tendons are cut free with fine scissors and placed in double-distilled water. Moving 1.5 cm toward the larger end of the tail, the procedure is repeated until the last of the tail is used. The tendons are teased apart with small forceps to loosen up clumps, and at the same time removing blood vessels and any other adherent nontendon connective tissue.

The tendons are extracted using 150 mL of sterile 0.1% acetic acid for each gram of tendons for 5 d at 4°C with daily agitation. The dissolved tendons are centrifuged in tissue culture tubes (10,000 rpm, 1 h), and the supernatant harvested. The acid extract is dialyzed (dialysis tubing #8-667D, Fisher Scientific) against 50 vol of sterile double-distilled water for 18 h at 4°C. The collagen is removed from the dialysis bags, aliquoted into sterile containers, tested for sterility in soy broth, and stored at 4°C.

2. Application of collagen to dishes: The detailed procedure for collagen coating Aclar dishes (see Section 6.1.) is given below; appropriate modifications can be made for other culture dishes. Aclar dishes (Bunge and Wood, 1973) are sterilized in 80% alcohol, dried, and transferred to a Petri dish. Two to three drops (on a dish of approx 22 mm in diameter) of dialyzed collagen are spread evenly over the bottom, using a sterile disposable Pasteur pipet flamed to close the tips and bent to the shape of a hockey stick. Avoiding delay, the freshly spread collagen is exposed to ammonia vapor for 2 min. The dishes are rinsed once or twice with sterile double-distilled water, drained, and allowed to dry. Because the collagen may be in fact more adhesive without these rinses, both methods should be tried. When thus dried, the dishes have the advantage of being able to be used to seed cells in a confined region, because the dried collagen is not easily wettable. Thus, a drop of feed will stand up as a bubble confining the neurons to the collagen area beneath. Utilizing this technique, cultures are obtained that are intermediate between disaggregated neuronal culture and explant cultures. Thus, several thousand neurons can be deposited in the disaggregated state, but confined to the center of the dish. The next day, the entire dish surface is made wet and the culture refed. Over the next few days, the neurons partially reaggregate and develop a neuritic outgrowth that eventually fills the remainder of the dish. This preparation thus has both a disaggregated neuronal and a purely neuritic domain in the same culture dish.

If a particularly adhesive collagen surface is desired, then a second layer of collagen is added after drying the first ammoniated layer, as mentioned above. Another 1–2 drops of collagen are then added, gently spread, and allowed to dry. Suspensions of disaggregated cells may be added directly to the air-dried layer without prior wetting (see above). For explants, wet the dishes first using Leibovitz medium (L-15), which is then removed and replaced by 3–4 drops of the desired medium.

The double-layered collagen substratum has been very useful in the culture of either disaggregated or explanted SCG neurons. Disaggregated neurons may not attach or grow well on the ammoniated collagen alone. Although explants will grow on ammoniated collagen, their rate of growth is slower, and after several weeks, they tend to detach from the substrate. Furthermore, neurite growth and nonneuronal cell migration from explants is not only age dependent, but also substrate dependent. Thus, E15 sympathetic ganglia explants on ammoniated collagen have neurites with accompanying nonneuronal cells. On air-dried collagen (double-layered as described above), the neurites have but a few nonneuronal cells and grow slower. These results, plus those of others (for review, *see* Roufa et al., 1986), serve to alert an investigator to the possible effects of both substratum and neuronal age on neuronal growth and differentiation.

FURTHER READING

Bunge, M. B., Johnson, M. I., Ard, M. D., and Kleitman, N. (1987), Factors influencing the growth of regenerating nerve fibers in culture, in: *Progress in Brain Research*, Seil, F. J., Herbert, E., and Carlson, B. M., eds., Elsevier, vol. 71, pp. 61–74.

Bunge, M. B., Bunge, R. P., Carey, D. J., Cornbrooks, C. J., Eldridge, C. F., Williams, A. K., and Wood, P. M. (1983), Axonal and nonaxonal influences in Schwann cell development, in: *Developing and Regenerating Vertebrate Nervous Systems*, Coates, P., Markwald, R., Kenny, A., eds., Alan R. Liss, New York, pp. 71–105.

Bunge, R. P. (1986), The cell of Schwann, in *Diseases of the Nervous System*, Saunders, New York, pp. 153–162.

Bunge, R. P., Bunge, M. B., and Eldridge, C. E. (1985), Linkage between axonal ensheathment and basal lamina production by Schwann cells. *Ann. Rev. Neurosci.* **9**, 305–328.

Bunge, R. P., Johnson, M., and Ross, C. D. (1978), Nature and nurture in the development of the autonomic neuron. *Science* **199**, 1409–1416.

Eldrige, C. F., Cornbrooks, C. J., Chiu, A. Y., Bunge, R. P., and Sanes, J. R. (1986), Basal lamina-associated heparan sulfate proteoglycan in the rat peripheral nervous system: characterization and localization using monoclonal antibodies. *J. Neurocytol.* **15**, 37–51.

Higgins, D. and Burton, H. (1982), Electrotonic synapses are formed by fetal rat sympathetic neurons maintained in a chemically-defined culture medium. *Neuroscience* **7**, 2241–2253.

Johnson, M. I. and Argiro, V. (1983), Techniques for preparation of sympathetic ganglion cultures. *Methods Enzymol.* **103**, 334–347.

Ratner, N., Bunge, R. P., and Glaser, L. (1985), A neuronal cell surface heparan sulfate proteoglycan is required for dorsal root ganglion neuron stimulation of Schwann cell proliferation. *J. Cell Biol.* **101**, 744–754.

SPECIFIC REFERENCES AND NOTES

Argiro, V., Bunge, M. B., and Johnson, M. I. (1984), Correlation between growth cone form and movement and their dependence on neuronal age. *J. Neurosci.* **4**, 3051–3062.

Bornstein, M. B. (1958), Reconstituted rat-tail collagen used as a substrate for tissue cultures on coverslips. *Lab. Invest.* **7**, 134–137.

Bottenstein, J. E. and Sato, G. H. (1979), Growth of a rat neuroblastoma cell line in serum-free supplemented media. *Proc. Natl. Acad. Sci. USA* **76,** 514–517.

Bray, D. (1970), Surface movements during the growth of single explanted neurons. *Proc. Natl. Acad. Sci. USA* **65,** 905.

Brockes, J. P., Fields, K. L., and Raff, M. C. (1979), Studies on cultured rat Schwann cells. I. Establishment of purified populations from cultures of peripheral nerve. *Brain Res.* **165,** 105–118.

Bruckenstein, D. A. and Higgins, D. (1988), Morphological differentiation of embryonic rat sympathetic neurons in tissue culture. II. Serum promotes dendritic growth. *Dev. Biol.* **128,** 337–348.

Bunge, R. P. and Wood, P. (1973), Studies on the transplantation of spinal cord tissue in the rat. I. Development of a culture system for hemisections of embryonic spinal cord. *Brain Res.* **57,** 261–276.

Bunge, R. P. and Wood, P. M. (1987), Tissue culture studies of interactions between axons and myelinating cells of the central and peripheral nervous system. *Prog. Brain Res.* **71,** 143–152.

Crain, S. (1976), *Neurophysiologic Studies in Tissue Culture.* Raven Press, New York.

Eagle, H. (1959), Amino acid metabolism in mammalian cell cultures. *Science* **130,** 432–437.

Eldridge, C. F., Bunge, M. B., and Bunge, R. P. (1989), Differentiation of axon-related Schwann cells *in vitro*: II. Control of myelin formation by basal lamina. *J. Neurosci.* **9,** 625–638.

Eldridge, C. F., Bunge, M. B., Bunge, R. P., and Wood, P. M. (1987), Differentiation of axon-related Schwann cells *in vitro*. I. Ascorbic acid regulates basal lamina assembly and myelin formation. *J. Cell Biol.* **105,** 1023–1034.

Harrison, R. G. (1907), The living developing nerve fiber. *Anat. Rec.* **1,** 116–118.

Hild, W. (1957), Myelinogenesis in cultures of mammalian central nervous tissue. *Z. Zellforsch.* **46,** 71–95.

Iacovitti, L., Johnson, M. I., Joh, T. H., and Bunge, R. P. (1982), Biochemical and morphological characterization of sympathetic neurons grown in chemically defined medium. *Neuroscience* **7,** 2225–2240.

Johnson, E. M., Rich, K. M., and Yip, H. K. (1986), The role of NGF in sensory neurons *in vivo*. *TINS* **9,** 33–37.

Johnson, M. I., Paik, K., and Higgins, D. (1985), Rapid changes in synaptic vesicle cytochemistry after depolarization of cultured cholinergic sympathetic neurons. *J. Cell Biol.* **101,** 217–226.

Kleitman, N. and Johnson, M. I. (1989), Rapid growth cone translocation on laminin is supported by lamellipodial not filopodial structures. *Cell Motil. Cytoskel.* **13,** 288–300.

Kleitman, N., Wood, P., Johnson, M. I., and Bunge, R. P. (1988), Schwann cell surfaces but not extracellular matrix support neurite outgrowth from embryonic rat retina. *J. Neurosci.* **8,** 653–663.

Leibovitz, A. (1963), The growth and maintenance of tissue-cell culture in free gas exchange with the atmosphere. *Am. J. Hyg.* **78,** 173–180.

McCarthy, K. and de Vellis, J. (1980), Preparation of separate astroglial and oligodendroglial cell cultures from rat cerebral tissue. *J. Cell Biol.* **85,** 890–902.

Meiri, K., Johnson, M. I., and Willard, M. (1988), Distribution and phosphorylation of the growth-associated protein, GAP-43, in regenerating sympathetic neurons in culture. *J. Neurosci.* **8,** 2571–2581.

Murray, M. M. (1965), Nervous tissue *in vitro*, in: *Cells and Tissues in Culture,* vol. 2, Wilmer, E. N., ed., Academic, New York, pp. 373–455.

Patterson, P. H. (1978), Environmental determination of autonomic neurotransmitter functions. *Ann. Rev. Neurosci.* **1,** 1–17.

Peterson, E. R. and Murray, M. R. (1955), Myelin sheath formation of avian spinal ganglia. *Am. J. Anat.* **96,** 319.

Porter, S., Clark, M. B., Glaser, L., and Bunge, R. P. (1986), Schwann cells stimulated to proliferate in the absence of neurons retain full functional capability. *J. Neurosci.* **6,** 3070–3078.

Roufa, D., Bunge, M. B., Johnson, M. I., and Cornbrooks, C. J. (1986), Variation in content and function of non-neuronal cells in the outgrowth of sympathetic ganglia from embryos of differing age. *J. Neurosci.* **6,** 790–802.

Roufa, D. G., Johnson, M. J., and Bunge, M. B. (1983), Influence of ganglion age, nonneuronal cells and substratum on neurite outgrowth in culture. *Dev. Biol.* **99,** 225–239.

Tropea, M., Johnson, M. I., and Higgins, D. (1988), Glial cells promote dendritic development in rat sympathetic neurons *in vitro*. *Glia* **1,** 380–392.

Wood, P. (1976) Separation of functional Schwann cells and neurons from normal peripheral nerve tissue. *Brain Res.* **115,** 361–375.

Wood, P. M. and Bunge, R. P. (1986), Myelination of cultured dorsal root ganglion neurons by oligodendrocytes obtained from adult rats. *J. Neurol. Sci.* **74,** 153–169.

Wood, P. M. and Williams, A. K. (1984), Oligodendrocyte proliferation and CNS myelination in cultures containing dissociated embryonic neuroglia and dorsal root ganglion neurons. *Dev. Brain Res.* **12,** 225–241.

Chapter Five

Chick Spinal Somatic Motoneurons in Culture

Bernhard H. J. Juurlink

1. INTRODUCTION

Cultures enriched in spinal somatic motoneurons are increasingly used as a test system for the detection of factors that are trophic or toxic for motoneurons (e.g., Schnaar and Schaffner, 1981; Calof and Reichardt, 1984; Dohrmann et al., 1986, 1987; McManaman et al., 1989, 1990; Juurlink et al., 1991a). Motoneurons in such cultures are obtained from embryonic spinal cord. There are basically two approaches whereby one can obtain cultures highly enriched in spinal motoneurons. One approach takes advantage of the fact that peripheral terminals of motoneurons can take up fluorescent labels and retrogradely transport these labels to the somas. Spinal cords can then be dissociated and labeled motoneurons isolated using a fluorescence-activated cell sorter (e.g., Calof and Reichardt, 1984; Schaffner et al., 1987); this approach is labor-intensive and yields small numbers of neurons, of which only about 80% are labeled motoneurons. There are also questions concerning the effects of the tracer on the motoneurons (Smith et al., 1986). The second approach takes advantage of the fact that the buoyant density of motoneurons is significantly different from that of the other neural cell populations; here motoneurons are separated from other cell populations by centrifuging cells through a density gradient (Schnaar and Schaffner, 1981; Dohrmann et al., 1986). This approach has the advantages that, technically, it

Protocols for Neural Cell Culture, 2nd Ed. • Eds.: S. Fedoroff and A. Richardson • Humana Press, Inc., Totowa, NJ

is much simpler than the fluorescence-activated sorting method and much larger numbers of motoneurons can be isolated. The cultures established from this latter approach are free of nonneuronal cells and are comprised of about 95% motoneurons as determined by calcitonin gene-related peptide immunocytochemistry (Juurlink et al., 1990). This is the procedure described in this chapter.

2. ISOLATION OF THE CHICK EMBRYOS

2.1. Materials

Fertile eggs (Hamilton and Hamburger [1951] stages 29–30, Carnegie stage 19 [Butler and Juurlink, 1987]), 6 d incubation (12).
Ethanol (70%).
Box of tissue paper or small squares of gauze.
Probe, sharp.
Forceps, sterile ($3\frac{1}{2}$ in.) (2).
Forceps, curved sterile ($4\frac{1}{2}$ in.) (1).
Egg carton.
Waste receptacle.
Petri dishes, sterile (60 mm).
Holding medium.

2.2. Procedure

1. Candle eggs and select eggs with viable embryos.
2. Place eggs blunt end up (i.e., air sac end up) in an egg carton or other holder placed adjacent to the laminar flow hood. Do not remove more than six embryos at one time.
3. Using tissue paper or gauze, wash the egg surface with 70% ethanol. This cleans the shell, but does not completely sterilize it.
4. Using a sharp probe, poke a hole through the shell at the blunt end.
5. Use one pair of $3\frac{1}{2}$ in. forceps to remove the egg shell. This is initiated by placing one tine of the forceps through the hole just made, and then closing the forceps and breaking off part of the egg shell. This should be done by holding the egg at an angle over the waste receptacle such that the broken bit of shell falls into the waste receptacle rather than into the air space. One then continues to nibble the egg shell away until the shell surrounding the air space is completely removed. The forceps may then be resterilized by placing in 70% ethanol.
6. Use the second set of $3\frac{1}{2}$ in. forceps to peel away the shell membrane. This is done by grasping the membrane at the edge of the air space and gently pulling toward the other edge. The embryo surrounded by the chorioallantoic membrane is now exposed to view.

7. Gently pierce the chorioallantoic membrane with one tine of the curved forceps and hook it around the neck of the embryo. Partially close the forceps and slowly lift the embryo out of the shell. The embryo is still attached to the extraembryonic membranes (amnion, yolk sac, allantois, and chorion), and if the embryo is slowly lifted out of the egg, these membranes will tear, thus freeing the embryo. However, if the embryo is lifted too quickly, the neck of the embryo will rupture. Place the embryo into the 60-mm sterile Petri dish containing holding medium.

3. ISOLATION OF SPINAL CORDS

3.1. Materials

Sterile wax dissecting dish.
Insect pins, stainless-steel, #1 (Polyscience, Niles, IL) (3).
Forceps, small curved, sterile.
Forceps, #5 microdissecting (2).
Dissecting microscope.
Holding medium.
Test tube rack.
Test tube.
Pasteur pipet, sterile cotton plugged with curved fire-polished tip.
Small rubber bulb.

3.2. Preparation of Materials

1. Sterile forceps can be placed on elevated surfaces on either side of the dissecting microscope. This is very convenient for dissection; however, ensure that the forceps' tines do not contact any surface.
2. Place holding medium into the dissecting dish.
3. Place the test tube at a slant in the test tube rack situated near the dissecting microscope. Insert the rubber bulb onto end of the Pasteur pipet and wet the pipet by drawing and expelling the holding medium. Use the test tube as a holding container for the pipet.
4. Place 5 mL of holding medium into a 60-mm Petri dish and place the dish adjacent to dissecting microscope.

3.3. Removal of Spinal Cord

1. Hook one tine of the small curved forceps around the neck of the embryo, lift embryo, and place into dissecting dish.
2. Pin embryo ventral (belly) surface down:
   a. Place one pin through the hindbrain.
   b. Grab one leg with forceps, pull taut, and pin leg.

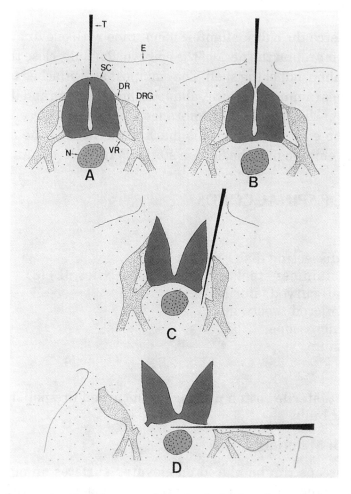

Fig. 1. Cartoon demonstrating the procedure for isolating the spinal cord from an embryo. **(A)** A tine (T) of a pair of forceps is used to cut the skin along the dorsal midline from the hindbrain to the tail, thus exposing the spinal cord to direct view. DR = dorsal root of spinal nerve, E = epidermis, N = notochord, SC = spinal cord, VR = ventral root of spinal nerve. **(B)** A forceps' tine is used to cut the roof of the spinal cord, causing the spinal cord to open up in the manner of a book. **(C)** The meninges and DRG are separated from the spinal cord by rubbing the forceps along the lateral surface of the spinal cord. **(D)** After cutting the spinal at its junction with the hindbrain, the forceps are used to separate the spinal cord from the notochord.

        c. Grab second leg, pull to the side, and pin. The head and the feet of the embryo should form the corners of a triangle.

    3. Using the two microdissecting forceps, remove the spinal cord as follows (note also Fig. 1):

        a. One pair of forceps is used to steady the embryo while a tine of the other pair is used to tear through the skin along the dorsal midline from the hindbrain to the tail. Using a tine of the forceps, free the skin from the underlying tissues along either side of the dorsal midline; this exposes the spinal cord to view.

b. Use the tine of a pair of forceps to cut the roof of the spinal cord, exposing the central canal. This causes the entire length of the spinal cord to open up like a book.

c. Rub a tine of the forceps along the outer surface of one side of the spinal cord and then that of the other side. If done properly, this separates the meninges and dorsal root ganglia (DRG) from the spinal cord.

d. Use the forceps to cut the spinal cord cranially at its junction with the hindbrain and caudally in the sacral region.

e. The notochord is separated from the spinal cord by sweeping the ventral surface of the spinal cord with forceps. Now lift the spinal cord away from the embryo. With practice, the spinal cord can be isolated free of meninges and DRG using this procedure. If some DRG are still present, it is essential that these be removed before proceeding any further.

4. Use the wetted Pasteur pipet to transfer the spinal cord to the holding medium.

5. After six spinal cords have been isolated, another six embryos can be removed from the eggs, spinal cords removed, and so forth, until sufficient spinal cords have been collected.

4. ISOLATION OF MOTONEURONS

4.1. Materials

Centrifuge tubes, polystyrene, sterile (15-mL).

Stomacher Lab Blender 80™ (Seward Medical UAC House, London, England, distributed in Canada by Baxter Corp., Mississauga, ON, Canada) set at 160 double kicks/min.

Whirl-pak™ bag (Nasco, New Hamburg, ON, Canada, distributed in Canada by Baxter Corp.), sterile, 10 cm wide, marked 8.5 cm from the bottom.

Pasteur pipets, sterile cotton plugged with fire-polished curved tips.

Serological pipets, cotton plugged, 5 mL.

Serological pipets, cotton plugged, 10 mL.

Ice.

Refrigerated centrifuge.

Trypsin solution (1.0%).

Deoxyribonuclease (DNase) solution (2.0%).

Bovine serum albumin (BSA) solution (3.5%).

Metrizamide solution (6.4%).

Dulbecco's Modified Eagle's Medium/Ham's nutrient mixture F-12 (DMEM/F12).

Puck's solution containing 15 mM sodium bicarbonate and 2 mM sodium pyruvate.

Tissue culture dishes, sterile (60 mm).

4.2. Procedure

1. Place spinal cords into a 60-mm Petri dish containing 5 mL Puck's bicarbonate solution. Add 125 µL of 1.0% trypsin (final trypsin concentration of 0.025%), and incubate for 30 min in an incubator containing an atmosphere of 5% CO_2 in air and maintained at 37°C.
2. Carefully aspirate the trypsin solution and resuspend spinal cords in 5 mL DMEM/F12. Place spinal cords and DMEM/F12 into sterile tube.

Note: From this point until cells are planted into culture, whenever possible, keep all solutions and cells at 0–4°C.

3. Allow spinal cords to settle for 5 min and decant DMEM/F12. Add 15 mL DMEM/F12–0.02% DNase and place spinal cords plus medium into Whirl-pak bag.
4. Place the lower 8.5 cm of the Whirl-pak bag into Stomacher Lab Blender™ adjusted to 160 double-kicks/min. Disaggregate spinal cords for 2 min.
5. Remove cell suspension from the Whirl-pak bag and place into test tube. Keep the test tube cold and upright. Allow fragments to settle for 10 min. Collect fragment-free cell suspension, place into centrifuge tube, and centrifuge (4°C) at 180g for 10 min.
6. Decant pellet and resuspend cell pellet in 5 mL DMEM/F12–0.02% DNase.
7. Carefully layer the cell suspension on top of 5 mL 3.5% BSA contained in a centrifuge tube. Centrifuge (4°C) for 15 min at 100g. This procedure results in much of the debris present in the cell suspension being trapped in the BSA cushion.
8. Decant the supernatant and resuspend the pellet in 5 mL DMEM/F12–0.02% DNase. Carefully layer cells on top of 5 mL 6.4% metrizamide. This is done by laying the metrizamide-containing tube on ice at an angle of approx 30°. The cell suspension is taken up with a Pasteur pipet, and with the tip of the pipet about 1 cm from the metrizamide solution surface, the cell suspension is slowly allowed to run down the tube and over the surface of the metrizamide. Once the cell suspension is layered on top of the metrizamide, the centrifuge tube is held upright and the interface between the cell suspension and the metrizamide is very slightly intermixed with gentle movements of the tip of a curved Pasteur pipet.
9. Place tube into centrifuge (4°C), and centrifuge at 500g for 30 min.
10. A band of cells is readily visible at the interface of the medium and metrizamide solution; this band consists of motoneurons. The remaining spinal cells have entered the metrizamide solution. Remove the motoneuron fraction using a Pasteur pipet. Dilute cells in 10 mL of DMEM/F12–0.02% DNase and centrifuge at 180g for 10 min. Discard supernatant and resus-

pend cells in 1.0 mL growth medium (*see* Section 7.2.) containing 0.02% DNase. This last procedure removes the residual metrizamide present in the motoneuron fraction.

11. Determine the cell density of this final cell suspension using a hemocytometer. Each spinal cord should yield approx 1.5×10^5 motoneurons.

5. PLANTING OF MOTONEURONS

5.1. Materials

Poly-D-lysine-coated round (12-mm) glass coverslips (German glass recommended), sterile (optional).
Poly-D-lysine-coated 35-mm Petri dishes.
100-mm plastic microbiological Petri dishes.
DNase (2.0%).
Growth medium.

5.2. Establishing Motoneuron Cultures

1. Dilute cell suspension to 4×10^4 cells/mL growth medium containing 0.02% DNase. This results in a very low cell density in the cultures; however, cells can be planted at higher densities. Plant 1.5 mL of cell suspension into each 35-mm Petri dish, or plant 150 μL cell suspension onto each glass coverslip (final cell densities are approx 60 cells/mm^2). Place cultures into an incubator containing a humidified atmosphere of 5% CO_2 in air.

Note: The glass coverslips should be in a hydrophobic 100-mm microbiological Petri dish, which tends to keep the medium on the coverslips.

2. After 1 h, place the coverslips into 35-mm Petri dishes containing 1.5 mL of growth medium and return to the incubator.

3. After 1 d, feed the cultures with fresh growth medium, and feed twice a week thereafter.

6. DESCRIPTION OF CULTURES

By 1 d of culture, 75% of the neurons planted are alive and putting forth neurites. Of these, half will survive to 8 d of culture (Juurlink et al., 1991b). At this time, the neurons are large cells with one long axon and numerous dendrites coming off the soma (Fig. 2). After 1 mo, 20% of the neurons are still alive. Approximately 95% of the neurons are motoneurons (Juurlink et al., 1990). If one observes glial cells in these cultures, it is because cell aggregation was not prevented in the steps between spinal cord disaggregation and cell planting; this suggests either that the cells were not kept cold during this time or that the DNase was not active.

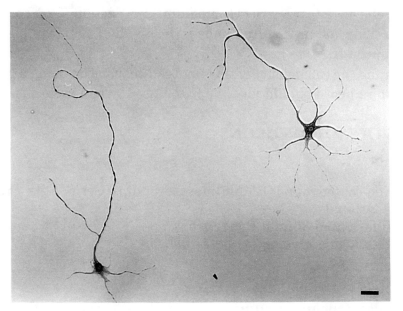

Fig. 2. Micrograph of a 12-d culture demonstrating two motoneurons stained for neurofilament protein. Bar = 40 μm.

7. APPENDIX

7.1. Dissection Material

1. Instrument cleaning and sterilization
   a. After use, soak instruments in 7X™ detergent and clean using a nylon brush. Rinse well with hot water followed by 70% ethanol. Allow to dry and store.
   b. Before use, sterilize instruments and insect pins by placing in a plastic beaker containing 70% ethanol.
2. Dissecting dish: A convenient dissecting dish can be prepared by pouring a molten mixture of three parts regular blue dental inlay wax (Sybron Corporation, Romulus, MI) and one part paraffin (melting point of 56°C) into a glass 60-mm Petri dish. The dish can be sterilized for use by dry heat at 250°F for 2 h. The 60-mm dish is a convenient size, since one can manipulate the position of the dish under the dissecting microscope using the fifth fingers and at the same time manipulate the dissecting instruments using the first and second fingers. The wax is not brittle, thus ensuring that the wax surface remains smooth despite repeated pinnings of embryos. The blue color of the wax also aids in visualizing the white tissues of the embryo when appropriate illumination is used. After use, the wax dish can be washed

using 7X detergent and nylon brush. After air-drying, the wax surface can be refinished by using the flame of a Bunsen burner to melt the wax. Once cooled, the dissection dishes can be sterilized by filling with 70% ethanol. The alcohol is removed prior to use, and the dish is allowed to dry in a laminar flow hood.

7.2. Preparation of Media

1. DMEM/F12: This can be obtained in powder form from Gibco-BRL (Burlington, Ontario, Canada; 12500-047). Prepare as per instructions that come with the medium package. This medium is buffered with 15 mM HEPES and 14 mM sodium bicarbonate. In an atmosphere of 5% CO_2, this medium attains a pH of 7.2.

2. Medium supplements:
   a. Transferrin:
      i. Dissolve 50 mg transferrin (Sigma T-4515) in 100 mL DMEM/F12.
      ii. Sterilize by filtration and store in small aliquots at –20°C.
   b. Selenium:
      i. Dissolve 5.2 mg sodium selenite in 10 mL DMEM/F12 and filter sterilize.
      ii. Take 1.0 mL of this and dilute in 99 mL DMEM/F12 (final concentration is $3 \times 10^{-6}M$).
      iii. Store at –20°C in small aliquots.
   c. Progesterone:
      i. Dissolve 3.1 mg progesterone in 10 mL 95% ethanol and filter sterilize.
      ii. Take 200 μL of this and dilute in 99.8 mL DMEM/F12 (final concentration is $2 \times 10^{-6}M$).
   d. Insulin:
      i. Dissolve 5 mg insulin in 10 mL DMEM/F12. Acidify this solution with 1M HCl (the solution will be an orange-yellow) and filter sterilize.
      ii. This solution can be stored at 4°C for up to 1 mo.
   e. Pyruvate:
      i. Dissolve 0.176 g pyruvic acid in 10 mL DMEM/F12 (i.e., 200 mM).
      ii. Filter-sterilize and store in aliquots at –20°C.
   f. Potassium chloride:
      i. Dissolve 7.455 g KCl in DMEM/F12 and make up to 100 mL (i.e., 1.0M KCl).
      ii. Filter-sterilize and store at 4°C.

3. Chemically defined growth medium: To 94 mL DMEM/F12 add 1.0 mL each of the progesterone, transferrin, selenium, insulin, pyruvate, and KCl stock solutions. This chemically defined component thus contains $3 \times 10^{-8}M$ selen-

ite, $2 \times 10^{-8}M$ progesterone, 5 µg/mL transferrin, and 5 µg/mL insulin. An additional 10 mM KCl (final concentration of 14 mM) is also present.

4. Complete growth medium: To 95 mL of the above chemically defined medium, add 5 mL heat-inactivated horse serum. In addition, add muscle extract (*see* Section 7.3.) to a final concentration of 50 µg protein/mL medium.

5. Heat-inactivated horse serum:
   a. Aliquot horse serum into sterile 15-mL test tubes with screw caps. Loosen the caps and place test tubes for 30 min in a water bath maintained at 56°C.
   b. Allow tubes to cool in a laminar flow hood, tighten caps, and store at –80°C.

6. Holding medium: This medium consists of DMEM/F12 containing 1.0 mM NaHCO$_3$ and 15 mM HEPES, pH 7.2, as buffer plus 5% heat-inactivated horse serum. Since this medium is buffered with HEPES, it will maintain a pH of 7.2 in an air atmosphere.

7.3. Preparation of Muscle Extract

1. Muscle extract is prepared as outlined by Dohrmann et al. (1986). Muscle is collected from hindlimbs of 18-d-old chick embryos and frozen at –80°C before being homogenized with a Polytron™ in 4 vol of extraction buffer, i.e., for each gram of muscle extract, add 4 mL extraction buffer.
   a. Preparation of extraction buffer: The extraction buffer consists of 10 mM Tris-HCl, pH 7.5, containing 1 mM EDTA, 1 mM N-ethylmaleimide, 1 mM benzamidine, and 2 mM phenylmethylsulfonyl fluoride.
      i. To 120 mL of triple-distilled water, add 0.188 g Tris-HCl, 0.048 g EDTA, 0.025 g benzamidine-HCl, and 0.031 g N-ethylmaleimide.
      ii. Take 98 mL of this solution and place in a 250 mL Erlenmeyer flask. While vortexing the solution, add 2 mL of 100 mM phenylmethyl-sulfonyl fluoride dissolved in absolute ethanol.
   Note: Caution should be used in the preparation and use of the extraction buffer, since many of the chemicals in this buffer are extremely toxic.

2. Let the homogenate stand at 4°C for 1 h; then centrifuge at 15,000g for 1 h, determine the protein concentration, and store in small aliquots at –80°C until ready to be used in the culture medium.

7.4. Preparation of Solutions Used in Isolating Spinal Cords

1. Bicarbonate containing Puck's solution: To 98.5 mL Puck's solution (a calcium magnesium-free balanced salt solution), add 1.5 mL 1.0M NaHCO$_3$. In a 5% CO$_2$ atmosphere, this solution containing 15 mM NaHCO$_3$ will attain a pH of 7.2.

2. Trypsin (1.0%):

   a. Add 1 g trypsin (Gibco-BRL, Gaithersburg, MD, 1:250) to 100 mL Puck's
      solution. Allow to dissolve (not all of the trypsin goes into solution).
   b. Filter through a set of filters ranging in pore size from 5 to 0.2 μm.
   c. Aliquot and store at –20°C.
3. DNase (2.0%):
   a. Add 200 mg crude deoxyribonuclease I (Sigma DN-25) to 10 mL DMEM/F12.
   b. Filter-sterilize and store at –20°C in small aliquots.
4. DMEM/F12–0.02% DNase: Add 0.4 mL 2.0% DNase to 39.6 mL DMEM/F12
   (final DNase concentration is 0.02%).
5. BSA (3.5%): Add 0.875 g BSA to the surface of 25 mL DMEM/F12. Do not
   stir. Allow the BSA to go into solution, and then filter-sterilize.
6. Metrizamide stock solution (38%):
   a. Dissolve 38 g metrizamide in 50 mL triple-distilled water and bring vol-
      ume up to 100 mL. Filter-sterilize.
   Note: Because of the varying water content of the metrizamide powder, the
      actual content of metrizamide may deviate from 38%; therefore, the actual
      density of the metrizamide solution should be determined by measuring
      the refractive index.*
   b. Keep this solution at 4°C in the dark.
7. Metrizamide working solution (6.4%): Place 1.01 mL 38% metrizamide in a
   sterile polystyrene centrifuge tube, add 4.99 mL DMEM/F12, and mix well.
   Keep the capped tube on ice.

7.5. Preparation of Culture Substrata

1. Poly-D-lysine stock solution: Prepare a stock solution of 1 mg/mL poly-D-lysine
   in triple-distilled water, filter-sterilize, and store in small aliquots at –20°C
   until ready to use.
2. Preparation of coverslips: Round coverslips 12 mm in diameter are a convenient surface for growing motoneurons. Clean such coverslips by soaking in
   acetone and then air-dry. Sterilize the coverslips by heating at 190°C for 3 h.
3. Poly-D-lysine coated culture substrata:
   a. Petri dishes:
      i. Dilute stock poly-D-lysine solution in sterile triple-distilled water to
         50 μg/mL (i.e., add 1.0 mL stock solution to 19 mL water).

---

*The refractometer is calibrated with distilled water and a saturated NaCl solution.
The refractive index of distilled water is 0%, whereas saturated NaCl is 29.6% at 20°C.
Appropriate instructions are provided with the refractometer.

   ii. Place 1.5 mL of this solution in each 35-mm Petri dish. After 2 h,
        remove fluid, wash with sterile triple-distilled water, and allow Petri
        dishes to dry. Such dishes are usable for a period of several weeks.
   iii. If dishes are prepared just prior to planting cells, they should be
        washed with DMEM/F12.
   b. Glass coverslips: Place coverslips into 100-mm microbiological plastic Petri
       dishes and add 150 µL of diluted (50 µg/mL) poly-D-lysine solution to
       each coverslip. After 2 h, remove the fluid, wash the coverslips with ster-
       ile triple-distilled water, and allow to dry.
Note: Coverslips are placed into microbiological Petri dishes, because these
   dishes are hydrophobic and this tends to ensure that the aqueous solution
   stays on the coverslip rather than spilling onto the surface of the Petri dish.
   Substrata can also be coated with polyornithine.

FURTHER READING

Butler, H. and Juurlink B. H. J. (1987), *An Atlas for Staging Mammalian and Chick Embryos*,
   CRC Press, Boca Raton, FL, p. 218.
Calof, A. L. and Reichardt, L. F. (1984), Motoneurons purified by cell sorting respond to two
   distinct activities in myotube-conditioned medium. *Develop. Biol.* **106,** 194–210.
Dohrmann, U., Edgar, D., and Thoenen, H. (1987), Distinct neurotrophic factors from skeletal
   muscle and the central nervous system interact synergistically to support the survival of
   cultured embryonic spinal motor neurons. *Develop. Biol.* **124,** 145–152.
Dohrmann, U., Edgar, D., Sendtner, M., and Thoenen, H. (1986), Muscle-derived factors that
   support survival and promote fiber outgrowth from embryonic chick spinal motor neurons
   in culture. *Develop. Biol.* **118,** 209–221.
Hamburger, V. and Hamilton, H. L. (1951), A series of normal stages in the development of the
   chick embryo. *J. Morph.* **88,** 49–92.
Juurlink, B. H. J., Munoz, D. G. and Devon, R. M. (1990), Calcitonin gene-related peptide identifies
   spinal motoneurons *in vitro. J. Neurosci. Res.* **26,** 238–241.
Juurlink, B. H. J., Munoz, D. G., and Devon, R. M. (1991a), Muscle derived trophic factors promote
   the survival of motoneurons *in vitro* only when serum is present in the growth medium.
   Int. J. Neurosci. **58,** 249–254.
Juurlink, B. H. J., Munoz, D. G., and Ang, L. C. (1991b), Motoneuron survival in vitro: effects of
   pyruvate, a-ketoglutarate, gangliosides and potassium. *Neurosci. Lett.* **133,** 25–28.
McManaman, J., Crawford, F., Clark, R., Richker, J., and Fuller, F. (1989), Multiple neurotrophic
   factors from skeletal muscle: demonstration of effects of basic fibroblast growth factor and
   comparisons with the 22-kilodalton choline acetyltransferase factor. *J. Neurochem.* **53,**
   1763–1771.
McManaman, J. L., Oppenheim, R. W., Prevette, D., and Marchetti, D. (1990), Rescue of
   motoneurons from cell death by a purified skeletal muscle polypeptide: effects of the ChAT
   development factor, CDF. *Neuron* **4,** 891–898.

Schaffner, A. E., St. John, P. A. and Barker, J. L. (1987), Fluorescence-activated cell sorting of embryonic mouse and rat motoneurons and their long term survival *in vitro*. *J. Neurosci.* **7**, 3088–3104.

Schnaar, R. L. and Schaffner, A. E. (1981), Separation of cell types from embryonic chicken and rat spinal cord: characterization of motoneuron enriched fractions. *J. Neurosci.* **1**, 204–217.

Smith, R. G., Vaca, K., McManaman, J., and Appel, S. H. (1986), Selective effects of skeletal muscle extract fractions on motoneuron development *in vitro*. *J. Neurosci.* **6**, 439–447.

Chapter Six

Neural Cells in Microcultures

In Vitro Biological Assays for Neuroactive Agents

Marston Manthorpe

1. INTRODUCTION

The purpose of this chapter is to introduce the reader to standard procedures for preparing microcultures of neural cells for quantification. The chick embryo was chosen as the source of neural tissue because embryos can be conveniently grown in the laboratory in large, replicate numbers with defined developmental stages and because chicken embryos are used by many laboratories as the routine source of many different peripheral and central nervous system tissues.

Presently available quantitative assays of viable neural cell number involve the presentation of serial dilutions of samples containing a neuroactive agent to disaggregated monolayer cultures and subsequent microscopic counts of surviving cells. These assays require:

1. The determination of the number of individual surviving cells within a defined fractional area of each culture and calculation of total cell number per culture;
2. Manually plotting the number of cells per culture vs test sample dilution; and
3. Calculation of the half-maximally effective sample dilutions and, thus, of the test sample titer in half-maximal "activity units"/mL. The disadvantages of these assays are that they are time-consuming (requiring about 1 h to count the viable cells in 96-wells of a microtiter plate), somewhat subjective

Protocols for Neural Cell Culture, 2nd Eds.: • Ed.: S. Fedoroff and A. Richardson • Humana Press, Inc., Totowa, NJ

(in scoring certain cells as "surviving" vs "dead"), and tedious (in plotting individual sample titration curves and titer calculation).

Mosmann (1983) reported a rapid colorimetric assay for lymphocyte cell survival and growth in 96-well microplate cultures. This assay involves supplying the cultures with a tetrazolium salt, 3-(4,5-dimethylthiazol-2-yl)-2,5-diphenyl tetrazolium bromide (MTT), which is reduced to an insoluble blue formazan product by living cells, but not by dying cells or their lytic debris. The blue product is then solubilized by the addition of an alcoholic solution, and color intensity is measured using a multiwell scanning spectrophotometer ("ELISA reader"). The optical density (OD) of the solution in the microwell is directly proportional to the number of viable lymphocytes present. Mosmann used the assay for the determination of cell numbers in the range of 10^2–10^5 cells/culture. Here, we have modified this technique for use in determining chick forebrain cell numbers per culture well.

2. PREPARATION OF CHICK EMBRYOS FOR CULTURING

2.1. Materials

> Fertile eggs (approx 8 d incubation), Hamburger and Hamilton (1951) stage 34.
> Ethanol (70%) in squeeze bottle.
> Ethanol (70%).
> Utility forceps, 15 cm in length (2).
> Forceps, curved, 10 cm in length.
> Beaker with double-lined plastic disposable bag, 600 mL.
> Sterile 100-mm plastic Petri dishes (2).
> Sterile 100-mm glass Petri dish.
> Hanks' balanced salt solution (BSS), 75 mL.

2.2. Procedure

1. Candle the eggs to select viable embryos. If there is no spontaneous movement of the embryo or no clearly defined blood vessels are seen, discard the egg.
2. Clean the egg shell surface.
   a. Stand eggs in the test tube holder with the air sac up (blunt end up).
   b. Using the 70% ethanol, wash the surface of the egg.

   Note: The shell is considered cleaned but not sterile. Therefore, avoid contact between shell and embryo.
3. Sterilize instruments: Sterilize two pairs of utility forceps and one pair of curved forceps by immersing them in 70% alcohol and drying them in air inside the laminar flow hood. When dry, put the instruments into a sterile glass Petri dish and keep the ends covered with the lid.

4. Add approx 15–20 mL Hanks' BSS to two plastic 100-mm Petri dishes.
5. Remove embryos from the eggs.
   a. With the sterile utility forceps, crack the shell at the top of the egg. Hold the egg over the 600-mL beaker and peel off the broken shell to expose the air sac and its underlying chorioallantoic membrane. Take care not to rupture the membrane. Carefully remove any pieces of shell that fall on the membrane.
   b. With the second pair of sterile utility forceps, remove the chorioallantoic membrane. Start at the edge and move around the circumference, trying to avoid contact between any small pieces of shell and the subjacent vascular membrane. With sterile curved forceps, break the vascular connections between the embryo and the membrane. Then using one tine of the forceps, hook the embryo under the neck and lift it gently into a sterile plastic Petri dish containing Hanks' BSS.
   Note: Stage the embryos according to Hamburger and Hamilton (1951). Use only stage 34 embryos.
   c. Decapitate the embryo by using the curved forceps and transfer the head to the second plastic Petri dish containing Hanks' BSS. Repeat for each embryo and combine up to 10 heads in one dish.
6. Clean work area before proceeding further.

3. REMOVAL OF FOREBRAIN

3.1. Materials

Petri dishes, sterile (100 mm), each containing chick embryo heads.
Petri dish, sterile, plastic (100 mm).
Hanks' BSS.
Petri dish, sterile, glass (100 mm).
Small eye forceps.
Angled fine watchmaker's forceps (2).
Scalpel handle and blade.
Sterile capped plastic test tube containing 5–8 mL Puck's balanced salt solution (Puck's BSS).
Pasteur pipet, cotton-plugged, siliconized, sterile (tip: fire-polished).
Ethanol (95%).
Binocular dissecting microscope.

3.2. Procedure

1. Preparation:
   a. Add approx 15–20 mL Hanks' BSS to the 100-mm plastic Petri dish.

    b. Sterilize instruments by immersing them in 70% alcohol (*see* Section 2.2., step 3). When sterile, put the instruments into a sterile glass Petri dish, and keep the ends covered with the lid.

2. Place the 100-mm plastic Petri dish containing the chick embryo heads on the stage of the dissecting microscope. Identify the structures. The forebrain (telencephalon) is the clearly visible, slightly flattened bilobed structure anterior to the larger, more easily visible bilobed optic lobes (which are immediately behind the eyes).

3. Using angled watchmaker's forceps, with the curved side down, insert the forceps under the eye, close the forceps, and remove the eye.

4. Carefully cut between the forebrain and optic lobes with the tips of the fine forceps. Cut in front of the forebrain through the fine ridge of cartilage in the forehead area. Cut under the lobes to free the forebrain from the orbits.

5. Remove the skull from the forebrain.

6. Carefully peel away and discard the meninges (containing many branching blood vessels) and other contaminating tissues that connect the two forebrain lobes together.

7. Cut the brain with an iridectomy or other sharp scalpel into about eight pieces per lobe.

8. Carefully transfer the tissue pieces from *only one* forebrain (the one that you believe was dissected most properly) with the fine forceps or Pasteur pipet (without crushing the tissue) into the capped plastic test tube containing 5–8 mL Puck's BSS.

4. DISAGGREGATION OF FOREBRAIN

4.1. Materials

Pasteur pipets, cotton plugged, siliconized, sterile, tips fire-polished (3).

Pasteur pipet, cotton plugged, sterile, siliconized, tips flame constricted to 1.0 mm inner diameter.

Trypsin (0.08%) in Puck's BSS (6 mL).

Hemocytometer and coverslip.

Trypan blue (0.4%).

Test tube, plastic, capped, sterile (15 mL).

Hand-held digital counter.

Hanks' BSS.

Culture medium (HEBM-P/G-N1–1.0% fetal bovine serum [FBS]; *see* Section 8.2.) (25 mL).

Water bath, 37°C.

Phase-contrast microscope.

4.2. Procedure

1. Incubate fragments in 5–8 mL Puck's BSS for 10 min in a 37°C water bath.
2. Carefully aspirate off the Puck's BSS and replace it with 5 mL 0.08% trypsin solution. Incubate the minced tissue in trypsin solution for 20 min in a 37°C water bath.
3. Remove trypsin by careful aspiration with a Pasteur pipet and wash tissue three times with 1.5 mL of culture medium by allowing the tissue to settle and carefully aspirating off the medium. Leave the tissue in the last wash of 1.5 mL culture medium.
4. Using the siliconized constricted Pasteur pipet, pass the tissue and the near-entire 1.5-mL culture medium through the pipet repeatedly until there are no intact tissue pieces visible (about 10–20 times).

   Note: Do not create air bubbles during this process! Air bubbles can be avoided by not expelling the last few microliters from the tip of the Pasteur pipet and by not drawing air bubbles into the tip during aspirations.

5. Determination of cell number:
   a. Prepare a sample from the cell suspension for counting with a hemocytometer. Dilute a 0.1-mL aliquot of the cell suspension with 1.7 mL Hanks' BSS. Add 0.2 mL trypan blue solution. This makes a cell dilution of 1:20.
   b. Fill the hemocytometer with the diluted cell suspension using a Pasteur pipet.
   c. Count the number of viable cells in at least one hemocytometer chamber (four squares). The use of trypan blue as a viability indicator is based on the ability of live, intact cells or viable cells to exclude the dye. Therefore, viable cells will appear unstained.
   d. Record the cell counts and calculate the number of cells/mL in the remaining 1.4 mL of cell suspension.
6. Dilute the cell suspension to 2.4×10^5 cells/mL (6×10^3 cells/25 μL) in culture medium in a volume of 10 mL.

5. MICROCULTURES

5.1. Materials

A/2 microplates (96-well) (Costar [Cambridge, MA], #3696) coated with poly-L-ornithine and laminin (2).
Culture medium (HEBM-PG-N1–1.0% FBS).
Multichannel microliter pipet.
Reagent reservoir, sterile.

Plastic tips, sterile.
Microplate template record sheets (2).
Test agent.

5.2. Procedure

1. Add 25 μL culture medium to all wells. The wells in column #1 then receive 25 μL of the test agent in culture medium to make a total of 50 μL. Then 25 μL is transferred from each well of column #1 to the corresponding wells of column #2 and the contents are mixed. This serial twofold titration is repeated for each set of wells up to column #11 and the last 25 μL discarded. Thus, the wells in the last column (#12) are controls without added test substance.
2. Mix the diluted cell suspension (2.4×10^5 cells/mL) and pipet 25 μL into each well of each microplate using a multichannel pipeter.
3. Place the two plates in a humidified 5% carbon dioxide 95% air incubator at 37°C for 4 d.

6. QUANTIFICATION OF VIABLE CELL NUMBERS

6.1. Materials

MTT (thiazolyl blue) dye solution, 5 mL.
Acid alcohol solution, 5 mL.
Logarithmic graph paper, four cycles.
Microplate spectrophotometer.
Standard inverted light microscope.

6.2. Selective Staining of Viable Cells with a Vital Dye

See previous section for preparation of cells for the bioassay.

1. Four hours before the end of the selected culture period, add 5 μL of the vital dye MTT to each well of one 96-well microplate.
2. Incubate the culture for an additional 4 h.
3. Dissolve the blue dye derivative in the wells created by the viable cells by adding 50 μL acid–alcohol and mixing by 10 aspirations/expirations using the multichannel pipet.
4. Determine the optical density of each well by using the microplate spectrophotometer set at a test wavelength of 570 nm, reference wavelength at 630 nm.

6.3. Evaluation of Cell Number by Multiwell Scanning Spectrophotometer

Instructions for operating the computerized microplate reader are given in the manuals accompanying the reader. Consult the manual for specific procedures.

6.4. Data Analysis

Plot the sample dilution on the logarithmic abscissa (x axis) and the average optical densities of the eight corresponding wells on the linear ordinate (y axis).

7. SELECTIVE IMMUNOSTAINING OF NEURONS IN MICROCULTURES

7.1. Materials

Fixing solution.
Blocking buffer.
Wash solution.
Saline.
Water.
Primary antibody to neurofilament protein in blocking buffer.
Peroxidase-conjugated secondary antibody in blocking buffer.
Chloronaphthol solution covered and stored in the dark.
Peroxide solution.
Plastic gloves.
Multichannel pipet.
Reagent troughs for pipets.

7.2. Fixation and Staining of Microculture

1. Add 100 µL of fixation solution to each well of the replicate plate (the one not used for MTT viability studies).

   Note: During all subsequent steps, never squirt solutions directly onto the well bottom, or you will tend to detach the cells. Rather, let the fluids run slowly down the well edges.

   Let the plate fix for 20 min at room temperature, remove the fixative by matting (flip the plate upside down into the waste bucket or sink and shake the solution out, then tamp the plate upside down onto a thick bed of clean paper towels), and replace with another 100 µL of fixation solution. Let fix another 20 min.

2. Remove the fixative by matting and add 100 µL of blocking buffer. Remove by matting and wash with 100 µL blocking buffer twice more. Allow the culture to incubate in the blocking buffer for 30 min to permeabilize the cells.

3. Remove the blocking buffer and add 50 µL of the primary antineurofilament antibody solution. Incubate the plate at 37°C for 1 h.

4. Remove the primary antibody and wash the wells three times with 100 µL washing solution.

5. Add 50 µL of secondary antibody and incubate at 37°C for 1 h.

6. Remove the secondary antibody and wash the wells as before three times with 100 μL washing solution. Wash a fourth time with saline.

7. Add peroxide to the stock chloronaphthol solution (Section 8.5.) and then add 100 μL chloronaphthol peroxide solution to each well. Store the plate in the dark at room temperature for 30 min. Replace the chloronaphthol with fresh chloronaphthol and observe under the microscope. Keep the plate in the dark, taking it out only occasionally to observe it under the microscope. When the neurons are at the desired staining intensity, replace the chloronaphthol with water, wash the culture with water a few times, and finally discard the water and allow the wells to dry. The neurons and their axons and growth cones, but not the glial cells and fibroblasts, should be stained dark brown.

7.3. Results

These stained plates can be used for counting the number of individual surviving neurons within a defined area and the results used for calculation of the total neuronal number per culture. The total neuronal number of both the control cultures and those treated with test substances should be determined.

8. APPENDIX

8.1. Hanks' and Puck's Balanced Salt Solutions: Stock Solution 10×

Component	Hanks' BSS	Puck's BSS
$CaCl_2$	1.4 g/L	0
KCl	4.0 g/L	4.0 g/L
KH_2PO_4	0.6 g/L	0.6 g/L
$MgCl_2 \cdot 6H_2O$	1.0 g/L	0
$MgSO_4 \cdot 7H_2O$	1.0 g/L	0
NaCl	80.0 g/L	80.0 g/L
$NaHCO_3$	See note	
$Na_2HPO_4 \cdot 7H_2O$	0.9 g/L	0.9 g/L
Glucose	10.0 g/L	10.0 g/L
Phenol red	0.1 g/L	0.1 g/L (10 mL of a 1% solution)

Note: Sodium bicarbonate is prepared as a solution containing 1.4 g $NaHCO_3$ in 100 mL triple-distilled water. It is sterilized by filtration through a 0.2-μm filter. Approximately 2.5 mL (0.35 g/L) of this sterile solution is added after dilution and before use to Puck's or Hanks' BSS.

1. Weigh out each chemical (except phenol red and sodium bicarbonate). Dissolve in 990 mL triple-distilled water.
2. Add 10 mL 1% phenol red (1 g/100 mL triple-distilled water). Mix.
3. Sterilize by filtration through a 0.2-μm filter.
4. For use, dilute 1:10 with sterile water or dilute and sterilize by filtration through 0.2-μm filter.

8.2. Eagle's Basal Medium (EBM) with Supplements (Eagle, 1955)

1. HEBM formulation
   a. Components   mg/L
      Inorganic salts
         $CaCl_2$ (anhyd.)   200.00
         KCl   400.00
         $MgSO_4$ (anhyd.)   97.67
         NaCl   6800.00
         $NaH_2PO_4 \cdot H_2O$ 140.00
      Other components
         D-glucose   1000.00
         Phenol red   10.00
      Amino acids
         L-Arginine · HCl   21.00
         L-Cystine · 2HCl   15.65
         L-Glutamine   292.00
         L-Histidine   8.00
         L-Isoleucine   26.00
         L-Leucine   26.00
         L-Lysine HCl   36.47
         L-Methionine   7.50
         L-Phenylalanine   16.50
         L-Threonine   24.00
         L-Tryptophan   4.00
         L-Tyrosine (disodium salt)   26.00
         L-Valine   23.50
      Vitamins
         Biotin   1.00
         D-Calcium pantothenate   1.00
         Choline chloride   1.00
         Folic acid   1.00
         i-Inositol   2.00

Nicotinamide	1.00
Pyridoxal HCl	1.00
Riboflavin	0.10
Thiamine HCl	1.00

   b. To the above formulation of Eagle's basal medium, add 5.0 g/L D-glucose and 2.2 g/L sodium bicarbonate. In addition, it is supplemented sterilely with 1.0% FBS and as indicated below with penicillin, glutamine, N1 mixture, and insulin (HEBM-P/G-N1–1% FBS).

2. Insulin:

   a. Weigh out 25 mg insulin.

   b. Add insulin to 10 mL HEBM containing PG.

   c. Acidify the insulin solution with drops of $1N$ HCl until the suspension is dissolved. (Solution will be clear yellow.)

   d. Sterilize by filtration through a 0.2-µm filter.

   e. Aliquot 0.5 mL/12 × 75 mm plastic tube.

   f. Store in the refrigerator at 4°C for up to 4 wk. **Do not freeze.**

3. Penicillin/glutamine (Pen/Glu or P/G): The solutions of penicillin and glutamine are made up so that each are 100 times the final concentration. They are then mixed together equally, so that they are in solution at 50 times the final concentration.

   a. Penicillin "G" potassium or penicillin "G" sodium:

Final concentration:	100 U/mL
Stock solution:	10,000 U/mL
Stock solution:	1,000,000 U/mL

        Example: 1585 U/g = 1,000,000 U/x

              630.9 mg = x

   b. L-Glutamine (mol wt 146.15):

Final concentration:	2 mM
Stock solution:	200 mM
Stock solution:	2.92 g/100 mL

   c. Procedure:

     i. The above solutions are diluted with isotonic saline (0.85%), which is made with double-distilled water.

    ii. Mix the two solutions together thoroughly for a total of 200 mL.

   iii. Sterilize by filtration through a 0.2-µm filter.

   iv. Aliquot 5.2 mL Pen/Glu/17 × 100 mm sterile opaque tube.

    v. Store by freezing at –20°C.

   Note: The volume of 5.2 mL Pen/Glu is sufficient for a 250 mL bottle of medium.

4. N1 Components (serum substitute)
    a. Preparation of N1 components:

Chemical	Weight	Volume	Solvent	Further manipulations
Transferrin Sigma T4515	25.00 mg	5 mL	HEBM-P/G	None
Putrescine Sigma P7505	80.55 mg	5 mL	HEBM-P/G	None
Progesterone Sigma P0130	3.145 mg	5 mL	95% ETOH	50 µL/10 mL HEBM-P/G
Sodium selenite ICN (Costa Mesa, CA) 201657	5.19 mg	100 mL	HEBM-P/G	0.5 mL/5 mL HEBM-P/G

   Note: This volume is sufficient for 18–20 tubes of N1 mixture as prepared below. A larger quantity may be made by increasing each component proportionally.

    b. Final N1 mixture (minus insulin): 25 mL

Transferrin	5 mL
Putrescine	5 mL
Progesterone	10 mL
Selenium	5 mL

    c. Procedure:
       i. Prepare chemical solutions as indicated in step a.
       ii. Combine chemical solutions as indicated in step b.
       iii. Sterilize by filtration through a 0.2-µm filter.
       iv. Aliquot 1.25 mL N1 mixture/12 × 75 mm tube.
       v. Store by freezing at –20°C for up to 2–3 wk.
    d. Preparation of HEBM-P/G-N1:
       i. Thaw one aliquot of N1 and add the 1.25 mL of N1 to 250 mL medium containing P/G.
       ii. Add 0.5 mL insulin solution to the N1, medium, P/G solution.
       iii. Store at 4°C for up to 3–4 d, but no longer than 5 d.
    Note: Final concentrations of each component in medium:

Transferrin	$6.25 \times 10^{-8}M$
Putrescine	$1.00 \times 10^{-4}M$
Progesterone	$2.00 \times 10^{-8}M$
Selenium	$3.00 \times 10^{-8}M$
Insulin	$8.30 \times 10^{-7}M$

5. FBS (1.0%): Add 0.1 mL to each 9 mL basal medium containing penicillin, glutamine, insulin, and N1.

8.3. Poly-L-Ornithine and Laminin-Coated Plates

1. Preparation of solutions:
   a. Poly-L-ornithine hydrobromide, mol wt 30,000–70,000 (Sigma [St. Louis, MO], catalog # P3655) should be stored desiccated at –20°C.
      i. 0.1 g poly-L-ornithine is added to 100 mL, pH 8.4, boric acid buffer to form a *stock* solution of 1.0 mg/mL.
      ii. Sterilize by filtration through a 0.2-µm filter.
      iii. Store at 4°C for up to 2 mo.
      iv. For use, dilute 10 mL poly-L-ornithine stock solution to a final volume of 100 mL with sterile distilled water to obtain a *working* solution of 0.1 mg/mL.
   b. Preparation of boric acid buffer:
      i. Make up an excess amount of 0.15M boric acid buffer: 1.159 g boric acid plus 0.75 g NaOH/125 mL distilled water.
      ii. Adjust pH to 8.4.
      Note: Test aliquots of the buffer for pH. Do *not* put the pH electrode into the entire buffer.
   c. Mouse laminin (EY Laboratories, Inc. [San Mateo, CA], Cat. #2404).
      i. Stock solutions should be reconstituted to approx 1 mg/mL in sterile phosphate buffered saline (PBS), pH 8.0. Store in 50-µL aliquots at 4 or –20°C, depending on manufacturer's instructions.
      ii. Dilute laminin immediately before use to a concentration of 10 µg/mL by the addition of sterile PBS.
2. Coating of 96-well A/2 microplates with poly-L-ornithine and mouse laminin:
   a. Add 25 µL working solution of poly-L-ornithine/microwell.
   b. Leave on for approx 30 min at room temperature.
   c. Remove poly-L-ornithine and add 25 µL sterile distilled water/well.
   d. Remove all the water with a suction pipet.
   e. Add 25 µL laminin/PBS solution/well.
   f. Incubate overnight at 37°C.
   g. Remove from incubator and freeze with laminin PBS solution.
   h. Store in Zip-Lock™ bags at –20°C.
3. Preparation of coated plates for culturing:
   a. Remove plate(s) from freezer and thaw in 37°C incubator.
   b. Remove laminin PBS solution and wash wells one time with media (optional).

c. **Do not allow the laminin-coated surface to dry out!**

8.4. Staining and Fixation for Quantification

1. MTT (thiazolyl blue) dye solution [3-(4,5-Dimethylthiazol-2-yl)-2,5-diphenyltetrazolium bromide] Sigma # M-2128:

Note: MTT is categorized as toxic and mutagenic. Use appropriate precautions.

   a. Working concentration is 1.5 mg/mL in culture medium (HEBM-P/G-N1–1.0% FBS).
   b. To make 50 3-mL aliquots at 1.5 mg/mL, weigh out 225 mg MTT, and dissolve in 150 mL medium.
      i. Weigh out quickly but carefully. This chemical is light-sensitive.
      ii. Add MTT to medium prewarmed to 37°C, and stir until the MTT is completely dissolved (10–15 min). Keep covered with aluminum foil to keep out light while the solution is being stirred.
      iii. Sterilize by filtration through a 0.2-μm filter in a hood with the lights out.
      iv. Aliquot 3 mL/12 × 75 mm polypropylene tube. Wrap tubes in foil or keep in light-tight box.
      v. Freeze at –20°C.
   c. To thaw: Place tube in a 37°C water bath.
2. Acid–alcohol solution
   a. Mix 6 mL concentrated HCl/L isopropanol.
   b. Store solution in a tightly capped 1-L plastic bottle. Solution is stable for 2 wk at room temperature.

8.5. Selective Immunostaining of Neurons in Microcultures

1. Fixing solution: Add 4 g paraformaldehyde to 100 mL PBS and add three drops 5N NaOH. Heat with stirring to dissolve. Cool to room temperature. Adjust the pH to 7.0–7.4 with 5N NaOH. Store at room temperature no longer than 2 d.
2. Blocking buffer: Add 1 g Tween 20 and 1 g bovine serum albumin (Sigma Chem. Co., Fraction V) to 1 L of PBS and mix to dissolve. Store at 4 or –20°C. Use at room temperature.
3. Wash solution: Dissolve 1 g Tween 20 and 9 g NaCl in 1 L of water. Use at room temperature.
4. Saline: Dissolve 9 g NaCl in 1 L of water. Store and use at room temperature.
5. Chloronaphthol solution: Add 50 mg 4-chloro-L-naphthol (Sigma #C8890) to 0.5 mL methanol to dissolve. Add the methanolic solution to a stirring solution of 100 mL saline (0.9 g NaCl/100 mL water). Cover and stir in the dark

1 h. Filter the saturated solution through a standard 0.2- or 0.4-μm filter. Keep in the dark at room temperature until use. Immediately before use, add 20 μL hydrogen peroxide solution (30%; Fisher #325). Make sure that the peroxide is relatively new, since this reagent will deteriorate on prolonged storage.

6. Antibodies:
    a. Mouse ascites fluid containing monoclonal antibody RT97 to neurofilament protein is diluted 1/100 in blocking buffer.
    b. Peroxidase-conjugated goat antimouse IgG antibody (Cappel, Durham, NC, Cat. 3211-0231) diluted 1/200 in blocking buffer.
    Note: The optimal concentration for use of each antibody should be determined by using a range of dilutions.

8.6. Method for Siliconizing Pasteur Pipets

1. Use a tall beaker to accommodate 9-in. Pasteur pipets (e.g., a pipet soaker).
2. Place pipets' tip up in a pipet basket (holes in the bottom).
3. Dilute Prosil-28™ (American Scientific Products) 1/100 with water.
4. Submerge the pipets in the solution, making sure the pipets are fully coated. Flush the basket up and down to eliminate bubbles in the tips.
5. Remove the basket to a siphon-type pipet washer and flush with deionized water several times, making sure the tips are not blocked by bubbles.
6 Place the pipets' tips up in foil-lined baskets and dry thoroughly in a drying oven.
7. Plug pipets with cotton balls (#1 size is available from dental supply houses) and autoclave in glass or paper holders for later use in the disaggregation of tissues.

8.7. Comments

1. Never let tissues dry out during dissection. Always keep them immersed in a balanced salt solution.
2. Minimize mechanical trauma:
    a. Teasing tissues apart is a very damaging procedure.
    b. Cutting tissues with very sharp instruments tends to break only cells contacting the instruments.
    c. For cutting, a tungsten needle in one hand and an iridectomy knife in the other make a good combination, provided they are very sharp and that you use them for cutting and not for teasing.
    d. A Pasteur pipet "charged" with dissecting medium is less traumatic than forceps for transferring tissues from one dish to another. Pipets break easily and care must be taken to:
        i.   Charge the pipet with 1 mL or less of dissecting medium.
        ii. Introduce the tip into the solution containing the tissue.
        iii. Expel a small amount of buffer.

  iv. Aspirate the tissue into the pipet tip and release the bulb completely before taking the tip out of the solution.

  Note: This procedure prevents bubble formation. If you are transferring tissue to a solid substrate (agar, plasma clot, and so on) you can control the position of the tissue within the pipet (close to the tip), thus reducing the amount of fluid that you add to the substrate.

3. If you have to dissect more than one animal and pool the tissues, there is no way to have all the tissues treated in exactly the same way—either some will wait longer before being taken out of the animal, or they will spend more time in BSS after being taken out of the animal. The procedure must be standardized. In routine work, you must determine exactly how long your dissection will take and come to depend on this same time for your experiments. Successive experiments must always use tissues and cells prepared as identically as possible.

4. Sometimes a concave surface is more practical than a flat one, especially if you have to collect small organs such as ganglia. A depression slide or watch glass contained within a Petri dish can be used.

5. Mistakes made during dissection frequently explain erratic experimental results.

  a. Before beginning an experiment, spend some time precisely defining the landmarks to be used during dissection. For instance, if you plan to use segments of spinal cord, remember that the different levels have a different structure and contain different cell types—be sure you recognize those levels. External landmarks, such as somites, vertebrae, ribs, and so forth, can be of help. If you collect ganglia, be sure to cut the nerve roots at the same level each time.

  b. The tissue that you plan to use will frequently be "contaminated" by unwanted tissues. Be sure to remove these contaminants. Sometimes further dissection will suffice (such as removing meninges from the spinal cord), but sometimes a brief enzyme treatment will be necessary.

  c. Blood left in tissues may alter the meaning of the cell counts and hemoglobin can be toxic to some cultured cells. Warm dissecting medium can help remove blood from the dissected tissue.

  d. Discard any piece of tissue the nature of which you are not absolutely certain. Remember this especially when you are under the pressure of such circumstances as not having as many embryos as you would wish. A smaller, yet meaningful, experiment is better than a larger, but useless one.

8.8. Tissue Culture Vessels and Cell Seeding Levels

Table 1 illustrates the differences in size of available vessels for monolayer cultures. Also shown are the cell plating requirements needed to obtain a modest cell

Table 1
Differences in Size of Available Vessels for Monolayer Cultures

Type of vessel	Diameter, mm	Total surface area, mm^2	Relative area	Seeding/well at 100 cells/mm^2
Roller bottle (250 mL)	N/A	85,000	6071	8,500,000
Roller bottle (144 mL)	N/A	49,000	3500	4,900,000
TC flask (1000 mL)	N/A	15,000	1071	1,500,000
TC flask (250 mL)	N/A	7,500	536	750,000
TC dish (100 mm)	84	5,541	396	554,000
TC flask (30 mm)	N/A	2,500	179	250,000
TC dish (60 mm)	52	2,124	152	212,400
Dish (35 mm)	32	804	57.4	80,400
TC plates (24 well)	16	201	14.4	20,100
Glass rings (10 mm)	10	78	5.6	7,800
Plates (96 well) (TC Microtiter)	6	28	2.0	2,800
A/2 96-well plates	4.5	14	1.0	1,400

density of 100 cells/mm^2. Although theoretically one should be able to generate equivalent cultures in different vessels plated with the same cell density (e.g., 100 cells/mm^2), other properties of the culture, such as medium volume, depth, and movements, as well as differences in the culture plastics, may tend to make the cultures unequivalent.

FURTHER READING

Eagle, H. (1955), Nutrition needs of mammalian cells in tissue culture. *Science* **122,** 501–504.

Hamburger, V. and Hamilton, H. L. (1951), A series of normal stages in the development of the chick embryo. *J. Morphol.* **88,** 49–92.

Manthorpe, M., Skaper, S. D., and Varon, S. (1981), Neuronotrophic factors and their antibodies: *In vitro* microassays for titration and screening. *Brain Res.* **230,** 295–306.

Manthorpe, M., Fagnani, R., Skaper, S. D., and Varon, S. (1986), An automated colorimetric microassay for neuronotrophic factors. *Dev. Br. Res.* **25,** 191–198.

Mosmann, T. (1983), Rapid colorimetric assay for cellular growth and survival: application to proliferation and cytotoxic assays. *J. Immunol. Meth.* **65,** 55–63.

Varon, S., Skaper, S. D., Barbin, G., Selak, I., and Manthorpe, M. (1984), Low molecular weight agents support survival of cultured neurons from the CNS. *J. Neurosci.* **4,** 654–658.

Chapter Seven

Construction and Use of Compartmented Cultures

Robert B. Campenot

1. INTRODUCTION

The compartmented culture method has numerous features that make it useful for studies of nerve fiber growth, among which are:

1. Distal neurites can be exposed to a different fluid and cellular environment than cell bodies and proximal neurites, which is useful for studies of trophic, ionic, and pharmacological regulation of growth;
2. Distal neurites can be removed (neuritotomy) and subsequently regenerate, which permits many useful approaches to the study of neurite growth and regeneration; and
3. Neurites can be chronically electrically stimulated during growth and regeneration.

Earlier versions of these procedures have been published (Campenot, 1979, 1992). The following protocol describes in detail the basic production of compartmented cultures and how to neuritotomize them. It is common practice to culture rat sympathetic neurons using L-15 culture media thickened with methylcellulose and containing nerve growth factor as described by Hawrot and Patterson (1979). Rat serum and ascorbic acid are supplied to compartments containing cell bodies, but omitted from culture medium given to neurites since this facilitates their adhesion to the substratum and their ability to grow in the face of medium changes (*see* Campenot, 1982). Media appropriate to the

Protocols for Neural Cell Culture, 2nd Ed. • Eds.: S. Fedoroff and A. Richardson • Humana Press, Inc., Totowa, NJ

particular neurons cultured should be used, and although methylcellulose appears to be important for the proper functioning of the compartmented system, the necessity for it has not been rigorously investigated. We use methyl cellulose 4000 cps (Sel-Win Chemicals, Ltd., Vancouver, British Columbia, Canada) at 1.5g/500 mL medium. A condenser modification of an inverted-phase contrast microscope that allows better visualization of the neurons is useful, but its description is beyond the scope of this protocol.

2. PREPARATION OF 35-MM TISSUE CULTURE DISHES

2.1. Materials

Tissue culture dishes, sterile plastic (35 mm).
Rat tail collagen solution, fresh, sterile.
Tissue-culture quality distilled water, sterile.
Pin rake (*see* Section 6.).
Tray for 12 cultures made from black Plexiglas™ (optional).

2.2. Collagen Coating of Dishes

Prepare a solution of rat tail collagen as described by Hawrot and Paterson (1979) using sterile technique. The shelf-life of collagen solution used for this purpose is 2 wk in the refrigerator. Collagen-coated culture dishes may be stored frozen indefinitely. "Bad" collagen will peel from tracks during scratching and produce an excessive amount of white powder. To coat culture dishes, dilute the collagen solution (four parts sterile, culture-quality distilled water to one part collagen solution for sympathetic neuron cultures; one part water to one part collagen solution for dorsal root ganglion [DRG] neuron cultures). Wet the floors of 35-mm tissue culture dishes by pouring enough solution into the first dish to fill it about half, and then pouring the solution from the first dish into the second dish and so forth. Replenish the solution as needed. This will leave behind a film sufficient to coat the floors of the dishes. Then air-dry the dishes with lids on overnight in a laminar flow hood.

2.3. Forming Collagen Tracks

Form the collagen tracks by scoring the collagen-coated floors of 35-mm tissue culture dishes with a pin rake. It is helpful to place the dish on a black Plexiglas background to permit visualization of the scratches as they are made. The tracks should be approx 20 mm long with the scratches positioned as indicated in Fig. 1A.

3. TEFLON DIVIDERS

3.1. Materials

Teflon™ dividers (Fig. 2A) machined from Teflon rod stock are commercially available (Tyler Research Instruments, Edmonton, Aberta, Canada).

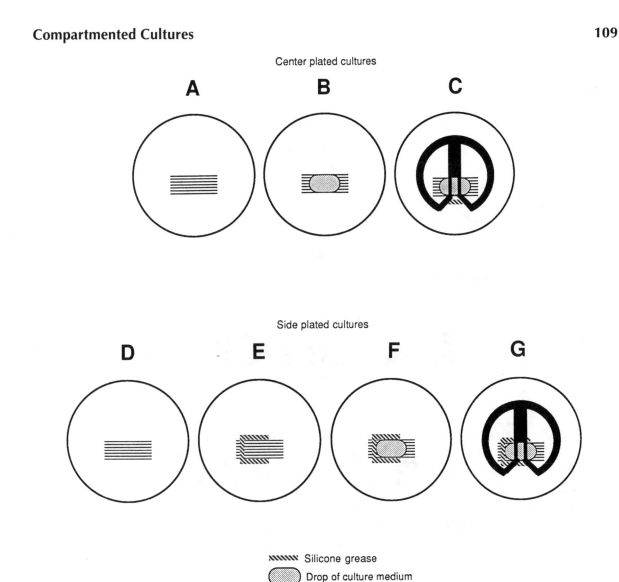

Fig. 1. Construction sequences for center and side-plated cultures.

3.2. Cleaning and Sterilization

1. Remove dividers from culture dishes with forceps and wipe off the silicone grease with a lint-free tissue. Place dividers in a beaker reserved for acid cleaning containing 70% ethanol until they are to be acid cleaned.
2. Pour off the ethanol, place beaker in a fume hood, and add clean sulfuric acid with Nochromix™ (Aldrich [Milwaukee, WI], #32, 869-3). Leave until dividers look pure white. (They can be left indefinitely in the acid without harm.)
3. Pour the acid back into its jug, catching the dividers in the funnel. Transfer them to a beaker. Rinse the dividers five times with culture-quality distilled

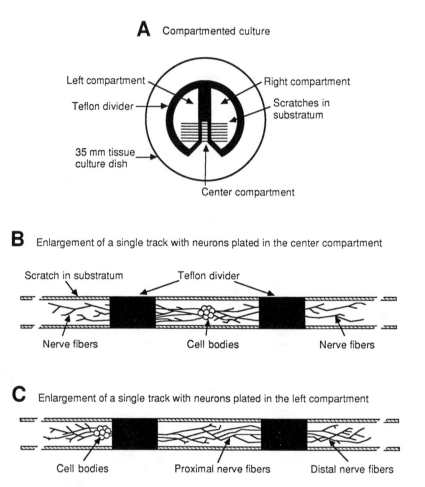

A Compartmented culture

Left compartment

Right compartment

Teflon divider

Scratches in substratum

35 mm tissue culture dish

Center compartment

B Enlargement of a single track with neurons plated in the center compartment

Scratch in substratum   Teflon divider

Nerve fibers   Cell bodies   Nerve fibers

C Enlargement of a single track with neurons plated in the left compartment

Cell bodies   Proximal nerve fibers   Distal nerve fibers

Fig. 2. Schematic of a compartmented culture chamber.

water to remove the acid and then boil them in the water for 1 h. Pour off the hot water and rinse again five times.

4. Using clean forceps, move the dividers to clean Petri dishes, taking with them as little water as possible. Autoclave them and dry them in an oven if necessary.

4. ASSEMBLING THE DISH AND DIVIDER

4.1. Materials

Collagen-coated and scratched tissue culture dishes (*see* Section 2.).
Culture medium.
Tray for 12 cultures made from black Plexiglas (optional).
Sterile Teflon dividers (*see* Section 3.).
Hemostat with right-angled jaws.
Stereo microscope set up in a sterile hood.

Fine forceps (dissection quality) (2 pairs).
Sterile silicone grease syringes (*see* Section 7.).

4.2. Procedure for Center-Plated Cultures

1. Assemble in a sterile hood equipped with a stereo microscope: a supply of sterile Teflon dividers, two pairs of forceps, a right-angle hemostat, and two sterile silicone grease syringes.

2. Under the stereo microscope, place a drop of methylcellulose-containing culture medium on the scratched region of the floor of each dish in order to wet the region where neurites will cross under the divider (Fig. 1B). Take care not to touch the pipet to the substratum.

3. Sterilize the hemostat. Remove a Teflon divider from the Petri dish by gripping the rim of the divider with sterile forceps. Transfer the divider to the sterile hemostat, clamping the divider by the solid septum. Lay the hemostat on its back on the work surface such that the divider is visualized under the stereo microscope. Apply silicone grease to the divider, taking care that the regions under which the neurites will cross receive a neat "rope" of grease.

4. Pick up a collagen coated pre-"scratched" culture dish, remove and set aside its lid, and invert the dish quickly so as not to disturb the drop of medium. Bring the dish into position over the divider and drop it in place (Fig. 1C). With a fine forceps, press on the dish bottom in the area of the solid septum and also around the rim to seat the grease. Do not press in the region where the neurites will cross. When the dish is properly seated (a judgment developed with experience), pick up the hemostat, turn it over, and release the dish so that it falls gently on the work surface. (Placing it on the surface can disrupt the seating of the divider.) Place a dab of grease at the entry of the slot (Fig. 1C), and calk any regions around the perimeter of the divider that did not seal properly. Place a drop of culture medium in each side compartment on the scratched region of the substratum and ensure that the full length of the scratched region is wetted with medium. This prevents drying at the edge of the original drop from damaging the substratum. Replace the cover of the dish.

5. Repeat steps 2–4 for each dish and then store trays of 12 dishes in the incubator as they are completed. After one or more hours in the incubator, fill the side compartments with culture medium.

4.3. Procedure for Side-Plated Cultures

1. Assemble in a sterile hood equipped with a stereo microscope: a supply of sterile Teflon dividers, two pairs of forceps, a right-angle hemostat, two sterile silicone grease syringes, and a sheet of black Plexiglas of sufficient size to serve as a tray for about 12 cultures.

2. Arrange 12 culture dishes on the black Plexiglas sheet. Under the stereo microscope, lay down a C-shaped perimeter of silicone grease in each dish as shown in Fig. 1E. Set the dishes in the incubator to allow the grease to settle for about 1 h.

3. After the grease perimeter has settled, place a drop of methylcellulose-containing culture medium on the scratched region of the floor of a dish within the C in order to wet the region where neurites will cross under the divider (Fig. 1F). Take care not to touch the pipet to the substratum.

4. Remove a Teflon divider from the Petri dish by gripping the rim of the divider with sterile forceps. Transfer the divider to the hemostat, clamping the divider by the solid septum. Lay the hemostat on its back on the work surface such that the divider is visualized under the stereo microscope. Apply silicone grease to the divider, taking care that the regions under which the neurites will cross receive a neat "rope" of grease.

5. Pick up a collagen-coated pre-"scratched" culture dish, remove and set aside its lid, and invert the dish quickly so as not to disturb the drop of medium. Bring the dish into position over the divider and drop it in place. (Fig. 1G). With fine forceps, press on the dish bottom in the area of the solid septum and also around the rim to seat the grease. Do not press in the region where the neurites will cross. When the dish is properly seated, pick up the hemostat, turn it over, and release the dish so that it falls gently on the work surface. With a dab of grease, calk any regions around the perimeter of the divider that did not seal properly. Place a drop of culture medium in the right compartment and ensure that the full length of the scratched region is wetted with medium. Replace the cover of the dish.

6. Repeat steps 3–5 for each dish and then store trays of 12 dishes in the incubator as they are completed. After one or more hours in the incubator, fill the center and distal compartments with culture medium.

5. PLATING THE NEURONS

5.1. Materials

Cell suspension.
Sterile syringe (1 mL) with 22-gage 1.5-in. needle (two are needed for side-plated cultures).

5.2. Procedure

1. Most commonly, sympathetic neurons dissociated from superior cervical ganglia of newborn rats are plated into the compartmented dishes; however, DRG neurons from rat embryos and other types of neurons have been used. Obtaining sympathetic neurons is carried out as described by Campenot and

Draker (1989) modified from Hawrot and Patterson (1979). The neurons from 20 ganglia are suspended in about 1.3 mL of L-15 CO_2 medium containing methylcellulose, nerve growth factor, rat serum, cytosine arabinoside, and vitamin C. For center-plated cultures, use 0.8 mL cell suspension/12 dishes and for side-plated cultures, use 0.5 mL/12 dishes. Allow 0.5 mL waste.

2. Transfer cell suspension to a 60-mm plastic Petri dish, tilted such that the fluid remains on one side, and load the cell suspension into a 1-mL syringe fitted with a 22-gage, 1.5-in. needle. For center-plated cultures, inject cell suspension into the center compartment slot of each dish. For side-plated cultures, remove residual medium from within the silicone grease perimeter, which will contain the neurons (Fig. 1G) by using an empty 1-mL syringe and needle. Then inject the cell suspension with care that it adheres to the Teflon divider. Also with side-plated cultures, use a syringe and needle to establish confluence between the medium in the center compartment slot and the medium in the outer perimeter of the center compartment. The next day, top up the cell-containing compartments with culture medium.

6. CONSTRUCTION OF PIN RAKE

6.1. Materials

Insect pins, size 1 (Carolina Biological Supply Co. [Burlington, NC], # 65-4331) (21).
Hot plate.
Dissecting microscope.
Aluminum sheet (about 3 × 3 × 1/2 in.).
Parafilm™.
Fine forceps.
5-Minute™ epoxy cement.
Phenolic or Plexiglas rod 7/16 in. diameter × 6 in.
Small handsaw.

6.2. Procedure

1. A pin rake can in principal be constructed from any type of pin. We typically use size 1 insect pins, which are approx 200 µm in diameter and produce collagen tracks about 200 µm wide.
2. Cut the heads off of the 21 size 1 insect pins.
3. Arrange a hot plate so that its surface may be viewed with a dissecting microscope. Place a piece of 1/2 in. thick aluminum sheet (about 3 × 3 in.) on the hot plate and melt a piece of Parafilm (about 2 × 2 in.) onto the surface of

the aluminum sheet to produce a sticky (not liquid) surface. The amount of heat required will be easily determined empirically. Make sure the Parafilm is positioned such that it comes right to one of the edges of the aluminum sheet.

4. Hold the back end of one of the pins with fine forceps. Embed a pin in the Parafilm such that the point is visible under the dissecting microscope and the back end extends over the edge of the aluminum plate. The pin may be pressed into the Parafilm with the side of the forceps. Place the next pin similarly, and locate it against the first pin with the points as even as possible. Continue placing pins until there are 21 pins, side by side, with their points as even as possible. Then, using the back end of the forceps as a straightedge, push against the points of the pins to move them slightly backward and, thus, even out the line of the points. In this way, the points can be made to line up almost perfectly straight. Turn off the hot plate.

5. Mix some 5-Minute epoxy cement and put several drops on the pins at about their midsection to cement them together. After the epoxy has set, lift the pin rake from the Parafilm.

6. A handle for the pin rake can be made from Plexiglas, or phenolic tubing or rod of about 7/16 in. diameter. A slot to accommodate the pins must be sawed in the end of the rod (tube) across the diameter and about $1\frac{1}{4}$ in. along the length. The back ends of the pins are then placed in the slot such that the points extend about 1/2 in. beyond the handle. Once positioned, the pins are glued in place with epoxy, and in a series of applications of epoxy, a cone is built up around the pins such that only about 1/8 in. of their ends extend beyond the epoxy.

7. The pin rake is cleaned and sterilized by wiping with a lint-free tissue soaked in 70% ethanol and then allowed to air-dry in the hood.

7. PREPARATION OF SILICONE GREASE SYRINGE

7.1. Materials

Dow Corning™ high-vacuum grease in 150-g tube.
Glass Luer-Lok™ syringe (1 mL).
Hypodermic needle (18-gage) with a squared off tip.
Scraps of vacuum tubing and ordinary rubber tubing.
Stiff, uninsulated wire.
Disposable syringe (10 mL).
Pliers.

7.2. Procedure

1. Apply silicone grease to the Teflon divider through a 1-mL glass, Luer-Lok syringe fitted with an 18-gage needle with a squared off tip. A needle about 2 cm long

works best. Because some force is required to squeeze the grease through the needle, it is beneficial to slip a 2-in. length of vacuum tubing over the barrel and to pad the plunger by taking a 3/4 in. length of rubber tubing of suitable diameter, cutting a hole in the side of the tubing midway between the ends, and slipping the head of the plunger through the hole. In this way, pressure can be applied with the first and second fingers crooked over the end of the vacuum tubing, encasing the barrel and the thumb pressing against the padded plunger.

2. To fill the applicator with silicone grease, first squeeze the grease from its tube into a 10-mL disposable syringe with no needle.

3. Remove the needle from the applicator syringe with pliers, and if there is grease remaining from previous applications, empty it by fully depressing the plunger. Then slowly (so as not to break the glass) withdraw the plunger completely and set it aside.

4. Hold the 10-mL syringe by the body in one hand, nipple up with the plunger resting on the lab bench. Hold the body of the applicator syringe in the other hand and place it over the nipple, holding it to make a tight seal. Press down with both hands to depress the plunger of the 10-mL syringe, and fill the 1-mL syringe about three-fourths full with silicone grease. Then insert the plunger into the 1-mL syringe and depress it until grease comes out of the nipple. Wipe with a lint-free tissue.

5. Sterilize the filled applicator syringe by dry heat with attention to the following details:

   a. Any air bubbles trapped in the applicator syringe can expand during heating and blow out the plunger. To prevent this, wire the plunger securely to the syringe by looping some ordinary stiff uninsulated wire over the end of the plunger and around the barrel of the syringe below the vacuum tubing. Bubbles will then harmlessly force grease out the needle.

   b. Applicator syringes need not be wrapped for heating, but should be placed in a pan or on aluminum foil to catch the exuded grease. Store the filled applicator syringe until needed.

6. Before using the applicator syringe, squeeze out some grease, wipe it away with a lint-free tissue, and then sterilize the exterior by dipping into 70% ethanol and allowing it to air-dry.

8. NEURITOTOMY

8.1. Materials

Sterile 3-mL disposable syringe with a 1.5-in., 22-gage needle.
Serum bottle containing sterile culture-quality distilled water.

Dissecting microscope set up in a sterile hood.
Sterile pipets and bulbs.
Sterile Pasteur pipet set up as an aspirator.

8.2. Procedure

1. Assemble in a sterile hood equipped with a stereo microscope, a sterile 3-mL syringe with needle, and a serum bottle containing distilled water.

2. Orient a three-compartmented culture under the dissecting microscope such that it is rotated 180° from the ordinary orientation. Remove the lid and aspirate the medium from the compartment(s) to be neuritotomized. Using the 3-mL syringe, squirt the substratum bearing the neurites moderately vigorously until the compartments fill with water. Do not squirt directly at the silicone grease barrier. Aspirate the water and repeat squirting two more times. Then aspirate the water and supply the desired medium to the compartments. Cover the culture dish.

FURTHER READING

Campenot, R. B. (1979), Independent control of the local environment of somas and neurites, in *Methods in Enzymology*, vol. 28, Jakoby, W. B. and Pastan, I. H., eds., Academic, New York, pp. 302–307.

Campenot, R. B. (1982), Development of sympathetic neurons in compartmentalized cultures I. Local control of neurite growth by nerve growth factor. *Dev. Biol.* **93,** 1–12.

Campenot, R. B. (1992), Compartmented culture analysis of nerve growth, in *Cell–Cell Interactions: A Practical Approach* (Stevenson, B., Paul, D., and Gallin, W., eds.), IRL, Oxford, UK, pp. 275–298.

Campenot, R. B. and Draker, D. D. (1989), Growth of sympathetic nerve fibers in culture does not require extracellular calcium. *Neuron* **3,** 733–743.

Hawrot, E., and Patterson, P. H. (1979), Long-term cultures of dissociated sympathetic neurons, in *Methods in Enzymology*, vol. 28, Jakoby, W. B. and Pastan, I. H., eds., Academic, New York, pp. 574–584.

Chapter Eight

Astrocyte and Oligodendrocyte Cultures

Ruth Cole and Jean de Vellis

1. INTRODUCTION

The study of glial cell development and function has been considerably enhanced by the development of methods to culture oligodendrocytes and astrocytes from central nervous system tissue. A primary mixed glial culture, primarily composed of astrocytes, oligodendrocytes, and some microglia, is obtained when newborn disaggregated cerebral brain cells from newborn rat are plated at high cell density (2×10^5/cm^2) in serum-supplemented media (McCarthy and de Vellis, 1980). At low cell density (e.g., 5×10^4 cells/cm^2), few oligodendrocytes develop and the culture consists largely of astrocytes. At high cell density, phase-dark process-bearing cells appear by 4 d and stratify into clusters and individual cells above the bedlayer of cells. The bedlayer consists of astrocytes rich in glial filaments. This observation led to the development of the shaking procedure that results in the selective removal of the process-bearing cells from the underlying astrocytes (McCarthy and de Vellis, 1980). Thus, highly purified cultures of astrocytes and oligodendrocytes can be obtained from the same piece of brain tissue (Fig. 1). The microglia are removed first from the mixed culture by a 6-h preshake before the oligodendrocyte lineage cells are removed. At the time of harvesting the process-bearing cells from the 7–9-d-old cultures, the cells are largely immature, containing progenitor cells and immature oligodendrocytes (Holmes et al., 1988). If the process-bearing cells are placed in a serum-free chemically defined medium, <4% of the cells express astrocyte markers, such as glial fibrillary acidic

Protocols for Neural Cell Culture, 2nd Ed. • Eds.: S. Fedoroff and A. Richardson • Humana Press, Inc., Totowa, NJ

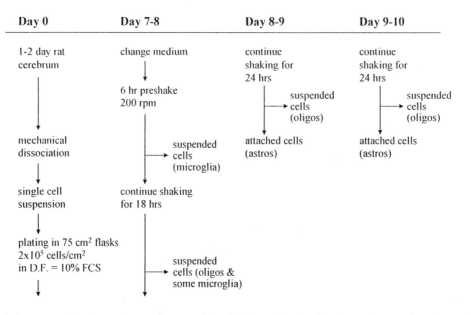

Day 0	Day 7-8	Day 8-9	Day 9-10

Fig. 1. Diagram for the preparation and isolation of oligodendrocytes and astrocytes from cultures of cerebral hemispheres from early postnatal rats.

protein (Saneto and de Vellis, 1985). In fetal-bovine-serum-supplemented medium, 25–35% of the cells express glial fibrillary acidic protein. The bedlayer cells can be maintained as pure astrocyte cultures by keeping the flasks shaking slowly to keep removing dividing oligodendrocyte progenitors and microglia. This primary culture of astrocytes can be used to set up pure cultures of secondary astrocyte cultures in serum or serum-free media (Morrison and de Vellis, 1981,1984). Astroglial and oligodendroglial cell lines have been developed from the cultures described above (Bressler et al., 1982; Bressler and de Vellis, 1985).

2. PREPARATION OF NEWBORN RATS FOR CULTURING

2.1. Materials

Newborn rats, P 1–2 d.
Sponges, sterile (4 × 4) (6).
Disposable towels, double thickness, sterile (3).
Ethanol (70%)
$4\frac{1}{2}$-oz Containers containing 80 mL of 70% ethanol (2).
Petri dishes, 35 mm (5).
Dulbecco's Modified Eagle's Medium/Ham's F-12 (DME/F12), serum free (10 mL).
Operating scissors, $5\frac{1}{2}$ in., straight.
Microdissecting scissors, 4 in., straight (2).
Microdissecting forceps (2).

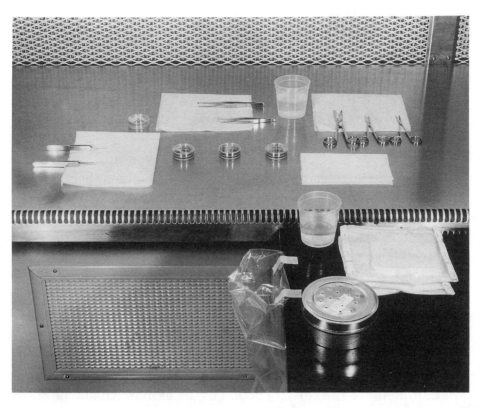

Fig. 2. Arrangement of work space for dissection of cerebral hemispheres from newborn rat.

Tissue forceps, $5\frac{1}{2}$ in.
Curved forceps, fine.
Plastic bag.

2.2. Procedure for Dissection

1. Clean the area for dissection with 70% ethanol and set up instruments in an array that logically follows the dissection procedure (Fig. 2).
   a. Place a $4\frac{1}{2}$-oz container filled with 70% ethanol next to container of pups.
   b. Place sterilized towels in an area next to a plastic bag for disposal of beheaded pups.
   c. Place the three sterile scissors on sterile towels next to another $4\frac{1}{2}$-oz container with 70% ethanol.
   d. Also near this container of ethanol, place tissue forceps and fine curved forceps on sterile toweling.
   e. Place fine microdissecting forceps on sterile gauze.
   f. Fill three 35-mm Petri dishes with $2\frac{1}{2}$-mL of DME/F12 (serum-free). One empty 35-mm Petri dish is used to dissect both cerebra and one for disposal of the remaining brain tissue.

2. Removal of the brain:
   a. After sacrificing the newborn pups by carbon dioxide inhalation, dip them into 70% ethanol, allowing the thumb and forefinger also to be immersed.
   b. Using a pair of sterile operating scissors and holding the body of the rat, decapitate the head onto a sterile towel. The scissors are dipped in ethanol and returned to the sterile towel with the other scissors. The rat's body is disposed of in the plastic bag.
   c. With the cut portion of the head facing you and with the head lying flat on the surface of the sterile towel, use a pair of microdissecting scissors to cut the skin at the midline of the head. Begin cutting from the base of the head and cut to the mid-eye area. The scissors are dipped in ethanol and returned to the sterile towel with the other scissors. These scissors are used only for procedures b and c. The skin is folded back by pulling the loose skin forward using the index finger and thumb and held open.
   d. The second pair of microdissecting scissors is utilized to cut the skull at the midline fissure. The scissors are dipped in ethanol and returned to the sterile towel.
   e. Using the thumb and forefinger, hold and apply "slight" pressure to the skull. Remove the raised portion of the skull with sterile tissue forceps.
   f. The brain is then removed by running the curved forceps along the bottom and sides of the brain calvarium from the olfactory lobes to the posterior of the midbrain. The freed brain is then placed into a 35-mm Petri dish containing 2½ mL of DME/F12 serum-free medium.
   g. Repeat step 2, a–f, for each pup, placing all the brains into the same Petri dish.
3. Removal of the cerebral hemispheres:
   a. Remove one brain from the 35-mm Petri dish to the inverted lid of a 35-mm Petri dish, and remove the cerebral hemispheres as follows:
      i. Using one pair of the microdissecting forceps, steady the brain at the median fissure. Using the second pair of microdissecting forceps, gently cut the tissue along the median fissure and pull one cerebral hemisphere away from the rest of the brain.
      ii. Remove the cerebral hemisphere by pinching it against the Petri dish surface. Remove the other hemisphere in a similar manner. Make sure that the olfactory lobes are no longer attached.
      iii. Immediately immerse the cerebral hemispheres in serum-free medium contained in another sterile 35-mm Petri dish. Repeat step a, i–iii for each pup.

Note: Hemispheres from 15–20 pups are usually collected.

b. Use the same microdissecting forceps that were used to remove cortices to remove meninges. Place a hemisphere onto the inverted lid of a second Petri dish. While using one pair of forceps to hold the hemisphere steady, pull off the meninges with the second pair of microdissecting forceps. The meninges can be easily teased away from the hemisphere by beginning with an exposed corner of the membrane on the outer surface and gently pulling the meninges off. The removed meninges are blotted onto a piece of sterile gauze.

c. Place the hemisphere piece into a fresh Petri dish containing serum-free medium. Repeat this process (steps b and c) until all the cerebral hemisphere pieces are free of meninges and blood vessels.

d. Dip both forceps in ethanol, allow to drain, and place on sterile towels.

3. PREPARATION OF GLIAL CELL CULTURES—NITEX™ BAG METHOD

The Nitex bag method was developed by Lu et al. (1980). The procedure is done in a laminar flow hood.

3.1. Materials

Petri dish, plastic, 100 mm.
DME/F-12 containing 10% fetal bovine serum (DME/F12 10% FBS) (75 mL).
Hanks' balanced salt solution (BSS) (25 mL).
Nitex (No. 210) bag, $1\frac{1}{2} \times 3$ in.
Forceps (2).
Glass rod, $7 \times 5/32$ in., sterile.
Beaker covered with 130 μm Nitex mesh or Cellector™ sieve with a 140-μm mesh (#100) and a sterile $4\frac{1}{2}$-oz container (Falcon #4014).
Beaker covered with 230 μm Nitex mesh or Cellector sieve with a 230-μm mesh (#60) and a sterile $4\frac{1}{2}$-oz container (Falcon #4014).
Centrifuge tube, 50 mL, sterile.
Flask, 75 cm^2.
Flask, 25 cm^2.
Hemocytometer.
Pasteur pipet.
Hand-held digital counter.
Microscope.

3.2. Disaggregation of Brain Tissue

1. Add 15 mL DME/F12 10% FBS to a 100-mm sterile Petri dish. Place the Nitex bag in this dish and hold the mouth of the bag open with sterile forceps.

2. Pour or pipet the tissue pieces into the bag. Close the bag with sterile forceps and immerse it in the medium in the Petri dish.

3. Use the sterile glass rod to tease the tissue through the mesh of the Nitex bag. Light strokes are used to prevent cell damage.

4. When teasing is completed, hold the closed bag upright with forceps above the Petri dish containing the screened cell suspension and rinse 10 mL of medium down the side of the bag. The combined cell suspension is then removed and filtered through the Nitex 230-µm covered beaker or Cellector Sieve, 230 µm, #60, which has first been wetted with 1 mL of Hanks' BSS to allow the fluids to flow through properly.

5. Next, filter the cell suspension through the Nitex 130-µm covered beaker or Cellector Sieve, 140 µm, #100. Collect the cell suspension in a 50-mL centrifuge tube.

6. Centrifuge the resulting filtrate at 200g for 5 min at room temperature. Resuspend the pellet in 10 mL culture medium.

7. Determination of cell number:

   a. Prepare a sample from the cell suspension for counting with a hemocytometer.

   b. Dilute 0.1 mL of the suspension with 1.9 mL Hanks' BSS. This is a cell dilution of 1:20. Since this is a total cell count, no trypan blue dye is required.

   c. Fill the hemocytometer with the diluted cell suspension using a Pasteur pipet.

   d. Count the number of cells in at least one hemocytometer chamber (four squares).

8. Dilute the cell suspension in DME/F12 10% FBS. Plate 15×10^6 cells/75 cm^2 culture flask in a total volume of 10 mL or 5×10^6 cells/25 cm^2 culture flask in a total volume of 5.0 mL.

9. Gas the flask with 5% carbon dioxide and incubate at 37°C with the lid tightly closed or incubate in a 5% CO_2, 95% air incubator without gassing procedure and lid loosened.

Note: Care should be taken not to disturb the flasks for 2 d. Movement of flasks during this initial 2-d period reduces cellular attachment. Culture medium is changed after d 2 and every other day thereafter.

4. ISOLATION OF ASTROCYTES AND OLIGODENDROCYTES

4.1. Introduction

The initial cortical cell cultures should be cultured for 7–9 d. Periods shorter than this are not sufficient for stratification of astrocytes and oligodendrocytes. Periods longer than this can result in clustering of astrocytes above the bed layer. On subsequent isolation of oligodendrocytes, the clustered astrocytes break up and contaminate the oligodendrocyte preparation. We have found that the oligodendrocytes tend to adhere more strongly the longer they remain in mixed culture, making the shaking process less efficient.

4.2. Materials

DME/F12 10% FBS.
Hanks' BSS.
Puck's BSS (15 mL).
30-µm Nitex mesh-covered beakers or Cellector Sieve, 25 µm, #500.
Versene (EDTA) solution (10 mL).
2.5% Trypsin solution (2 mL).
Centrifuge tubes, 15 mL (2).
Lab-Line Junior orbit shaker in a dry 37°C incubator (A layer of packing foam will help insulate the flasks from the heat generated by the shaker.).
Tissue culture dishes, 35 mm (4).

4.3. Method for Isolation of Oligodendrocytes and Astrocytes

1. Oligodendrocytes
   a. At the end of the 7–9-d culture period, phase-dark process-bearing cells are observed to approximate a confluent phase-gray bed layer of cells. Change the culture medium, close and tighten the plastic culture lids, and place the flasks on a rotary shaker.
   b. Shake flasks at 200 rpm with a 1.5-in. stroke diameter at 37°C for 6 h.
   c. Remove flasks from the rotary shaker, change medium (the discarded medium usually contains dividing astrocytes and macrophages), and return them to the rotary shaker for 18 h.
   d. After 18 h, remove the cell suspension and filter through a Nitex 30-µm mesh covered beaker (Cellector Sieve, 25 µm, #500). Collect the filtrate in a tube for counting.
   e. Determine the cell number by enumerating the cells using a hemocytometer (0.1 mL of cell suspension plus 1.9 mL of diluent for a 1:20 dilution). Plate 4×10^5 cells in a volume of 1.5 mL/35-mm Petri dish.
   f. Additional oligodendrocytes can be harvested by replenishing the culture media and shaking the flasks for an additional 24 and 48 h, with fewer cells but more purified oligodendrocytes being harvested at each interval.
2. Astrocytes:
   a. At the desired number of oligodendrocytes harvests, replenish the media and place the flasks on a rotary shaker at 100 rpm, until fewer than 10

phase dark cells per microscope field (100X) are observed. Replenish the media every 2 d.

b. Purified cultures can subsequently be subcultured by utilizing a Versene-trypsin wash. Remove all media from the flasks and wash the cells with 5 mL of a Versene (EDTA) solution (*see* Section 5.4.). Pour off and wash the cells with 2.0 mL/flask of a 2.5% trypsin solution, making sure that all the cells have been bathed. Pour off and incubate the flasks at 37°C, until the cells are completely disaggregated and run freely when the flask is inverted, usually 5–10 min.

c. Resuspend the cells in 8 mL DME/F12 10% FBS. Remove cells to a centrifuge tube and centrifuge for 5 min at 80*g*. Aspirate off old media and discard. Resuspend the pellet in 10 mL fresh culture media.

d. Determine the cell number by hemocytometry and plate 4×10^5 cells/35-mm Petri dish.

Note: As cells are passaged in culture, they change in biochemical and immunological properties and we do not use astrocytes past the initial passage.

5. APPENDIX

5.1. Dulbecco's Modified Eagle's Medium with High Glucose (DME)/Ham's F-12

DME/F-12 is prepared by mixing DME and F-12 in a 1:1 ratio (v/v). Then add 1.2 g/L sodium bicarbonate and 15 m*M* HEPES. Filter through a 0.2-μm filter. The medium is completed with 10% FBS.

1. DME formulation (Dulbecco and Freeman, 1959; Morton, 1970):

Components	mg/L
Inorganic salts:	
$CaCl_2$ (anhyd.)	200.00
$Fe(NO_3)_3 \cdot 9H_2O$	0.10
KCl	400.00
$MgSO_4$ (anhyd.)	97.67
NaCl	6400.00
$NaH_2PO_4 \cdot H_2O$	125.00
Other components:	
D-glucose	4500.00
Phenol red	15.00
Amino acids:	
L-Arginine · HCl	84.00

L-Cystine · 2HCl	62.57
L-Glutamine	584.00
Glycine	30.00
L-Histidine HCl · H_2O	42.00
L-Isoleucine	05.00
L-Leucine	105.00
L-Lysine HCl	146.00
L-Methionine	30.00
L-Phenylalanine	66.00
L-Serine	42.00
L-Threonine	95.00
L-Tryptophan	16.00
L-Tyrosine (disodium salt)	104.20
L-Valine	94.00

Vitamins:

D-Calcium pantothenate	4.00
Choline chloride	4.00
Folic acid	4.00
i-Inositol	7.20
Nicotinamide	4.00
Pyridoxal HCl	4.00
Riboflavin	0.40
Thiamine HCl	4.00

2. F-12 Nutrient mixture formulation (Ham, 1965):

Inorganic salts:	mg/L
$CaCl_2 · 2H_2O$	44.00
$CuSO_4 · 5H_2O$	0.00249
$FeSO_4 · 7H_2O$	0.834
KCl	223.60
$MgCl_2 · 6H_2O$	122.00
NaCl	7599.00
$NaHCO_3$	1176.00
$Na_2HPO_4 · 7H_2O$	268.00
$ZnSO_4 · 7H_2O$	0.863

Other components:

D-glucose	1802.00
Hypoxanthine	4.10

Linoleic acid	0.084
Lipoic acid	0.21
Phenol red	1.20
Putrescine 2HCl	0.161
Sodium pyruvate	110.00
Thymidine	0.73

Amino acids:

L-Alanine	8.90
L-Arginine HCl	211.00
L-Asparagine H_2O	15.01
L-Aspartic acid	13.30
L-Cystine HCl H_2O	35.12
L-Glutamic Acid	14.70
L-Glutamine	146.00
Glycine	7.50
L-histidine HCl H_2O	20.96
L-Isoleucine	3.94
L-Leucine	13.10
L-Lysine HCl	36.50
L-Methionine	4.48
L-Phenylalanine	4.96
L-Proline	34.50
L-Serine	10.50
L-Threonine	11.90
L-Tryptophan	2.04
L-Tyrosine	5.40
L-Valine	11.70

Vitamins:

Biotin	0.0073
D-Ca pantothenate	0.4800
Choline chloride	13.9600
Folic acid	1.300
i-Inositol	18.000
Niacinamide	0.0370
Pyridoxine HCl	0.0620
Riboflavin	0.0380
Thiamine HCl	0.3400
Vitamin B_{12}	1.3600

5.2. Nitex Mesh-Covered Beakers

1. Suppliers of Nitex Mesh
   a. B. & S. H. Thompson & Co. Ltd.
      140 Midwest Road
      Scarborough, Ontario
      M1P 3B3 Canada
   b. B. & S. H. Thompson & Co. Ltd.
      8148 Chemin Devonshire
      Ville Mont Royal, Quebec
      H4P 2K3 Canada
   c. Tetko
      420 Sawmill River Road
      Elmsford, NY
      10523 USA
2. Preparation of mesh: Nitex mesh is soaked in a large container of triple-distilled water. The water is changed three times. The mesh is then coiled into a large beaker and dried in a drying oven at 65°C.
3. Preparation of Nitex mesh-covered beakers:
   a. Materials:
      50 mL beaker.
      7 cm Square of Nitex mesh.
      8 cm Squares of aluminum foil, masking tape, and autoclave tape.
   b. Procedure:
      i. Place the square of Nitex mesh on the beaker and tape all four corners down using masking tape.
      ii. Cut autoclave tape to about 1 cm wide and long enough to encircle the beaker.
      iii. Wrap the tape securely over the mesh just under the lip of the beaker. The mesh should not be very taut. It is preferable to avoid taping the mesh to the beaker, since the tape is difficult to remove for washing.
      iv. Remove the masking tape from the corners of the mesh.
      v. Cover the beaker with two layers of aluminum foil.
      vi. Place a small piece of autoclave tape in the center of the foil cover. Autoclave at 30 min, wrapped setting.

5.3. Cellector Tissue Sieves

For the filtration of cell suspensions, Cellector tissue sieves may be used in place of Nitex mesh-prepared beakers. The sieve is first sterilized with the selected screen in place. The sieve is then placed into a sterile cup (4½ oz—Falcon #4014), and the tissue suspension is poured into it, allowing the liquid to flow through by gravity only. Forcing the suspension through can result in damage to cell membranes. Any remaining cells are rinsed into the sterile container with medium or a balanced salt solution. The Cellector, complete, including 85-mL pan, glass pestle, key, and nine screens (#1985-85000) with various replacement screens, is available from Bellco Glass, Inc. (Vineland, NJ).

5.4. Versene Solution

Component	Amount
NaCl	8.0 g
KH_2PO_4	0.2 g
KCl	0.2 g
Na_2HPO_4	1.15 g
EDTA (disodium salt)	0.2 g

1. Preparation of Versene:
   a. Dissolve in 1000 mL of distilled H_2O.
   b. Dispense in convenient amounts and sterilize by autoclaving at 120°C for 15 min.

5.5. Alternate Disaggregation Method: Stomacher Blender

1. Materials: 50 mL centrifuge tubes, Lab-Blender Bag with 80-mL capacity, Cellector sieve with 230-μm screen (#60), Cellector sieve with 140-μm screen (#100), $4\frac{1}{2}$ oz sterile containers (2) (Falcon #4014), DME/F12 10% FBS (60 mL), and Stomacher Blender attached to a variable transfer set at 80 V.
2. Disaggregation:
   a. Carefully pipet the tissue/media suspension into a sterile blender bag and add enough media to bring the total amount in the bag to 50–60 mL.
   b. Place the bag into the Stomacher Blender with about 2 cm of the bag visible above the closed door.
   c. The blender should be attached to a variable transformer that is set at 80 V. This setting controls the speed of the blender paddles and prevents the disruption of the cell membranes.
   d. Blend the tissue for 2.5 min and remove the bag with the cell suspension to the hood.
   e. Pour the cell suspension into the #60 sieve, allowing it to filter by gravity only.
   f. Pour this filtrate into the #100 sieve, again allowing the cells to flow by gravity only. Wash the adhering cells through the screen with 10 mL complete media.
   g. Centrifuge the cell suspension at 80*g* for 5 min.

h. Pour off the supernatants, resuspend the cells in DME/F12 (approx 100 mL/10 brains), and prepare a 1:100 dilution of cells for counting in a hemocytometer.

i. Dilute the cell suspension in DME/F12 10% FBS and plate at 15×10^6 cells/75 cm^2 culture flask in a total volume of 10–11 mL.

j. Incubate at 37°C in a humidified 5% CO_2 incubator with the lid tightly closed.

5.6. Optimal Plating Densities

1. The optimal plating density for oligodendrocytes is as follows:
   a. 5×10^6 cells/75 cm^2 flask.
   b. 1×10^5 cells/well in 2.0 cm^2 24-well culture plate.
   c. 4×10^5 cells/35-mm Petri dish.
   d. 4×10^4 cells/well in 0.32 cm^2 96-well culture plate.
2. The optimal plating density for astrocytes is as follows:
   a. 1×10^6 cells/75 cm^2 culture flask.
   b. 2×10^4 cells/2.0 cm^2 24-well culture plate.
   c. 4×10^5 cells/35-mm Petri dish.

FURTHER READING

Bressler, J. P. and de Vellis, J. (1985), Neoplastic transformation of newborn rat astrocytes in culture. *Brain Res.* **348,** 21–27.

Bressler, J. P., Cole, R., and de Vellis, J. (1982), Neoplastic transformation of newborn rat oligodendrocytes in cultures. *Cancer Res.* **43,** 709–715.

Butler, H. and Juurlink, B. H. J. (1987), *Atlas for Staging Mammalian and Chick Embryos.* CRC, Boca Raton, FL.

Dulbecco, R. and Freeman, G. (1959), Plaque formation by the polyoma virus. *Virology* **8,** 396–397.

Ham, R. G. (1965), Clonal growth of mammalian cells in a chemically defined synthetic medium. *Proc. Natl. Acad. Sci. USA* **53,** 288–293.

Holmes, E., Hermanson, G., Cole, R., and de Vellis, J. (1988), Developmental expression of glial-specific mRNAS in primary cultures of rat brain visualized by *in situ* hybridization. *J. Neurosci. Res.* **19,** 389–396, 458–473.

Lu, E. J., Brown, W. J., Cole, R., and de Vellis, J. (1980), Ultra-structural differentiation and synaptogenesis in aggregating rotation cultures of rat cerebral cells. *J. Neurosci. Res.* **5,** 447–463.

McCarthy, K. D. and de Vellis, J. (1980), Preparation of separate astroglial and oligodendroglial cell cultures from rat cerebral tissue. *J. Cell Biol.* **85,** 890–902.

Morrison, R. S. and de Vellis, J. (1981), Growth of purified astrocytes in a chemically defined medium. *Proc. Natl. Acad. Sci. USA* **78,** 7205–7209.

Morrison, R. S. and de Vellis, J. (1984), Preparation of a chemically defined medium for purified astrocytes, in *Methods for Serum-Free Culture of Neuronal and Lymphoid Cells,* Sato, G., Sirbasku, D., and Barnes, D., eds., Liss, New York, pp. 15–22.

Morton, H. J. (1970), A survey of commercially available tissue culture media. *In Vitro* **6,** 89–108.

Saneto, R. P. and de Vellis, J. (1985), Characterization of cultured rat oligodendrocytes proliferating in a serum free chemically defined medium. *Proc. Natl. Acad. Sci. USA* **82,** 3509–3513.

Saneto, R. P. and de Vellis, J. (1987a), Neuronal and glial cells: cell culture of the central nervous system, in: *Neurochemistry: A Practical Approach*, Turner, H. J. and Bachelard, H. S., eds., IRI, pp. 27–63.

Saneto, R. P. and de Vellis, J. (1987b), The use of primary oligodendrocyte and astrocyte cultures to study glial growth factors, in: *Neuronal Factors,* Perez-Polo, J. R., ed., CRC, Boca Raton, FL, pp. 175–195.

Chapter Nine

Generation of Mouse Astroglia and Microglia Cultures from Mouse Neopallium

Sergey Fedoroff and Arleen Richardson

1. INTRODUCTION

Newborn rats or mice are generally used as the source of tissue for glial cultures. Only about 1% of cells survive the cell disaggregation process and culture environment, and neurons that survive die within the first few days of culturing. Terminally differentiated cells, which can no longer divide, are overgrown by the proliferating, immature cells. As a result, the cells in culture are mainly immature cells and therefore cultures are very plastic. How the cultures will develop and which cell types, i.e., astroglia, oligodendroglia, ependymal cells, or microglia, will enrich the culture, depends on the culture medium and the physical conditions under which the cells are grown. In addition to varying the components of a chemically defined medium or adding or removing serum from the medium, it is possible to add to the cultures growth factors and/or cytokines in pure recombinant form, or as soluble products in medium conditioned by cells, that produce and secrete the factors. (The latter is considerably cheaper). The addition of such factors to cultures can have dramatic effects. It should be noted that such factors may affect more than one cell type and may initiate different effects in different cells. The factors may interact with other factors synergistically, additively, or in an inhibitory way. Moreover, their half-life is short. This subject is extremely complex and beyond the scope of this book.

Protocols for Neural Cell Culture, 2nd Ed. • Eds.: S. Fedoroff and A. Richardson • Humana Press, Inc., Totowa, NJ

In this chapter we outline a procedure for initiation of neopallial cell cultures and their development into astroglia-enriched cultures that can be used to form nearly pure microglia cultures. The next chapter describes a procedure that uses neopallial cell cultures to produce oligodendroglia.

Neopallium (cerebral cortex and underlying white matter) yields cells that, when cultured in chemically defined medium with added serum, produce highly enriched cultures of astroglia. Colony stimulating factor-1 (CSF-1), which is required for the development, survival, and differentiation of microglia, is mainly produced in the central nervous system by astroglia. It is also secreted by astroglia into the medium in cultures. We therefore describe a simple protocol originally developed by Hao et al. (1991) that uses well-established, confluent astroglia cultures to produce better than 99% pure cultures of microglia.

2. ASTROGLIA CULTURES

2.1. Preparation of Newborn Mouse For Dissection of Neopallium

1. Materials:
   Mouse, newborn.
   Forceps, curved, 12 cm (2).
   Forceps, straight, blunt, 14 cm.
   Forceps, Irex #5 (2).
   Forceps, fine curved, 10 cm.
   Scissors, large, 15 cm.
   Scissors, straight, 10 cm.
   Scissors, curved, 10 cm.
   Sterile wax dissecting dish.
   Needles, 25-gage, sterile.
   Ethanol, 70% in Coplin jar.
   Petri dishes, glass, sterile, 100 mm (3).
   High-sucrose phosphate buffer.
2. Preparation of materials
   a. Place several discrete drops of high-sucrose phosphate buffer around the periphery of the Petri dish. (One cerebral hemisphere will be placed in each drop). In the center of the Petri dish, place a number of drops of high-sucrose phosphate buffer, in which the neopallia will be collected.
   b. Sterilize all instruments. When the instruments have been sterilized, place them into two sterile glass Petri dishes and keep the ends covered with a lid.

3. Preparation of newborn mouse
   a. Deeply anesthetize a newborn mouse with Halothane™ or Metofane™.
   b. Using forceps, pick up the mouse and briefly submerge it in the container of 70% alcohol.
   c. Using the large scissors, decapitate the mouse so that the head falls onto the wax dissecting dish.
   d. Using a sterile needle, pin the head through the nose, dorsal side up, to the wax dish (Fig. 1A).

2.2. Dissection of the Cerebral Hemispheres

1. Using sterile curved forceps and curved scissors, remove the skin over the dorsal surface of the skull. This is easily accomplished by beginning the cut ventral to the ears, continuing toward the snout, then across the head just above the eyes and finally back toward the neck, and at the same time, gently pulling the skin from the skull with forceps (Fig. 1A).
2. Using straight sterile scissors, divide the skull and cerebral hemispheres from posterior to anterior, that is, by bringing the bottom blade of the scissors up through the brain. Do not cut down initially through the skull, because the pressure will mutilate the soft brain tissue (Fig. 1A).
3. Remove the cerebral hemispheres.
   a. Using a pair of sterile curved forceps, grasp the muzzle of the mouse and squeeze gently. This serves to hold the head in place as well as to open the skull.
   b. Next, using the fine curved forceps, lift the brain out of the skull and place each hemisphere into a drop of medium in the sterile Petri dish.
   c. Using the Irex forceps, remove the delicate, almost transparent meninges. Begin at the olfactory bulbs and peel it off by pulling gently posteriorly. Try to avoid tearing the meninges.
   d. Pinch off the cerebellum (Fig. 1B) and olfactory bulb from the cerebral hemispheres (Fig. 1C,D) using the Irex forceps.

2.3. Disection of the Neopallium

1. Place the cerebral hemisphere with the ventral surface facing up (Fig. 1D). Scoop out the basal ganglia using the fine forceps. With the removal of the basal ganglia, a bowl-shaped hemisphere is left (Fig. 1E).
2. Remove the hippocampus using the Irex forceps (Fig. 1E). The remaining part of the hemisphere is neopallium (Fig. 1F).
3. Transfer each neopallium into the drops in the center of the Petri dish.
4. Cut each neopallium into two or three fragments.

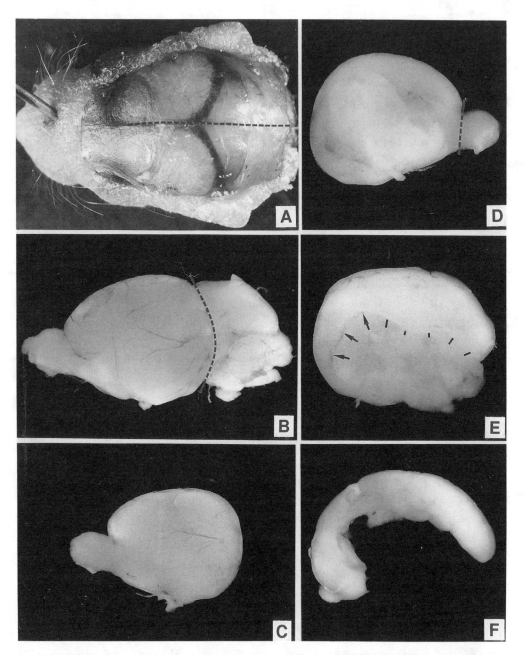

Fig. 1. Dissection of newborn mouse neopallium. **(A)** Pinning of head through nose using sterile needle. **(B)** Removal of the skin. **(C)** Midline cut through skull and brain. **(D)** Newborn brain (no midline cut) showing cerebral hemispheres and cerebellum. **(E)** Cerebral hemispheres (no midline cut). **(F)** One cerebral hemisphere (dorsal view). **(G)** The same cerebral hemisphere (ventral view). **(H)** Bowl-shaped hemisphere after the removal of basal ganglia. Arrows depict the site of dissection to remove hippocampus. **(I)** Isolated neopallium.

2.4. Preparation of Cultures

1. Materials:

    Beaker covered with 75 μm Nitex™ mesh.
    Pasteur pipet, sterile, with bent tip.
    Rubber bulb to fit Pasteur pipet.
    Centrifuge tube, 50 mL, sterile.
    Puck's balanced salt solution (Puck's BSS).
    Tissue culture flask, 75 cm².
    Medium, mMEM containing 5% HS (30 mL).

2. Disaggregation of neopallia:

    a. Place fragments of neopallia on top of 75 μm Nitex mesh, which is stretched over a beaker.

    b. Place a few drops of growth medium over the neopallia to keep them moist.

    c. Gently roll the fragments of neopallia over the mesh using the back side of a curved Pasteur pipet and at the same time, add medium that has been taken up in the curved Pasteur pipet. Avoid adding air bubbles. Add 5 mL medium/brain to the mesh and continue until the neopallia are completely disaggregated and the cells have passed through the mesh. Rinse the mesh with the medium.

    d. Remove the mesh and transfer the cells in the beaker to a centrifuge tube. Use a pipet to resuspend the cells.

    e. Determine the cell number:

        i. Prepare a sample from the cell suspension for counting in a hemocytometer using 0.05 or 0.1 mL of 0.3% Nigrosin as a viability indicator (viable cells exclude the dye) and 0.2 or 0.4 mL of cell suspension, respectively.

        ii. Fill the hemocytometer and count the number of viable cells in at least four squares of one chamber.

        iii. Calculate the number of viable cells/mL (*see* Chapter 16).

    Note: Usually, the brain of a newborn mouse should yield $2-3 \times 10^6$ viable cells.

3. Preparation of astroglia cultures:

    a. Before plating, make sure that the cells are well-suspended. Plate $3-5 \times 10^6$ viable cells in a 75 cm² tissue culture flask in a final volume of 12 mL mMEM, 5% HS.

    b. Incubate culture flasks in a 37°C highly humidified atmosphere containing 5% carbon dioxide in air.

    c. Feed cultures every 2–3 d for 10 d.

2.5 Comments

1. Instead of flasks, Petri dishes of various sizes can be used. A convenient way to prepare astroglia cultures is to place coverslips into a nonculture Petri dish and to plant cells as described above. The coverslips can be removed from the Petri dish at any stage of culturing and used for sequential analyses. Cells grown on coverslips are convenient for immunocytochemistry, histochemistry, morphometry, or electron microscopy.
2. When large numbers of astroglia are required for chemical analysis or for conditioning medium, large-sized flasks, roller bottles, or large flasks filled with beads to increase the surface area, can be used.

3. MICROGLIA CULTURES

3.1. Materials

Astroglial cultures medium, mMEM with 5% HS.
LM cell conditioned medium.
Hank's BSS.

3.2. Preparation of Highly Enriched Microglia Cultures

1. Prepare astroglia cultures as described in Section 2.4. and incubate 10–12 d.
2. Examine the cultures under the microscope to ensure that they have reached confluency.
3. Wash and refeed the cultures and incubate for another 10–12 d without medium change.
4. Remove the medium and wash cultures with Hanks' BSS. Repeat the washing until all dead and floating cells have been removed.
5. Refeed the cultures with mMEM with 5% HS and add 20% LM cell-conditioned medium. (This medium contains CSF-1). Incubate cultures at 37°C in a highly humidified atmosphere containing 5% CO_2 in air.

3.3. Subculturing of Microglia

The cultures of microglia (Fig. 2) can be used directly or subcultured. Microglia attach firmly to the substratum. To remove them from the substratum, microglia can be treated with 0.25% trypsin for 10 min at room temperature. The trypsin can be inhibited by the addition of medium containing serum or soy bean trypsin inhibitor (see Chapter 17). Transfer the cell suspension into another culture vessel.

A more gentle and more effective way to remove microglia from the substratum, without altering their cell surface antigenic characteristics, is the following procedure:

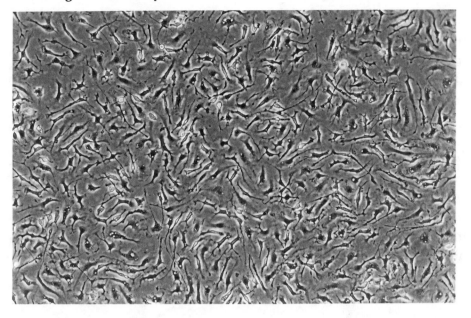

Fig. 2. Microglia isolated from neonatal mouse astroglia cultures.

1. Refrigerate a culture of microglia at 4°C for 10 min.
2. Remove medium and add cold (4°C) 0.01% versene.
3. Incubate culture for 10 min with versene at 4°C.
4. Gently triturate culture with a Pasteur pipet 30 times.
5. Transfer the cell suspension into a test tube and centrifuge at 200g for 5 min.
6. Remove the versene solution and resuspend microglia in fresh medium.

4. APPENDIX

4.1. Comments

1. Gebicke-Haerter et al. (1989) reported that bacterial lipopolysaccharide (LPS) present in culture medium inhibits the formation of brain macrophages. It should be noted that most commercially available fetal bovine serum contains some LPS (Northoff et al., 1986a,b) and thus may inhibit the formation of microglia. It is therefore advisable to use HS, which normally has no detectable LPS. Moreover, it is advisable to use the embryos of C_3H/HeJ mice, which are resistant to LPS.
2. This method for isolation of microglia from mouse neopallia-astroglia cultures can also be used to obtain microglia from rats or humans.
3. The first indication of the formation of microglia is the appearance of phase-dark cells with poorly defined, thick, cytoplasmic processes abutting the

underlying astroglia. A few days later, the phase-dark cells show cytoplasmic vacuoles and become attached to the substratum. Subsequently, they assume a morphology characteristic of ameboid cells (vacuoles, irregular shape, and pseudopodia) and eventually form process-bearing cells that resemble paronchymal, ramified microglia.

4.2. Solutions

1. Medium: MEM is modified to contain a fourfold concentration of vitamins, a double concentration of amino acids except glutamine, and 7.5 mM glucose (Gibco-BRL [Gaithersburg, MD], 90-5175). Before using the modified MEM for culturing, 5.2 mL of 1M sodium bicarbonate and 2.5 mL of 200 mM glutamine are added to 200 mL mMEM, and the pH adjusted to 7.2 by bubbling 5% carbon dioxide into the medium. The prepared modified MEM is supplemented with 5% HS.
2. Puck's BSS

    a.
Composition	g/L
NaCl	8.00
KCl	0.40
Na_2HPO_4 $2H_2O$	0.06
KH_2PO_4	0.06
Glucose	1.00
1% Phenol red	2.00 mL

    b. Procedure for making 1 L of Puck's BSS.
        i. Dissolve all components in order (except Phenol red) in a beaker containing 400 mL triple-distilled water.
        ii. Add phenol red to a 1 L volumetric flask. Add other components to the flask. Rinse beaker used for solutions with triple-distilled water and add to the volumetric flask. Add enough water to make the volume up to 1 L.
        iii. Stir on magnetic stirrer for 30 min (minimum time).
        iv. Filter through 0.2 μm filter.
        v. Label and store stock solution in refrigerator.
3. High sucrose phosphate buffer: This maintenance medium is for freshly dissected parts of the brain. It contains physiological ion concentrations (Na^+ and K^+), some buffering action and an energy source. Sucrose is the best compound for adjustment of osmolality, because it is neither taken up by the cells nor extracellularly degraded.

Component	g/L
NaCl	8.00
KCl	0.40
Na_2HPO_4	0.024
KH_2PO_4	0.03
Glucose	0.90
Sucrose	20.0

a. Dissolve chemicals in 1 L of high quality distilled water.
b. Sterilize by filtration through a 0.2 μm filter, aliquot, and store at 4°C.

4.3. Preparation of LM Cell Conditioned Medium

For the preparation of conditioned medium containing CSF-1, LM cells (ATCC catalog no. CCL-1.2) are used. The advantage of using LM cells is that they can grow well in suspension and in serum-free medium. By using suspension flasks, a large amount of conditioned medium can easily be prepared. LM cells can also be grown in large stationary flasks or roller bottles. The cells are grown in Medium 199 with 0.5% Bacto-peptone without the addition of serum. Suspension cultures are usually inoculated with 6×10^5 cells/mL and grown for a week or 10 d without feeding, or until they reach about 2×10^6 cells/mL. By then, the culture medium appears orange in color and cloudy because of the high cell concentration. The cells are allowed to settle, and the supernatant is removed and centrifuged at 1400 rpm for 15 min. The supernatant medium is then filtered through a stack of 1.2, 0.8, and 0.45 μm pore size filters and sterilized by filtration through a 0.2 μm-size filter. The sterile conditioned medium is aliquoted, labeled, and stored at –80°C. The conditioned medium can also be concentrated, using a stirred ultrafiltration unit and a YM-10 (>10,000 MW) filter (Amicon).

It is important that an aliquot of the conditioned medium be used for determination of the CSF-1 content in the medium, using the Radioceptor Assay (RRA) (Das et al., 1980, as modified by Hao et al., 1990). The biological activity of CSF-1 can be determined by using the MTT colorimetric population growth assay of 5/10.14 and DA1.K cells (Branch and Guilbert, 1986).

4.4. Nitex Mesh-Covered Beakers

See Chapter 8, Section 4.2., for suppliers of Nitex mesh and for the preparation of Nitex mesh-covered beakers.

4.5. Wax Dissecting Dishes

1. Preparation
   a. Take nine sticks of Kerr Brand Blue Inlay Casting Wax, Regular Type II (Sybron, Emeryville, CA), and break into pieces. Place wax pieces in 100-mm Petri dishes.
   b. Place the dishes containing the wax in a pan and sterilize by dry heat in an oven for 2 h at 250°F.
   c. The dishes may be allowed to cool overnight in the oven. If removed while hot, be careful not to tilt the dishes so that wax reaches the cover of the Petri dish.
   d. When cool, wrap wax dishes in aluminum foil and store until needed.
2. Cleaning used wax dissecting dishes:
   a. Clean the wax dissecting dishes by rinsing with water. Dry with a soft lint-free tissue.
   b. Wash the wax dishes with 70% ethanol and dry with a soft lint-free tissue. Close the lids and sterilize as above for new wax dishes.

FURTHER READING

Abd-El-Basset, E. and Fedoroff, S. (1995), Effect of bacterial wall lipopolysaccharide (LPS) on morphology, motility and cytoskeletal organization of microglia in cultures. *J. Neurosci. Res.* **41,** 222–237.

Abd-El-Basset, E. and Fedoroff, S. (1994), Dynamics of actin filaments in microglia during Fc receptor-mediated phagocytosis. *Acta Neuropathol.* **88,** 527–537.

Branch, R. D. and Guilbert, L. J. (1986), Practical in vitro assay systems for the measurement of hematopoietic growth factors. *J. Tissue Culture Methods* **10,** 101–108.

Das, S. K., Stanley, E. R., Guilbert, L. J. and Farman, L. W. (1980), Determination of a colony stimulating factor subclass by a specific receptor on a macrophage cell line. *J. Cell Physiol.* **104,** 359–366.

Frei, K., Siepl, C., Groscurth, P., Bodmer, S., and Fontana, A. (1988), Immunobiology of microglial cells. *Adv. Neuroimmunol. Ann. NY Acad. Sci.* **540,** 218–227.

Fedoroff, S. (1995), Development of microglia, in *Neuroglia*, Kettenmann, H. and Ransom, B. R., eds., Oxford University Press, pp. 162–181.

Fedoroff, S., Hao, C., Ahmed, J. and Guilbert, L. J. (1993), Paracrine and autocrine signalling in regulation of microglia survival, in *Biology and Pathology of Astrocyte-Neuron Interactions*, Fedoroff, S., Juurlink, B. H. J., and Doucette, R., eds., Plenum, New York, pp. 247–261.

Gebicke-Haerter, P. J., Baker, J., Schobert, A. and Northoff, H. (1989), Lipopolysaccharide-free conditions in primary astrocyte cultures allow growth and isolation of microglial cells. *J. Neurosci. Res.* **9,** 183–194.

Gehrmann, J., Matsumoto, Y. and Kreutzberg, G. W. (1995), Microglia: intrinsic immune effector cell of the brain. *Brain Res. Rev.* **20,** 269–287.

Giulian, D. and Bauer, T. J. (1986), Characterization of ameboid microglia isolated from developing mammalian brain. *J. Neurosci.* **6,** 2163–2178.

Hao, C., Richardson A., and Fedoroff, S. (1991), Macrophage-like cells originate from neuro-epithelium in culture: characterization and properties of the macrophage-like cells. *Int. J. Devl. Neurosci.* **9,** 1–14.

Hao, C., Guilbert, L. J. and Fedoroff, S. (1990), Production of colony-stimulating factor-1 (CSF-1) by mouse astroglia in vitro. *J. Neurosci. Res.* **27,** 314–323.

Hayes, G. M., Woodroofe, M. N., and Cuzner, M. L. (1988), Characterization of microglia isolated from adult human and rat brain. *J. Neuroimmunol.* **19,** 177–189.

Northoff, H., Gluck, D. Wolpl, A., Kubanek, B., and Galanos, C. (1986a), Lipopolysaccharide induced elaboration of interleukin-1 (IL-1) by human monocytes: Use for the detection of LPS in serum and influence of serum-LPS interactions. *Rev. Infect. Dis.* **9(Suppl. 5),** 599–602.

Northoff, H., Kabelits, D., and Galanos, C. (1986b), Interleukin 1 production for detection of bacterial polysaccharide in fetal calf sera and other solutions. *Immunol. Today* **7,** 126,127.

Perry, V. H. and Gordon, S. (1991), Macrophages and the nervous system. *Int. Rev. Cytol.* **125,** 203–244.

Rieske, E., Graeber, M. B., Tetzlaff, W., Czlonkowska, A., Streit, W. J., and Kreutzberg, G. W. (1989), Microglia and microglia-derived brain macrophages in culture: generation from axotomized rat facial nuclei, identification and characterization *in vitro. Brain Res.* **429,** 1–14.

Streit, W. J. (1995), Microglial cells, in *Neuroglia.* Kettenmann, H. and Ransom, B. R., eds., Oxford University Press, pp. 85–96.

Chapter Ten

Generation of Oligodendroblasts from Primary Cultures of Rat Neopallium

Bernhard H. J. Juurlink,
Shawn K. Thorburne, and Richard M. Devon

1. INTRODUCTION

Several distinct stages of differentiation have been described for the oligodendroglial lineage in vitro (Gard and Pfeiffer, 1990; Gard et al., 1995). These include the actively proliferating bipolar or tripolar oligodendroglial precursor cell, characterized by the presence of GQ1c and GD3 gangliosides in the plasmalemma. The oligodendroglial precursor cell differentiates into the multipolar oligodendroblast, a proliferative cell that has sulfatide but no galactocerebroside in its plasmalemma. The oligodendroblast differentiates into the mitotically quiescent oligodendrocyte, a cell characterized by the presence of galactocerebroside in its plasmalemma. These oligodendrocytes also express other myelin-associated proteins, such as myelin basic protein. When transplanted into the central nervous system (CNS) of hypomyelinating hosts, oligodendrocyte precursors migrate over considerable distances and give rise to large numbers of myelinating oligodendrocytes; oligodendroblasts migrate only short distances and give rise to far fewer myelinating oligodendrocytes (Warrington et al., 1993). When transplanted into the CNS, the mature oligodendrocyte will also myelinate axons (Duncan et al., 1992).

Protocols for Neural Cell Culture, 2nd Ed. • Eds.: S. Fedoroff and A. Richardson • Humana Press, Inc., Totowa, NJ

143

Dissection of cellular interactions that occur during myelination (or remyelination) of CNS axons requires access to large numbers of oligodendroglial cells. Currently, several methods are described in the literature for isolation of large numbers of oligodendroglial cells from the CNS. One approach is to isolate mature oligodendrocytes directly from adult brain tissue, using enzymatic dissociation of the nervous tissue followed by isolation of the oligodendrocytes through the use of differential centrifugation (Szuchet et al., 1980; *see also* Chapter 11) or differential centrifugation followed by fluorescence-activated cell sorting (Duncan et al., 1992). A second approach is to isolate oligodendroglial precursor cells from the immature brain and allow them to differentiate into mature oligodendrocytes in vitro. Oligodendroglial precursors can be separated from other brain cells using fluorescence-activated cell sorting (Behar et al., 1988) or immunopanning (Gard et al., 1993). A third approach takes advantage of the fact that primary glial cultures established from the immature brain are composed of a mixture of cell types, including precursor cells. Thus, oligodendroglial and astroglial cells develop in primary cultures established from the newborn rat cerebrum; the oligodendroglial cells can be separated from the astroglial cells using shearing forces (McCarthy and de Vellis, 1980; *see also* Chapter 8).

The approach used in this laboratory is a modification of a procedure initially described by Hunter and Bottenstein (1989, 1990; Louis et al., 1993) and takes advantage of the observation that conditioned medium obtained from B104 neuroblastoma cells contains one or more factors that will cause proliferation of oligodendroglial precursor cells. In this chapter, we demonstrate a technically simple procedure to directly isolate large numbers of oligodendroglial precursor cells from primary cultures of newborn rat neopallial cells. The predominant cell population isolated in the procedure described below is the oligodendrocyte precursor cell; this precursor can be induced to differentiate into the oligodendroblast and then into the oligodendrocyte.

2. ESTABLISHMENT OF PRIMARY RAT NEOPALLIAL CULTURES

2.1. Materials

Newborn rat (Wistar) pups (P1–P4).
Small chamber with lid for anesthesia.
Metafane (methoxyfluorane) anesthetic.
2% Iodine in 70% alcohol.
70% Alcohol.
Beakers, plastic (5).
Stainless steel #1 insect pins (Polyscience, Niles, IL) sterilized in 70% alcohol.
Scissors, $3\frac{1}{2}$ in., sterile.
Forceps, $3\frac{1}{2}$ in., sterile (2).

Forceps, $3\frac{1}{2}$ in., curved, sterile.
Watchmaker's forceps, sterile (4).
Scalpels, sterile (2).
Sterile wax dissecting dish.
Nylon mesh (75 μm) sterile covered beaker.
Primary culture growth medium.
Tissue storage medium.
Dissecting microscope.

2.2. Procedure

1. After sacrificing neonatal rats by overdosing with methoxyfluorane, sterilize the heads by dipping into iodine solution, followed by a rinse in 70% alcohol. Cut off the head of the rat pup and place into an empty sterile dish, ventral surface down.

2. Pin the head, ventral surface down, onto a wax dish using sterile stainless steel insect pins. Place pins through the snout and through the occipital bones on either side of the caudal part of the skull, making sure that the pins do not pierce the cerebrum. Slant the pins away from the head; this gives more room to maneuver during the dissection.

3. With two pairs of sterile $3\frac{1}{2}$ in. forceps, peel the skin off the head; make sure that the skin is well away from the roof and sides of the calvarium. The forceps can be returned to beaker of 70% alcohol.

4. With two pairs of fine watchmaker's forceps, remove the parietal bones from the region of the cerebral hemispheres. Do this by inserting the tips of one pair of forceps into the interparietal suture and separating the parietal bones by a gentle stroking movement; the other pair of forceps is used to steady the head by bracing the exposed skull bones. Do the same for the parietofrontal sutures and the parieto-occipital sutures. Then reflect the parietal bones laterally. These forceps can be returned to the beaker of 70% alcohol and reused.

5. With the remaining pair of sterile $3\frac{1}{2}$ in. forceps, gently stroke the cerebral hemispheres at their junction with the olfactory bulbs, thus separating the bulbs from the hemispheres; make sure that you do not use force, since you can enter the oral cavity very easily from this direction. With the same forceps, gently stroke through the midbrain, thus freeing the cerebral hemispheres from the hindbrain. Using the tines of the curved forceps to cradle the ventral surface of the forebrain, lift the forebrain and place into a Petri dish containing tissue storage medium.

6. With the second pair of sterile watchmaker's forceps, separate the two hemispheres of the cerebrum by opening the tips of the forceps and then closing them along the

sagittal sulcus. Using the tips of your forceps as scissors, remove the midbrain remnants and the thalamus. Remove the hippocampus. Separate the neopallium from the basal ganglia. Remove the meninges from the neopallium. Place the neopallium into growth medium. The neopallium can be transferred using forceps, by spreading the tines of the forceps slightly and using surface tension to hold the neopallium between the tines, or by using a wetted Pasteur pipet.

7. Dice the neopallium into small fragments of about 1 mm^3, using sterile scalpel blades. Then gently force these fragments through nylon mesh covering the top of a beaker; this is done by stroking with the side of a sterile pipet and occasionally washing the cells through the mesh with growth medium. Plant the cells into culture vessels and place into an incubator containing a humidified atmosphere of 5% CO_2 in air and maintained at 37°C. We routinely plant the cells obtained from the neopallia of one rat pup into four 100-mm tissue culture Petri dishes (Falcon #3003, obtained from VWR Scientific, Toronto, ON), i.e., about 800,000 viable cells/100-mm Petri dish. Total volume of the growth medium used per 100-mm Petri dish is 8 mL. Cultures are fed with growth medium after 2 d.

3. PREPARATION OF OLIGODENDROCYTE PRECURSOR CELL CULTURES

3.1. Materials

Oligodendroglial precursor medium with glucose (OPM-G).
Oligodendroglial precursor medium with no glucose (OPM).
Oligodendrocyte differentiation medium.
Puck's balanced salt solution (BSS).
Cell harvest medium.
Primary oligodendroglial planting medium.
Cell filtration tubes containing 15, 35, and 50 μm sterile nylon meshes.
Cotton-plugged, sterile Pasteur pipets.
Hemocytometer.
Petri dishes, tissue culture, polylysine-coated.

3.2. Procedure

1. After 5 d, primary cultures are placed on OPM-G and fed every 2 d with this same medium.
2. After 10–14 d of culture, the majority of cells are oligodendroglial precursors and cultures are ready for harvest (see Section 5.). The day before harvest, feed the cultures with OPM-G. The following day cultures are washed twice with Puck's BSS, then placed on harvest medium and maintained at 37°C in air (i.e., there should be no CO_2 in the incubator).

3. After 15–30 min, cell processes can be seen to retract. Use Pasteur pipet to gently swish harvest fluid over the entire surface of the dish; this should remove all adherent cells.

4. Filter cell suspension sequentially through 50, 35, and 15 μm nylon filters. This removes cell clumps, which contain the majority of nonoligodendroglial cells.

5. Centrifuge cells at 180g for 15 min at room temperature and resuspend in a small volume (1–5 mL) of primary oligodendroglial planting medium. Do a cell count and plant cells in primary planting medium into culture vessels coated with polylysine. We routinely plant 50,000 cells into 35-mm Petri dishes and 400,000 cells into 100-mm Petri dishes.

6. After cells have attached, the medium is replaced with the glucose-free OPM, a medium that contains lactate as the primary energy-yielding substrate. This medium acts as a selection medium for oligodendroglial precursors, since this is the only cell type that preferentially survives and proliferates with lactate as the primary energy source.

7. Cultures can be repeatedly subcultured as long as cells remain at the oligodendroglial precursor stage (see Section 5.); however, if cultures become too dense, the cells differentiate into oligodendroblasts and then into mature oligodendrocytes. One day before subculturing, cultures should be put on the glucose-containing OPM-G and then cells can be harvested using harvest medium. Since the cultures should be composed essentially of oligodendroglial precursor cells, there is no necessity to filter the harvested cells through nylon mesh filters. Cells can be centrifuged, resuspended in primary planting medium, and planted into polylysine-coated culture vessels. After cells have attached, the medium can be replaced with OPM-G (if cultures are not contaminated with nonoligodendroglial cells) or with OPM (if cultures have a significant nonoligodendroglial contamination).

8. Oligodendroglial precursor cell cultures can be placed on oligodendrocyte differentiation medium and be induced to differentiate into mature oligodendrocytes.

4. LONG-TERM STORAGE OF CELLS

4.1. Materials

Dulbecco's Modified Essential Medium (DMEM) containing 2 mM pyruvate.
Fetal bovine serum (FBS).
Dimethyl sulfoxide (DMSO).
Hemocytometer.
Cryogenic vials (Nalgene, obtained from VWR Scientific).
Cryo 1°C Freezing Container (Nalgene, obtained from VWR Scientific).

Freezer, −80°C.

Cryobiological storage container (VWR Scientific).

4.2. Procedure

1. After harvesting oligodendroglial precursors, resuspend in pyruvate-containing DMEM and count cells.
2. Dilute cells to 4×10^6 cells/mL using pyruvate-containing DMEM containing FBS, so that the final concentration of FBS is 10% (v/v).
3. Slowly add DMSO to the cell suspension to a final DMSO concentration of 10% (v/v). Place the cell suspension into cryogenic vials.
4. Place vials into the Cryo 1°C Freezing Container and then into the −80°C freezer. Although the cells can be maintained for several months at −80°C, for long-term storage, it is best that the vials be transferred to liquid nitrogen in the Cryobiological storage container.
5. To prepare cultures from frozen cells, thaw vials rapidly at 37°C, dilute cells into primary planting medium, perform a cell count, and plant cells as usual.

5. CULTURE DESCRIPTION

By 5 d after planting of cells into primary cultures, several distinct cell populations are evident when viewed with the phase contrast microscope, including a larger flat cell population and a smaller process-bearing cell population (Fig. 1). The flat cells contain glial fibrillary acidic protein and are, thus, astrocytic in nature; the majority of the process-bearing cells express the GQ1c and GD3 gangliosides on their cell membranes (Fig. 2) and thus are oligodendroglial precursor cells. If these cultures were allowed to develop in primary culture growth medium for an additional 5–10 d (e.g., Husain and Juurlink, 1995), they would be the same culture preparation as that described in Chapter 8.

Several changes soon become apparent once the cultures are placed on OPM-G medium. The astrocytic cell population tends to become detached from the substratum and form long cable-like structures that are in intimate association with the oligodendroglial lineage of cells (Fig. 2). This is followed by proliferation of the oligodendroglial lineage of cells, with subsequent migration of these cells over the Petri dish surface. Subsequent to this, the astrocytic cell population tends to become detached and float into the medium, whereas there is rapid proliferation of the oligodendroglial lineage of cells (Fig. 3).

To obtain highly enriched cultures of oligodendroglial cells lineage requires harvesting and filtering out cellular aggregates to end up with a single cell suspension of cells. The cell aggregates are composed mainly of oligodendroglial precursors and astrocytes. The majority of cells in the single cell suspension are oligodendroglial precursor cells; however, there are a few astrocytes and microglia present. These latter two cell populations require glucose in the OPM medium for their survival; thus, they can be selectively eliminated by leaving out glucose from the medium and having lactate as the principal energy substrate source. Harvesting results in damage of some cells, resulting in the release of DNA from the injured cells. DNA is sticky and causes cells to aggregate; hence, it is important to have DNase in the harvest medium, to have as high a yield as possible of single cells following filtration.

After 1 wk, a typical moderate density secondary culture (Fig. 4) is minimally contaminated by astrocytes, being comprised of $0.9 \pm 0.7\%$ glial fibrillary acidic protein-positive cells. The remaining cells are at early stages of differentiation in the oligodendroglial lineage; thus, $91.9 \pm 4.1\%$ of the cells express the GQ1c ganglioside, and $8.6 \pm 2.4\%$ of the cells express sulfatide, but no cells express galactocerebroside. Such secondary cultures can readily be subcultured, giving rise to tertiary, quartenary, and other cultures.

When cultures become more dense, an increasing proportion of the cells exhibit a multipolar morphology typical of the oligodendroblasts (Fig. 5); these cells express sulfatide. Mature oligodendrocytes can also be seen expressing galactocerebroside in such cultures. When these cultures are placed upon the medium described by Gard and Pfeiffer (1995), more than 95% of the cells differentiate into oligodendrocytes (Fig. 6) and express galactocerebroside, myelin basic protein, and other oligodendrocyte-specific macromolecules.

Two features of this procedure facilitate the obtention of large numbers of oligodendroglial cells. One feature takes advantage of factor(s), the number of which is unknown, present in conditioned medium obtained from B104 neuroblastoma cells. They actively promote the proliferation of oligodendrocyte precursor cells, while interfering with the survival and/or attachment of astroglial cells. The second feature of the procedure that results in obtaining cultures highly enriched in oligodendrocyte precursor cells is the substitution of glucose with lactate. Although oligodendrocytes and astrocytes require glucose for survival, oligodendrocyte precursors can survive and proliferate using lactate as their primary energy source. This suggests that the oligodendrocyte precursors are exclusively dependent on mitochondrial respiration for production of ATP. Metabolic studies are in agreement with this, demonstrating that oligodendrocyte precursors produce more CO_2 from lactate than do oligodendrocytes and astrocytes, and that anoxia does not increase glucose uptake in oligodendrocyte precursors, whereas there is an increase in glucose uptake during anoxia in astrocytes and mature oligodendrocytes (B. H. J. Juurlink and L. Hertz, unpublished observations).

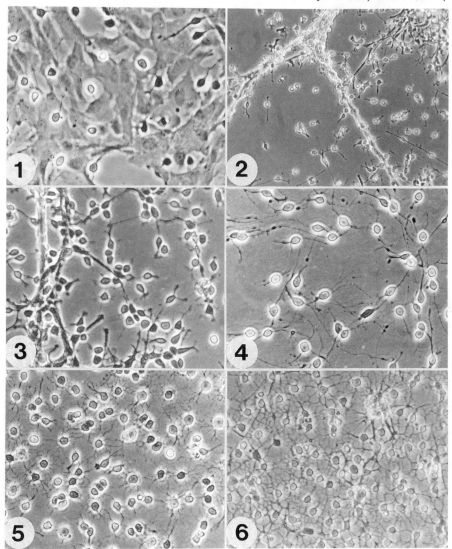

Fig. 1. Phase contrast micrographs (Figs. 1–6) of living glial cells in cultures derived from the newborn rat neopallium. The diameters of the white number-bearing disks represent 48 μm, except for Fig. 2, where the diameter of the white disk represents 96 μm. Five-day old culture grown using primary culture growth medium, demonstrating that the predominant cell populations consist of large flat astroglial cells and small process-bearing oligodendrocyte precursor cells.

Fig. 2. Ten-day-old culture grown for the last 5 d on oligodendrocyte precursor medium containing glucose. The astroglial cells are detaching from the substratum and forming cable-like structures. From these cables oligodendrocyte precursor cells migrate over the substratum.

Fig. 3. Twelve day-old culture demonstrating that oligodendrocyte precursor medium causes proliferation of the oligodendrocyte precursor cells.

Fig. 4. Secondary culture demonstrating oligodendrocyte precursor cells.

Fig. 5. Dense tertiary culture established from oligodendrocyte precursor cells. These cells exhibit the typical multipolar morphology of oligodendroblasts and express sulfatide.

If there is no glucose in the medium, oligodendrocyte precursor cells are readily damaged during subculturing, resulting in low cell survival. This increased fragility is likely related to lack of proper glycosylation of membrane proteins and lipids. Therefore, it is critical to feed cultures with glucose-containing medium 1 d prior to subculturing. Even if glucose is in the medium prior to harvesting the cells, we find much better survival of the cells if they are initially planted in a serum-containing medium (i.e., primary oligodendroglial planting medium). As soon as the cells are attached, they can be placed on a serum-free medium.

6. APPENDIX

6.1. Dissection Material

1. Instrument cleaning and sterilization:
    a. After use, soak instruments in 7X™ detergent (obtained from ICN Biomedicals, Aurora, OH), and clean using a nylon brush. Rinse well with hot water, followed by 70% ethanol. Allow to dry and store.
    b. Before use, sterilize instruments and insect pins by placing in a plastic beaker containing 70% ethanol.
2. Dissecting dish: Pour a molten mixture of three parts regular blue dental inlay wax (Sybron, Romulus, MI) and one part paraffin (melting point 56°C) into a glass 60-mm Petri dish. The dish can be sterilized for use by dry heat at 121°C (250°F) for 2 h. The 60-mm dish is a convenient size, since one can manipulate the position of the dish using the fifth digits and at the same time manipulate the dissecting instruments using the first and second digits. The wax is not brittle, thus ensuring that the wax surface remains smooth despite repeated pinnings. After use, the wax dish can be washed using 7X detergent and nylon brush. After rinsing in water, air-dry and refinish the wax surface, melting the surface using the flame of a Bunsen burner. Once cooled, the dissection dishes can be sterilized by filling with 70% ethanol. The alcohol is removed prior to use and the dish is allowed to air-dry in a laminar flow hood.

6.2. Preparation of Media

1. Stock Dulbecco's Modified Essential Medium (DMEM, this can be obtained in powder form from Gibco-BRL, Burlington, ON). We recommend Gibco-BRL

Fig. 6. *(opposite page)* This is a sister culture to that in Fig. 5. These cells have been placed on oligodendrocyte differentiation medium for the last 5 d and exhibit the complex morphology of oligodendrocytes. Such cells express oligodendrocyte-specific antigens, such as galactocerebroside, myelin basic protein, and proteolipid protein.

for all media, since we have had problems with powdered media obtained from other sources. Purchase the glucose-free, sodium bicarbonate-free, and glutamine-free form of DMEM (cat. no. 23800-048), since this gives one greater flexibility in controlling medium composition. Prepare as recommended by the manufacturer.

2. Working DMEM. Add glutamine to a final concentration of 2 mM. We buffer this medium with 14 mM sodium bicarbonate. In an atmosphere of 5% CO_2, this medium attains a pH of 7.2.

3. Primary culture growth medium: To 79 mL working DMEM, add 0.75 mL 1.0M glucose stock solution and 20 mL horse serum (Hyclone, Logan, UT).

4. OPM-G: To 82 mL working DMEM, add in the following order: 0.75 mL 1.0M glucose stock solution, 1.0 mL lactate stock solution, 1.0 mL TBS stock solution, 15 mL B104 conditioned medium, and 100 µL of the 5 mg/mL insulin stock solution.

5. OPM: To 83 mL working DMEM, add in the following order: 1.0 mL lactate stock solution, 1.0 mL TBS stock supplement solution, 15 mL B104 conditioned medium, and 100 µL 5 mg/mL insulin stock solution.

6. Primary oligodendroglial planting medium: To 93 mL working DMEM, add 0.75 mL glucose, 1.0 mL pyruvate, 5 mL fetal bovine serum (FBS), and 100 µL 5 mg/mL insulin stock solution.

7. DMEM/F12 Medium: This can be obtained in powder form (cat. no. 12500-047) from Gibco-BRL. Prepare according to manufacturer's instructions. This medium is buffered with 15 mM HEPES and 14 mM sodium bicarbonate. In an atmosphere of 5% CO_2, this medium attains a pH of 7.2.

8. Oligodendrocyte differentiation medium: To 98 mL of DMEM/F12 add 1.0 mL heat-inactivated FBS and 1.0 mL of oligodendrocyte conversion stock supplements.

9. B104 neuroblastoma defined medium: To 99 mL DMEM/F12, add 1.0 mL TPPS supplements and 100 µL 5 mg/mL insulin stock solution.

10. Medium supplements (obtained from Sigma, St. Louis, MO):
    a. Glucose: Dissolve glucose (cat. no. G 7021) in triple distilled water to a final concentration of 1.0M, filter sterilize, and store stock solution at 4°C.
    b. Pyruvate: Dissolve pyruvate (cat. no. P 5280) in stock DMEM and filter sterilize. Pyruvate is unstable, particularly in the presence of oxygen; therefore, store pyruvate solution in aliquots at –20°C and when thawed, use within 1 wk.
    c. Glutamine: Dissolve glutamine (cat. no. G 5763) in triple-distilled water to a final concentration of 200 mM, filter sterilize and store in aliquots at –20°C.
    d. Lactate: Dissolve L(+) lactate (cat. no. L 4338) in stock DMEM to a final concentration of 0.5M, filter sterilize, and store at 4°C.

e. Transferrin*-biotin-selenium (TBS) solution: Prepare a 100X stock solution containing 100 µg/mL transferrin (cat. no. T 1283), 3 µM sodium selenite (cat. no. S 5261), and 1 µg/mL D-biotin (i.e., 40 nM: cat. no. B 4639) in stock DMEM. Filter sterilize and aliquot in 5 mL volumes and store at –20°C. Once thawed, the stock solution is maintained at 4°C.

f. Transferrin-putrescine-progesterone-selenium (TPPS) solution: Prepare progesterone (cat. no. P 6149) initially as a 2 mM stock in ethanol. For preparation of 100 mL of a 100X TPPS stock solution, add to 99 mL stock DMEM the following: 100 µg/mL transferrin, 10 mM putrescine (cat. no. P 5780), 3 µM sodium selenite, and 1.0 mL of 2 mM progesterone in ethanol stock solution. Filter sterilize and store in appropriate (~5 mL) aliquots at –20°C. Once thawed the stock solution is maintained at 4°C.

g. Oligodendrocyte conversion supplements: To stock DMEM, add the following: triiodothyronine (1.5 µM; cat. no. T 5516), transferrin (100 µg/mL), sodium selenite (3.0 µM), D-biotin (1.0 µM), sodium pyruvate (200 mM), hydrocortisone hemisuccinate (1.0 mM; cat. no. H 2270). Filter sterilize and freeze in 1 mL aliquots. Prepare a 1.5 mM stock of triiodothyronine (T3) in alkaline stock DMEM and add 100 µL of stock T3 to 100 mL of 100X stock solution of oligodendrocyte conversion supplements.

h. Insulin: Prepare insulin (cat. no. I 1882) as indicated in an acidified fluid to a final concentration of 10 mg/mL and freeze in 0.5 mL aliquots. Thaw only once and dilute in acidified Puck's fluid (phenol red having a yellow color) to final concentration of 5 mg/mL.

i. HEPES buffer, pH 7.2: Dissolve 23.83 g N-2-hydroxyethylpiperazine-N'-2-ethanesulfonate, sodium salt (cat. no. H 9136) in 50 mL triple-distilled water. Adjust pH to 7.2 with 1M HCl. Make up to 100 mL and filter sterilize. Store in aliquots at 4°C protected from the light.

6.3. Preparation of Solutions Used in Harvesting Cells

1. Tissue storage medium: To 9.35 mL stock DMEM, add 0.075 mL 1.0M glucose stock solution, 0.5 mL horse serum, and 0.15 mL 1.0M HEPES buffer, pH 7.2.
2. Puck's BSS, a calcium- and magnesium-free BSS:
   a. Stock solution, 10X Puck's BSS:

NaCl	80.0 g
KCl	4.0 g
$Na_2HPO_4 \cdot 7H_2O$	0.9 g
KH_2PO_4	0.6 g
Glucose	10.0 g

*Any proteins (e.g., transferrin, insulin) added to serum-free medium will tend to attach to glass; therefore, always store protein-containing solutions in plastic containers.

Dissolve in 1000 mL triple distilled water and filter sterilize. **Note:** 20 mL of a 1% aqueous phenol red solution may also be added before making up to 1000 mL. Phenol red addition has the advantage that one has a visual indicator of solution pH.

b. Working solution, 1X Puck's BSS: Dilute stock solution 1:10 with sterile triple-distilled water.

3. Versene solution: Dissolve 0.2 g ethylenediaminetetra-acetic acid, disodium salt (EDTA or versene) in 1000 mL Puck's BSS (i.e., 0.6 mM), filter sterilize, and store at 4°C in aliquots of 50 mL.

4. Deoxyribonuclease (DNase) stock solution: Dissolve 4 g DNase (Sigma cat. no. DN-25) in 100 mL Puck's BSS (4% DNase stock solution), filter sterilize, and store in 1 mL aliquots at –20°C.

5. Harvest medium: Mix 10 mL Puck's BSS with 10 mL versene solution. To this add 0.2 mL 1.0M HEPES stock buffer solution, pH 7.2, 0.2 mL 200 mM stock pyruvate solution, 20 μL 5 mg/mL insulin stock solution, and 0.1 mL 4% DNase stock solution. **Note:** Antibiotics are not necessary for successful culture and are therefore not recommended; however, cultures are most easily contaminated when cells are harvested, therefore, one may wish to add antibiotics to the harvest medium.

6.4. Preparation of B104 Conditioned Medium

1. Grow B104 neuroblastoma cells (Schubert et al., 1974) to confluency using DMEM/F12 containing 10% FBS (v/v) as growth medium. We thank D. Schubert (Salk Institute, San Diego, CA) for the gift of B104 neuroblastoma cells. Convenient culture vessels are 100-mm tissue culture Petri dishes (Falcon #3003, VWR Scientific) or expanded surface roller bottles (Falcon #3079, obtained from VWR Scientific). The roller bottles have a 1500 cm^2 surface area available for cell growth; the 100-mm Petri dishes have a usable surface area of 75 cm^2. For the Petri dishes, use 8 mL medium and for the roller bottles use 100 mL medium.

2. Once cultures are confluent, cultures are washed with Puck's BSS and fed with B104 neuroblastoma-defined medium. To 100-mm Petri dishes add 8 mL medium and to roller bottles add 150 mL medium.

3. After 4 d, the conditioned medium is removed and cultures are fed with a fresh lot of B104 defined medium. Phenylmethylsulfonyl fluoride** (Sigma, cat. no. P 7626) is rapidly mixed into the conditioned medium to a final con-

---

**Prepared as a 1 mg/mL stock solution of phenylmethylsulfonyl fluoride in absolute ethanol. Store in aliquots at –20°C. Use caution in handling, since the compound is a potent protease inhibitor and highly toxic if ingested.

centration of 1 μg/mL. The conditioned medium is centrifuged at 2000*g* for 30 min, filter sterilized, and stored frozen in aliquots. Protein content of this conditioned medium ranges from 3.5–4.5 mg/mL. For short-term storage, use –20°C and for long-term storage use –80°C.

4. We routinely maintain B104 neuroblastoma cultures in 100-mm dishes as a source of cells for the preparation of new B104 neuroblastoma cultures for the purposes of collection of conditioned medium. These maintenance cultures are harvested using harvest medium.

6.5. Preparation of Cell Filtration Apparati

1. Beakers: Nylon meshes of differing pore sizes can be obtained from L. and S. H. Thompson (Montreal, Canada). Cut nylon mesh of 75-μm pore size into squares that fit over the mouths of 50-mL beakers. Use masking tape to fix the mesh in place. Enclose beaker in aluminum foil and autoclave. These meshed beakers are used in the preparation of primary cultures.

2. Filtration tubes: The apparatus consists of a polypropylene tube, open at the top and covered by a nylon mesh at the bottom. Remove the bottom of a 50-mL polypropylene centrifuge tube (VWR Scientific, cat. no. 21008-667), using a hot knife. Remove the cap from the tube and, using a hot cork borer, remove central disk of the cap. Cut nylon mesh into 4 cm squares, cover the top of the tube with the nitex, fix nylon in place by screwing on the cap, place in an autoclave bag, and autoclave. The original top of the tube now becomes the bottom of the filtration device. Prepare filtration devices with nylon meshes of the following pore sizes: 50, 35, and 15 μm.

6.6. Preparation of Culture Substrata

1. Poly-D-lysine stock solution: Prepare a stock solution of 1 mg/mL poly-D-lysine (Sigma, cat. no. P 6407) in triple-distilled water, filter sterilize, and store in aliquots at –20°C.

2. Wash coverslips made of German glass (Fisher Scientific, Nepean, ON, e.g., cat. no. 12-546) by soaking in acetone overnight, air-drying, and sterilizing by heating at 190°C for 3 h.

3. Poly-D-lysine-coated culture substrata: prepare on same day as usage.
   a. Petri dishes:
   b. Coverslips:
       i. Dilute stock poly-D-lysine in sterile triple-distilled water to 20 μg/mL.
       ii. Place 1.5 mL of this solution in each 35-mm Petri dish, or 7 mL of this solution into each 100-mm Petri dish.
       iii. After 2 h, wash dishes with Puck's BSS.

    i. Place coverslips into appropriate culture vessel and add diluted poly-D-lysine solution. Useful culture vessels are 100 mm microbiological Petri dishes. Coverslips are placed into microbiological Petri dishes, because these dishes are hydrophobic and this tends to ensure that the aqueous solution stays on the coverslip rather than spilling onto the surface of the Petri dish. Coverslips can then be washed and cells planted directly onto the coverslips.

    ii. After 2 h, wash with Puck's solution.

FURTHER READING

Behar, T., McMorris, F. A., Novotny, E. A., Barker, J. L., and Dubois-Dalq, M. (1988), Growth and differentiation properties of O-2A progenitors purified from rat cerebral hemispheres. *J. Neurosci. Res.* **21,** 168–180.

Duncan, I. D., Paino, C., Archer, D. R., and Wood, P. M. (1992), Functional capacities of transplanted cell-sorted adult oligodendrocytes. *Dev. Neurosci.* **14,** 114–122.

Gard, A. L. and Pfeiffer, S. E. (1990), Two proliferative stages of oligodendrocyte lineage (A2B5⁺O4⁻ and O4⁺GalC⁻) under different mitogenic control. *Neuron* **5,** 615–625.

Gard, A. L., Pfeiffer, S. E., and Williams II, W. C. (1993), Immunopanning and developmental stage-specific primary culture of oligodendrocyte precursors (O4⁺ GalC⁻) directly from postnatal rodent cerebrum. *Neuroprotocols* **2,** 209-218.

Gard, A. L., Williams, W. C., and Burrell, M. R. (1995), Oligodendroblasts distinguished from O-2A glial progenitors by surface phenotype (O4⁺GalC⁻) and response to cytokines using signal transducer LIFR beta. *Dev. Biol.* **167,** 596–608.

Hunter, S. F. and Bottenstein, J. E. (1989), Bipotential glial progenitors are targets of neuronal cell-line derived growth factors. *Develop. Brain Res.* **49,** 33–49.

Hunter, S. F. and Bottenstein, J. E. (1990), Growth factor responses of enriched bipotential glial progenitors. *Dev. Brain Res.* **54,** 235–248.

Husain, J. and Juurlink, B. H. J. (1995), Oligodendroglial precursor cell susceptibility to hypoxia is related to poor ability to cope with reactive oxygen species. *Brain Res.* **698,** 86–94.

Louis, J. C., Magal, E., Muir, D., Manthorpe, M., and Varon, S. (1993), CG-4, a new bipotential glial cell line from rat brain, is capable of differentiating in vitro into either mature oligodendrocytes or type-2 astrocytes. *J. Neurosci. Res.* **31,** 193–204.

McCarthy, K. D. and de Vellis, J. (1980), Preparation of separate astroglial and oligodendroglial cell cultures from rat cerebral tissue. *J. Cell Biol.* **85,** 890–902.

Schubert, D., Heinemann, S., Carlisle, W., Tarikas, H., Kines, B., Patrick, J., Steinbach, J. H., Culp, W., and Brandt, B. L. (1974), Clonal cell lines from the rat central nervous system. *Nature (Lond.)* **249,** 224–227.

Szuchet, S., Arnason, B. G. W., and Polak, P. E. (1980), Separation of ovine oligodendrocytes in two distinct bands on a linear sucrose gradient. *J. Neurosci. Methods* **3,** 7–19.

Warrington, A. E., Barbarese, E., and Pfeiffer, S. E. (1993), Differential myelinogenic capacity of specific developmental stages of the oligodendrocyte lineage upon transplantation into hypomyelinating hosts. *J. Neurosci. Res.* **34,** 1–13.

Chapter Eleven

Culture of Glial Cells from Human Brain Biopsies

Voon Wee Yong and Jack P. Antel

1. INTRODUCTION

Surgical resections of selected human brain areas to ameliorate intractable epilepsy provide opportunities to isolate, maintain, and examine nonmalignant human neural cells in vitro. Since these specimens tend to be from patients of early adulthood or older, neurons do not survive the isolation process; the cells extracted are thus of glial origin, and include oligodendrocytes, astrocytes, and microglial cells. In our laboratories, although the biopsy materials (frontal or temporal lobes and corpus callosum) are mostly from subjects undergoing surgery to treat intractable epilepsy, we have not found any differences in properties of cells from such surgery when compared to other types of resections, such as those used to treat vascular anomalies involving the brain. In the frontal and temporal lobe resections, tissue is removed either *en bloc* or by Cavitron™ ultrasonic aspiration (CUSA), which fragments the tissue into cubes of 2 mm on average. Corpus callosum tissue is always removed by CUSA.

Biopsy-derived human brain specimens offer several advantages over autopsy-derived materials. Being relatively fresh, the cell viability and yield are high (5–10 million cells/g wet wt of tissue; cell yield for autopsy specimens is at least an order of magnitude less). The success rate of bulk-isolating viable cells from biopsy specimens has been in the over 90% range. Another advantage offered by biopsy speci-

Protocols for Neural Cell Culture, 2nd Ed. • Eds.: S. Fedoroff and A. Richardson • Humana Press, Inc., Totowa, NJ

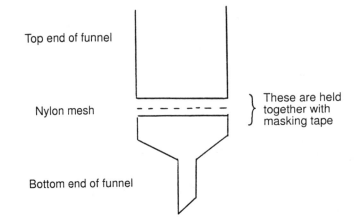

Fig. 1. Buchnel funnel nylon mesh assembly. The Buchnel funnel is a two-piece Nalgene™ polypropylene funnel (Fisher, 10-362 B or C) with the perforated filter cutout. This assembly is useful because the funnel can sit comfortably in 50-mL tubes during the filtration process.

mens is that blood samples, and the associated mononuclear cells, can be easily procured from the living patients and tested on cultured neural cells to assess autologous or heterologous immune reactivity.

2. PREPARATION OF CULTURED CELLS

2.1. Materials

Human brain tissue.
Scalpels (2).
Forceps (2).
Glass Petri dish, 100 mm.
Disposable plastic pipets with wide mouth (10 mL) (5).
Glass Pasteur pipets (2 mL) (2).
Phosphate-buffered saline (PBS), pH 7.4 (Unipath Ltd., Basingstoke, Hampshire).
Percoll (Pharmacia LKB, Piscataway, NJ, 17-0891-01).
Sterile 50-mL plastic conical tubes.
Glass bottle with cap (100 mL).
Magnetic stir bar.
Trypsin (2.5% stock solution) (Gibco-BRL, Gaithersburg, MD).
DNAse Type I (1 mg/mL stock) (Sigma, St. Louis, MO).
Water bath set at 37°C and placed on a magnetic plate.
Buchnel funnel with perforated plate removed, and containing a 132-μm nylon
    mesh (B. and S. H. Thompson & Co., Montreal, Quebec) (Fig. 1).
Polycarbonate tubes (40 mL).
Feeding medium (see Section 4.2.).
Poly-L-lysine-coated (10 μg/mL) Aclar™ 9-mm diameter coverslips.

Uncoated or poly-L-lysine-coated Falcon flasks (25 cm²).
Plastic dishes (60 mm).
Fetal bovine serum (FBS) (Gibco).

2.2. Sterilization of Instruments

Sterilize scalpels, forceps, and magnetic stir bar prior to use by immersing in 95% ethanol and then flaming. Autoclave Buchnel funnel nylon mesh, glass Petri dish and bottle, Pasteur pipets, and polycarbonate tubes, which have previously been wrapped in autoclave bags. All other sterile disposable materials are purchased from manufacturers.

2.3. Bulk Isolation of Mixed Human Glial Cells

1. CUSA bag specimens:
   a. Cut the top end of the CUSA bag with scalpel to expose the specimen.
   b. Using a 10-mL pipet, decant blood and transfer tissues either into 50-mL plastic tubes or, if the bulk of the specimen is over 2 mm³, into the 100-mm glass dish for further dicing with scalpels. After dicing, these samples are then transferred into 50-mL plastic tubes.
   Note: We prefer to have approx 20 mL of tissue suspension in each 50-mL tube so that subsequent PBS washes can be more effective.
2. *En bloc* specimens:
   a. Remove the blood vessels with forceps.
   b. Using scalpels, cut the tissue into chunks of <2 mm³. Transfer these cubes into 50-mL tubes.
   Note: We prefer to have approx 20-mL of tissue suspension in each 50-mL tube so that subsequent PBS washes can be more effective.
3. Washing the tissue:
   a. Add enough PBS to the 50-mL tube to make the volume up to 45 mL. Allow chunks to settle (10–20 s) and then remove the supernatant using a 10 mL wide mouth pipet.
   b. Wash tissue several times, as above, to remove contaminating blood. During these washes, use a glass Pasteur pipet to fish off visible capillaries and blood vessels.
   c. For an extremely bloody preparation, even after the PBS washes, overlay the specimen in PBS with a 50/30% Percoll gradient.
      i. Percoll gradient from top to bottom consists of 20 mL of brain suspension, 5 mL of 30% Percoll, and 5 mL of 50% Percoll.
      ii. Centrifuge the gradient at 1700g for 20 min.

> **Note:** The brain chunks remain above the 30% Percoll layer, whereas blood contaminants are trapped between the 30–50% Percoll layers.

    iii. Remove the brain suspension, dilute with PBS, and centrifuge at 70g for 10 min.

    iv. Repeat this wash twice to remove the Percoll.

4. Weighing the specimen (optional):
  a. Place the tissue into a weighed 50-mL plastic tube.
  b. Centrifuge the suspension at 200g for 10 min.
  c. Aspirate the supernatant. The tube containing the brain pellet is then weighed.

5. Trypsinization of the tissue:
  a. Place the brain into a 100-mL glass bottle to which is added PBS to make a total volume of 68 mL.
  b. Add 8 mL of trypsin (2.5% stock solution) to achieve a final concentration of 0.25%.
  c. Add 4 mL of DNase stock for a final concentration of 50 µg DNase/mL.
  d. Place a stir bar in the solution and cap the bottle.
  e. Incubate the enzyme brain suspension at 37°C in a water bath on a magnetic plate. The speed of the stirrer should be slow enough so that a conical vortex does not form at the top of the solution. Incubation times can range from 30 min to an hour, depending on the rate at which tissues are fragmented during this process.

6. Preparation of cell suspension:
> **Note:** Pipeting should be done gently to ensure high cell viability. Squirting of air bubbles into the cell suspension should be discouraged.

  a. Pass the cell suspension through the Buchnel funnel nylon mesh into one of six 50-mL plastic tubes each containing 1 mL of fetal bovine serum (FBS) to inactivate the trypsin.
  b. Add 20 mL of PBS to the filter and mechanically disrupt the fragments retained on the filter with a 10-mL pipet (horizontal motion of pipet on the filter) in order to yield further disaggregated cells. Repeat this process several times.
  c. After further disaggregation of the tissue, completely mix the cell suspension in the 50-mL tube with the serum, using a fresh 10-mL pipet (three strokes).
> **Note:** If large amounts of chunks are retained on the filter, these are collected and retrypsinized for 30 min (steps 5 and 6).

  d. Centrifuge the filtrate at 300g for 10 min.

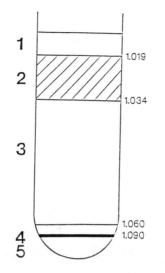

Fig. 2. Gradients following Percoll centrifugation. The numbers on the right of the diagram show the specific gravities of the gradient. The left panels are the following: Layer 1: PBS; Layer 2: myelin and cellular debris; Layer 3: viable cell layer; Layer 4: red blood cells; Layer 5: PBS.

 e. Aspirate most of the supernatant off, leaving behind 2 mL of the supernatant. Resuspend the pellet using a 10 mL wide mouth pipet in this medium.

 f. When the cells are suspended, add 5 pellet vol of PBS.

 g. Gradients (Fig. 2):

  i. Add 21 mL of this suspension to one of several 40-mL polycarbonate tubes each containing 9 mL of undiluted Percoll. The final concentration of Percoll is thus 30%.

  ii. Centrifuge the suspensions at 15,000g for 30 min in order to allow gradients to form.

  iii. Aspirate off the cell debris/myelin layer. Using a glass Pasteur pipet, transfer the viable cell layer to clean 50-mL plastic tubes. Discard the red cell layer.

 h. Transfer 15–20 mL of the viable cell layer to each 50-mL tube. Add enough PBS to make a total volume of 45 mL. Mix the suspension using a 10-mL pipet. Cap the tubes and centrifuge at 800g for 10 min.

 i. Aspirate the supernatant leaving 1 mL. Using a glass Pasteur pipet (the finer bore of glass pipets allows better resuspension of live cells at this stage), resuspend the pellet in the 1-mL supernatant.

 j. Cell suspensions from several tubes can be pooled into a single 50-mL plastic tube. Add 2 mL of feeding medium into each tube that contains the cell suspensions, twice, so that cells can be transferred with maximal yield into the pool.

k. Add enough feeding medium to make a total volume of 45 mL. Cap the
    tube and centrifuge at 300g for 10 min.

l. Again, aspirate the supernatant leaving 1 mL. Then resuspend the pellet
    with a glass Pasteur pipet. Add feeding medium (25 mL) and centrifuge
    at 70g for 10 min. Repeat this process twice.

Note 1: The lower centrifugation speed at this point allows the majority of
viable cells to settle while keeping cellular debris in the supernatant.

Note 2: This protocol is essentially similar to that described by Kim (Kim et
al., 1983; Kim, 1985) for autopsy-derived human brain specimens.

7. Cultures:

a. Resuspend the cell pellet in feeding medium to a density of 2×10^6 to
    4×10^6 cells/mL. Plate these cells directly onto 10 µg/mL poly-L-lysine-
    coated Aclar fluorocarbon plastic 9-mm coverslips (*see* Section 3.1.) at a
    density of 5×10^4 cells/coverslip in 50 µL vol (mixed cell population), or
    into uncoated Falcon flasks (10×10^6 cells/flask) for further separation of
    cell types.

b. Incubate the cultures in humidified incubators at 37°C pulsed with an
    atmosphere of 5% CO_2 and 95% air.

3. SEPARATION OF OLIGODENDROCYTE, ASTROCYTE, AND MICROGLIA POPULATIONS

3.1. Enriched Oligodendrocyte Preparation

Oligodendrocytes derived from adult brains adhere relatively poorly to tissue
culture plastic when compared to astrocytes or microglia cells. (The poor adherence
increases with advancing age of human subjects.) Thus, 24 h after initial cell plating
in uncoated Falcon flasks, floating cells, most of which are oligodendrocytes, can be
removed with glass Pasteur pipets. At this stage, the percentage of oligodendrocytes
tends to be approx 70–80%. These cells are centrifuged (70g, 10 min), resuspended,
and plated on poly-L-lysine-coated coverslips at a seeding density of 5×10^4 cells/
coverslip. Alternatively, to enrich further for oligodendrocytes, the floating cells
removed can be replated onto another set of 25-cm^2 uncoated Falcon flasks for
another 24 h (5×10^6 cells/flask in 5 mL medium). The floating cells are then collected to give oligodendrocyte preparations of about 90% purity.

3.2. Microglia and Astrocyte Mixed Populations

1. Following removal of oligodendrocytes, add 5 mL of feeding medium to each
    flask. These adherent cells (microglia and astrocytes) are kept undisturbed
    in the 37°C incubator to allow them to develop morphologically.

a. These cells can be removed from the flask at any stage during the incubation to yield a mixed astrocyte and microglia preparation. Removal from flasks is achieved by aspirating off the feeding medium and then effecting four changes of PBS to remove completely trace amounts of feeding medium. The cells are then incubated with 0.05% trypsin in 4 mL of PBS at 37°C for 15 min. Although astrocytes will be dislodged after the trypsin treatment, most microglia cells remain adherent. To dislodge all cells, the sealed flask is knocked strongly against the palm of the hand once. One hundred microliters of FBS are then added to each flask to inactivate the trypsin. The floating cells are collected into a 50-mL plastic tube using a glass pipet. Each flask is washed twice with PBS to remove cells maximally, and is centrifuged at 300*g* for 10 min. The pellet is resuspended with feeding medium and centrifuged at 70*g* for 10 min. This process is repeated twice.

b. Cells are then seeded on poly-L-lysine coated coverslips at a density of 5×10^3 to 5×10^4 cells/coverslip.

3.3. Separation of Microglia and Astrocyte Populations

1. Following removal of oligodendrocytes, adherent cells are left for 1–2 wk to allow cells to develop morphologically. To further separate microglia from astrocytes, another differential adhesion protocol is employed; this takes advantage of the observation that the microglia cells have very strong adherence to plastic when compared to astrocytes. The following procedure allows separation of the microglia and astrocyte populations.

    a. Remove the feeding medium and add 5 mL of fresh medium.

    b. Tightly seal the caps of the Falcon flasks and place them on a rotary shaker, 150 rpm, at room temperature for 5 h.

    Note: During this process, most astrocytes and some microglia cells are floated off.

    c. Remove the floating cells and wash the flask twice with feeding medium to maximize removal of floating cells.

    d. Centrifuge the cell suspension at 160*g* for 10 min and replate the cells.

2. At best, such preparations contain up to 70% astrocytes, the rest being microglia cells. We presently cannot purify astrocytes beyond 70% purity, even though magnetic separation (allowing the rapidly phagocytosing microglia cells to ingest magnetic beads), and chemical treatments for eliminating microglia from rodent glia cultures (leucine-methyl ester and silica ingestion) (Thiele et al., 1983; Giulian and Baker, 1986) were used.

3. For microglia enrichment, the adherent cells following flotation are retrypsinized as described above. Such preparations routinely yield microglia purity of over 90% (Williams et al., 1992).

4. APPENDIX

4.1. Preparation of Poly-L-Lysine-Coated Coverslips or Flasks

1. Washing coverslips:
   a. Soak Aclar™ 9-mm diameter plastic fluorocarbon coverslips (supplied by S. Kim, University of British Columbia, Vancouver, BC) overnight in a 6N HCl solution in a glass beaker capped with a piece of cotton gauze.
   b. Wash off the HCl with running tap water (30 min) and decant the water off.
   c. Use several washes of absolute ethanol to sterilize the coverslips, which are then left overnight in absolute ethanol.
   d. Decant the absolute ethanol, transfer the coverslips into sterile 60-mm plastic dishes, and dry them in a laminar flow hood.
   e. When the coverslips are dry, wash them twice with sterile water and then leave overnight (or for at least 30 min) in a 10 µg/mL poly-L-lysine (Sigma P 1524, mol wt >400,000) solution in water.
2. To use the coverslips, transfer them through two 60 mm dishes of water and finally into the bottom of dry 60 mm plastic dishes (15 coverslips placed apart from each other and apart from the walls of each dish). Aspirate off excess fluid and allow the coverslips to dry for an hour in the laminar flow hood. These coverslips are then ready for plating cells.
3. For coating of 25-cm² flasks, add 5 mL of 10 µg/mL poly-L-lysine solution for 30 min. Aspirate off the solution, wash the flask twice with sterile water, and allow to dry.

Note 1: For cultures seeded onto coverslips as 50 µL droplets, we routinely flood these after 48 h; flooding consists of the addition of 3 mL of feeding medium into each 60-mm dish so that all coverslips are entirely submerged in feeding medium.

Note 2: Cells growing on coverslips are used mostly for immunohistochemical experiments. Cells seeded onto poly-L-lysine-coated flasks provide the larger samples that are needed for biochemical experiments.

4.2. Notes on Cultured Human Adult Glial Cells

1. Feeding medium: An adequate feeding medium for adult human glial cells in culture is Eagle's Minimum Essential Medium (Gibco 330-1430 AJ) supplemented with 5% FBS, 1 mg/mL dextrose, and 20 µg/mL gentamicin (all

ingredients from Gibco, Grand Island, NY). This medium can allow some cells to survive for up to 8 mo in vitro (the longest time period examined). Higher amounts of serum in the feeding medium have not conferred any advantage to cell viability or development, in our experience. Cells need only to be refed once a week.

2. Cell yield: Per gram wet weight of tissue, total cell yield is between 5 and 10 million. This is considerably higher than from freshly sacrificed adult rodent brains using the same isolation process where cell yield ranges from 1–3 million/g wet wt and from autopsy human brain specimens (with an average interval of 12 h from death to start of cell isolation) where cell yield averages 0.5 million/g. Of the cells bulk-isolated from human brain biopsies, approx 25% tend to be oligodendrocytes. The remaining cells are a mixture of microglia and astrocytes. This ratio between microglia and astrocytes is extremely variable, and can be as low as 10% for microglia or as high as 95%. Presently, we have not been able to correlate the amount of microglia cells to patient diagnosis, the site of brain resection, the amount of gliosis in the resected specimen, or the age of the patient.

3. Plating requirements:
   a. When plated on coverslips, astrocytes and microglia require relatively low seeding density for survival or to develop morphologically. Thus, on a 9 mm diameter surface, a seeding density of as low as 5×10^3 is sufficient. We routinely employ a plating density of 1×10^4 cells/9-mm coverslip.
   b. The seeding requirement for oligodendrocytes is more stringent. At seeding density below 1×10^4/9-mm coverslip, survival is poor. At 1×10^4 or 2.5×10^4 plating density, morphological differentiation (process formation) is slow. We routinely plate oligodendrocytes at seeding density of at least 5×10^4 cells/coverslip.

4. Immunohistochemical characterization of cultures (Fig. 3): We employ routine immunofluorescence to characterize the types of cells present in culture (McLaurin et al., 1995). For oligodendrocytes, the expression of galactocerebroside on the cell surface is used; surface expression of Leu-M5, a monocyte marker, is used to identify microglia in addition to their bipolar morphology and avid phagocytic activity. An antibody to glial fibrillary acidic protein following fixation of cells is employed to label astrocytes.

5. What about fibroblasts? Unlike the adult rodent brain, fibroblasts do not become a contaminating problem for adult human brain cells isolated by trypsin digestion, except at longer-term cultures. We do not observe fibroblasts (cytoplasmic fibronectin immunoreactivity) in cultures until approx 3–4 wk postisolation. No explanation is readily apparent for the inability of

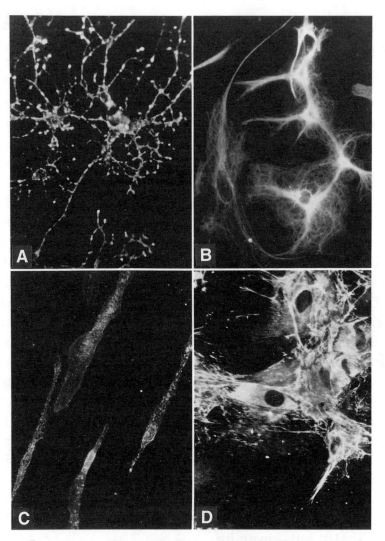

Fig. 3. Immunofluorescence characterization of cells from cultures of adult human brain tissue. (A) Galactocerebroside-positive oligodendrocytes. (B) GFAP-positive astrocytes. (C) Leu-M5-positive microglia cells. (D) Fibronectin-positive fibroblasts.

human brain fibroblasts to thrive in the early culture periods following trypsin disaggregation when compared to cultures from the adult rodent brain. However, if we were to explant human brain tissues without trypsin treatment (adhering fragments of 0.5 mm^3 or less to a surface and then collecting cells that migrate out of the explant), then the majority of cells are invariably fibroblasts, in our experience. We do not routinely use this explant technique because of the high yield of fibroblasts and the low yield of glia cells.

To suppress fibroblast growth in longer-term cultures of cells from adult human brain biopsies isolated by trypsin digestion, we use a chemically defined serum-free medium (DM5) supplemented with 10 μ*M* cytosine arabinoside. This is initiated at 2 wk postisolation, and the cytosine arabinoside is added and withdrawn for 3-d periods.

Constituents of DM5: Eagle's Minimum Essential Medium, pH 7.4 (Gibco 330-1430 AJ):

Bovine serum albumin (Sigma Fr V)	0.1%
MEM nonessential amino acids, (Gibco 320-1140 AG)	100.0 μ*M*
Dextrose	1.0 mg/mL
Gentamicin	20.0 μg/mL
Insulin	0.5 U/mL
Hydrocortisone	50.0 n*M*
Human transferrin	50.0 μg/mL
Selenium	30.0 n*M*
Tri-iodo-L-thyronine	30.0 n*M*
HEPES buffer	1.0 m*M*
Sodium pyruvate	1.0 m*M*

DM5 may be stored for 2 mo at −20°C or for 2 wk at 4°C.

6. Characteristics of adult human glial cells in culture:

a. Oligodendrocytes: Under phase-inverted microscopy, these cells have a phase bright round cell body of approx 8–15 μm in diameter. When examined for possible capability to proliferate, we have found that galactocerebroside-positive cells do not incorporate bromodeoxyuridine (a thymidine analog and an index of proliferation) under any conditions. We have assessed the rate of process formation by these cells and have noted that this is dependent on seeding density as mentioned. However, this is variable among different preparations, even when seeded at the same seeding density; it is influenced mainly, but not exclusively, by the age of the human subjects: The younger the patient, the better the process-extending capability of the oligodendrocytes. The extent of process formation can be enhanced by treatment of these cells with biologically active phorbol esters (4b-phorbol-12,13-dibutyrate and phorbol-12-myristate-13-acetate) (Yong et al., 1991a, 1994); again, although the majority of oligodendrocytes will enhance process formation after phorbol ester treatment, there is variability in the rate among preparations. In addition to galactocerebroside, adult human oligodendrocytes express the following markers as detected by immunohistochemistry: 2',3'-cyclic nucleotide phosphophydrolase, myelin basic protein, proteolipid protein, and myelin-associated glycoprotein.

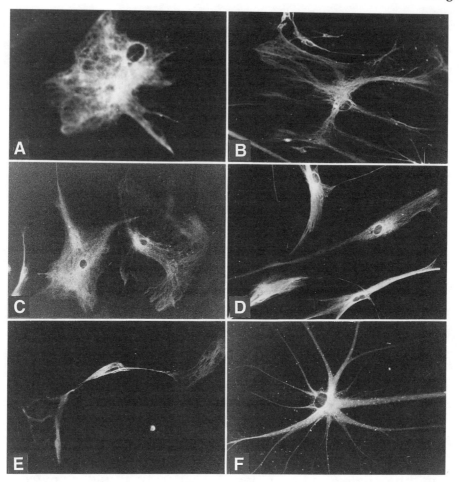

Fig. 4. GFAP immunofluorescence of adult human astrocytes demonstrating the heterogeneity in morphology of cells in culture *(continued)*.

b. Astrocytes: Unlike the well-described flat and process-bearing morphology of rodent astrocytes, adult human astrocytes from biopsy materials are extremely heterogenous in morphology. They range from a flat-fibroblastic form to process-bearing cells with little soma cytoplasm; the majority of astrocytes are intermediate in form (Fig. 4) (Yong et al., 1990). Based on morphology, we have been unable to characterize adult human astrocytes into the Type 1 and 2 forms that have been described for rodent astrocytes in vitro by Raff et al. (1983); none of the adult human astrocytes express the polysialoganglioside A2B5. However, we have found that the process-bearing adult human astrocytes are more likely than the flat forms to express major histocompatibility complex (MHC) antigens (Class I and II) in 5% FBS feeding medium; in contrast to this, adult or neonatal

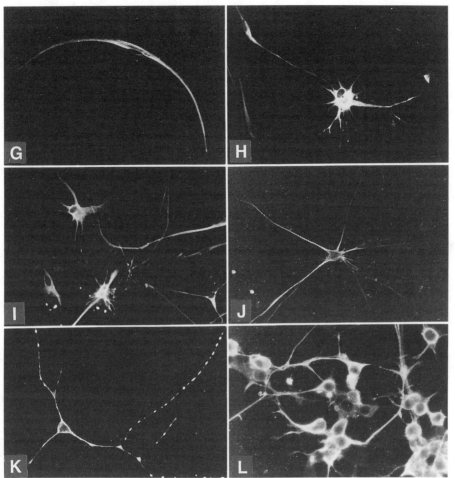

Fig. 4. *(continued)*.

rodent astrocytes do not express MHC antigens when isolated and cultured under identical conditions (Yong et al., 1990, 1991b). Adult human astrocytes can undergo proliferation, but the extent is comparatively low. When pulsed with bromodeoxyuridine for 48 h in the 5% FBS-containing feeding medium, approx 2% of adult human astrocytes will incorporate bromodeoxyuridine (Yong et al., 1991c). In contrast, approx 20% of adult rat astrocytes will incorporate the proliferation label under the same conditions.

c. Microglia: The morphology of adult human microglia tends to be bipolar upon morphological differentiation, although some preparations of human biopsies will present with microglia that are round and ameboid-like. These cells, after 1 wk in culture, are of larger size and have greater autofluorescence than immediately ex vivo microglia, as assessed by flow cytometry analyses. Some degree of "activation" does occur even under basal culture conditions. Further activation, measured both by cell surface antigen expression (MHC molecules and CD14) and cytokine production (TNF-α, IL-1, and IL-6), can be induced with γ-interferon and liposaccharide. We are reasonably satisfied that microglia cells from human brain biopsies are not merely monocytes from blood contaminants during the cell isolation process. In studies where the properties of microglia cells are compared with monocytes isolated from peripheral human blood, we have observed that, although microglia cells have high survival rate and plating efficiency (attachment factor) on poly-L-lysine coverslips, monocytes do not. In addition, monocytes tend to remain rounded in morphology, except at longer-term culture (after at least 2 wk) when some can assume a bipolar form. In contrast, the majority of microglia undergo morphological differentiation within 4 d in vitro. Microglia do express the CD45 molecule characteristic of cells of hematopoietic origin but al levels less than those found on blood monocytes. Almost none of the cells in our microglia cultures are CD45[hi], indicating little if any contamination by blood or blood vessel elements (Becher and Antel, submitted).

7. Are there precursor cells in adult human brain cultures? We have not explored this issue exhaustively, but have noted that a high percentage (50% on average, but can be as high as 80%) of cells (excluding microglia) express the 04 antigen, a marker that is found on certain Type II astrocytes and oligodendrocytes; the 04 antigen is also expressed by precursor cells of the 0-2A lineage. Using human biopsy-derived materials, Armstrong et al. (1990) have reported the presence of precursor cells of the 0-2A lineage in vitro, by the criteria that these cells are 04-positive, but lack expression of galactocerebroside or glial fibrillary acidic protein. It is thus likely that a proportion of cells from adult human biopsies are precursor cells for oligodendrocytes and astrocytes. In our experience, >90% of cells expressing the oligodendrocyte precursor molecule recognized by the antibody A007 also express myelin basic protein, when examined within 2 d of isolation (Prabhakar et al., 1995).

5. ACKNOWLEDGMENTS

We thank our colleagues whose contributions have resulted in the above chapter: Seung U. Kim, Sue Prabhakar, Burkhart Becher, Luke Oh, Kenneth Williams, Trevor Tejada-Berges, Amit Bar-Or, and Fiona P. Yong. We acknowledge the valuable contribution of Seung U. Kim (University of British Columbia, Vancouver), who initially taught us the techniques of neural cell culture.

FURTHER READING

Armstrong, R., Dorn, H., Kufta, C. V., and Dubois-Dalcq, M. (1990), Do oligodendrocyte precursor cells persist in adult human CNS? 20th Annual Meeting of the Society of Neuroscience, St. Louis, Abstract 402.12.

Barna, B. P., Chou, S. M., Jacobs, B., Yen-Lieberman, B., and Ransohoff, R. M. (1989), Interferon-b impairs induction of HLA-DR antigen expression in cultured adult human astrocytes. *J. Neuroimmunol.* **23,** 45–55.

Giulian, D. and Baker, T. J. (1986), Characterization of ameboid microglia isolated from developing mammalian brain. *J. Neurosci.* **6,** 2163–2178.

Kim, S. U. (1985), Antigen expression by glia cells grown in culture. *J. Neuroimmunol.* **8,** 255–282.

Kim, S. U., Sato, Y., Silberberg, D. H., Pleasure, D. E., and Rorke, L. (1983), Long-term culture of human oligodendrocytes. Isolation, growth and identification. *J. Neurol. Sci.* **62,** 295–301.

McLaurin, J., Antel, J. P., and Yong, V. W. (1995), Immune and non-immune actions of interferon-β-1b on primary human neural cell. *Multiple Sclerosis* **1,** 10–19.

Norton, W. T., Farooq, M., Chiu, F. C., and Bottenstein, J. E. (1988), Pure astrocyte cultures derived from cells isolated from mature brain. *Glia* **1,** 403–414.

Prabhakar, S., D'Souza, S., Antel, J. P., McLaurin, J., Schipper, H. M., and Wang, E. (1995), Phenotypic and cell cycle properties of human oligodendrocytes in vitro. *Brain Res.* **672,** 159–169.

Raff, M. C. (1989), Glial cell diversification in the rat optic nerve. *Science* **243,** 1450–1455.

Raff, M. C., Abney, E. R., Cohen, J., Lindsay, R., and Noble, M. (1983), Two types of astrocytes in cultures of developing rat white matter: differences in morphology, surface gangliosides, and growth characteristics. *J. Neurosci.* **3,** 1289–1300.

Szuchet, S. and Yim, S. H. (1984), Characterization of a subset of oligodendrocytes separated on the basis of selective adherence properties. *J. Neurosci. Res.* **11,** 131–144.

Szuchet, S., Stefansson, K., Wollmann, R. L., Dawson, G., and Arnason, B. G. W. (1980), Maintenance of isolated oligodendrocytes in long-term culture. *Brain Res.* **200,** 151–164.

Thiele, D. L., Kurosaka, M., and Lipsky, P. E. (1983), Phenotype of the accessory cell necessary for mitogen-stimulated T and B cell responses in human peripheral blood: delineation by its sensitivity to the lysosomotrophic agent, L-leucine methyl ester. *J. Immunol.* **131,** 2282–2290.

Williams, K., Bar-Or, A., Ulvestad, E., Olivier, A., Antel, J. P., and Yong, V. W. (1992), Biology of adult human microglia in culture: comparisons with peripheral blood monocytes and astrocytes. *J. Neuropath. Exp. Neurol.* **51,** 538–549.

Yong, V. W., Kim, M. W., and Kim, S. U. (1989), Human glial cells and growth factors, in: *Myelination and Demyelination: Implications for Multiple Sclerosis,* Kim, S. U., ed., Plenum, New York, pp. 29–48.

Yong, V. W., Cheung, J. C. B., Uhm, J. H., and Kim, S. U. (1991a), Age-dependent decrease of process formation by cultured oligodendrocytes is augmented by protein kinase C stimulation. *J. Neurosci. Res.* **29,** 87–99.

Yong, V. W., Yong, F. P., Ruijs, T. C. G., Antel, J. P., and Kim, S. U. (1991b), Expression and modulation of HLA-DR on cultured human adult astrocytes. *J. Neuropath. Exp. Neurol.* **50,** 16–28.

Yong, V. W., Moumdjian, R., Yong, F. P., Ruijs, T. C. G., Freedman, M. S., Cashman, N., and Antel, J. P. (1991c), γ-Interferon promotes proliferation of adult human astrocytes in vitro and reactive gliosis in the adult mouse brain in vivo. *Proc. Natl. Acad. Sci. USA* **88,** 7016–7020.

Yong, V. W., Yong, F. P., Olivier, A., Robitaille, Y., and Antel, J. P. (1990), Morphologic heterogeneity of human adult astrocytes in culture: correlation with HLA-DR expression. *J. Neurosci. Res.* **27,** 678–688.

Yong, V. W., Dooley, N. P., and Noble, P. G. (1994), Protein kinase C in cultured adult human oligodendrocytes: a potential role for isoform α as a mediator of process outgrowth. *J. Neurosci. Res.* **39,** 83–86.

Chapter Twelve

Colony Cultures

Sergey Fedoroff and Arleen Richardson

1. INTRODUCTION

Colony cultures are based on the assumption that single viable cells can attach to the substratum, divide, and form a progeny of cells that constitute a cell colony. Colony cultures can be initiated either from the original disaggregated cell suspension made directly from animal tissue, or from primary or secondary cultures. When large numbers of viable cells are plated/cm² of substratum, on culturing, a confluent layer of cells forms. When a small number of cells are plated/cm² of substratum, then single, discrete cell colonies form. Colonies, especially ones initiated directly from tissues, are not necessarily uniform. The morphology and size of the colony depends on the kinds of cells plated, the degree of their differentiation, the cell generation time, the composition of the medium, the type of substratum, and the physical conditions. In practice, disaggregated tissue yields a variety of cells of varying degrees of maturity, resulting in heterogeneity in colony size and morphology. Colony cultures from secondary cultures usually have more uniform colonies.

Generally, only a small percentage of the cells from disaggregated tissue attach to a substratum and form progeny. The older the tissue, the smaller the percentage of colony-forming cells. The estimate of the percentage of cells in a given cell population that can form colonies in culture is called the plating efficiency. Colony cultures are very effective for determination of plating efficiency, for standardization of culture media and various reagents, for semiquantitative growth and toxicity assays, and for cell lineage studies.

Protocols for Neural Cell Culture, 2nd Ed. • Eds.: S. Fedoroff and A. Richardson • Humana Press, Inc., Totowa, NJ

2. PREPARATION OF NEWBORN MOUSE FOR DISSECTION OF NEOPALLIUM

2.1. Materials

Mouse, newborn.
Forceps, curved, 12 cm (2).
Forceps, straight, blunt, 14 cm.
Forceps, Irex #5 (2).
Forceps, fine curved, 10 cm.
Scissors, large, 15 cm.
Scissors, straight, 10 cm.
Scissors, curved, 10 cm.
Sterile wax dissecting dish.
Needles, 25-gage, sterile (1/mouse).
Ethanol, 70% in Coplin jar.
Petri dishes, glass, sterile, 100 mm (3).
High sucrose phosphate buffer (10 mL).

2.2. Preparation

1. Place several discrete drops of high sucrose phosphate buffer around the periphery of the Petri dish. (One cerebral hemisphere will be placed in each drop). In the center of the Petri dish, place a number of drops of high sucrose phosphate buffer, in which the neopallia will be collected.
2. Sterilize all instruments. When the instruments have been sterilized, place them into two sterile glass Petri dishes and keep the ends covered with a lid.

2.3. Preparation of Newborn Mouse

1. Deeply anesthetize a newborn mouse with Halothane™ or Methofan™.
2. Using forceps, pick up the mouse and briefly submerge it in the container of 70% alcohol.
3. Using the large scissors, decapitate the mouse so that the head falls onto the wax dissecting dish.
4. Using a sterile needle, pin the head through the nose, dorsal side up, to the wax dish (*see* Fig. 1A, Chapter 9).

2.4. Dissection of the Cerebral Hemispheres

1. Using sterile curved forceps and curved scissors, remove the skin over the dorsal surface of the skull. This is easily accomplished by beginning the cut ventral to the ears, continuing toward the snout, then across the head just above the eyes and finally back toward the neck, and at the same time, gently pulling the skin from the skull with forceps (*see* Fig. 1A, Chapter 9).

2. Using straight sterile scissors, divide the skull and cerebral hemispheres from posterior to anterior, that is, **by bringing the bottom blade of the scissors up through the brain. Do not cut down initially through the skull,** because the pressure will mutilate the soft brain tissue (*see* Fig. 1A, Chapter 9).

3. Remove the cerebral hemispheres:
   a. Using a pair of sterile curved forceps, grasp the muzzle of the mouse and squeeze gently. This serves to hold the head in place as well as open the skull.
   b. Next, using the fine-curved forceps, lift the brain out of the skull and place each hemisphere into a drop of medium in the sterile Petri dish.
   c. Using the Irex forceps, remove the delicate, almost transparent meninges. Begin at the olfactory bulbs and peel the meninges off by pulling gently posteriorly. Try to avoid tearing the meninges.
   d. Pinch off the cerebellum (*see* Fig. 1B) and olfactory bulb from the cerebral hemispheres (*see* Fig. 1C, D, Chapter 9) using the Irex forceps.

2.5. Dissection of the Neopallium

1. Place the cerebral hemisphere, ventral surface facing up (*see* Fig. 1D, Chapter 9). Scoop out the basal ganglia using the fine forceps. With the removal of the basal ganglia, a bowl-shaped hemisphere is left (*see* Fig. 1E, Chapter 9).
2. Remove the hippocampus using the Irex forceps (*see* Fig. 1E, Chapter 9). The remaining part of the hemisphere is neopallium (*see* Fig. 1F, Chapter 9).
3. Transfer each neopallium into the drops of high sucrose phosphate buffer in the center of the Petri dish.
4. Cut each neopallium into two or three fragments.

3. PREPARATION OF COLONY CULTURES

3.1. Materials

Beaker covered with 75-μm Nitex™ mesh.
Pasteur pipet, sterile, with bent tip.
Rubber bulb to fit Pasteur pipet.
Centrifuge tube, 50 mL, sterile.
Puck's balanced salt solution (BSS).
Medium, modified Eagle's Minimum Essential Medium (mMEM) containing 5% horse serum (HS), 30 mL.
Tissue culture Petri dish, sterile 100 mm.

3.2. Disaggregation of Neopallia

1. Place fragments of neopallia on top of 75 μm Nitex mesh, which is stretched over a beaker.

2. Place a few drops of growth medium over the neopallia to keep them moist.

3. Gently roll the fragments of neopallia over the mesh using the back side of a curved Pasteur pipet and, at the same time, add medium, that has been taken up in the curved Pasteur pipet. Add 5 mL medium/brain to the mesh and continue until the neopallia are completely disaggregated and the cells have passed through the mesh.

4. Remove the mesh and transfer the cells in the beaker to a centrifuge tube. Use a pipet to resuspend the cells.

5. Determine the cell number:
   a. Prepare a sample from the cell suspension for counting in a hemocytometer, using 0.05 or 0.1 mL of 0.3% Nigrosin as a viability indicator (viable cells exclude the dye) and 0.2 or 0.4 mL of cell suspension, respectively.
   b. Fill the hemocytometer and count the number of viable cells in at least four squares of one chamber.
   c. Calculate the number of viable cells/mL (*see* Chapter 16).
   Note: Usually, the brain of a newborn mouse should yield $2–3 \times 10^6$ viable cells.

3.3. Colony Cultures

1. Before plating, make sure that the cells are well-suspended. Plate 1.25×10^3 to 2.5×10^3 viable cells per cm^2.

2. It is important that the cells are randomly distributed within the culture vessel. To achieve this, place a hand flat on the culture vessel and move the vessel forward and backward several times, then the same number of times from side to side. **Never** use a circular motion, to avoid centrifugal distribution of the cells.

3. Adjust the amount of medium per dish, if necessary. (For a 35-mm dish, use 1.5 mL; 60-mL dish, 3.0 mL; 100-mL dish, 6.0 mL).

4. Incubate culture dishes in a 37°C highly humidified atmosphere, containing 5% carbon dioxide in air.

5. After 3 d of incubation, wash out cell debris and nonattached cells, using fresh prewarmed medium.

6. Incubate cultures for 10 d without disturbance.
   Note: Cultures may be incubated without medium change, because of the small cell inoculum, which does not deplete the medium of required nutrients.

4. COMMENTS

1. For colony cultures, the first 24–48 h of culturing are critical. During this time, small cell aggregates may form, especially if the inoculum is too large

or if the culture vessels are disturbed. Sometimes the vibration of the incubator fan or vibrations in the building are enough to upset the random distribution of cells. Aggregates are also more likely to form in cultures derived from young embryos than from those of older embryos or neonatal animals. Thus, it is important, that for at least the first 3 d, that the cultures should not be disturbed.

2. The number of colonies formed depends on the number of viable cells initially plated as well as on the age of the animal. A plating efficiency obtained from cells of newborn mice is higher than that obtained from those of older mice.

3. The colony cultures are much more sensitive to culture conditions than are cultures initiated from a large inoculum. It is therefore important to provide conditions under which the pH and osmolarity of the medium are as constant as possible during the culture period. pH can be maintained by careful control of the carbon dioxide in air atmosphere and bicarbonate concentrations in the medium. Providing sufficient humidity to prevent evaporation of the medium prevents changes in osmolarity.

4. The compactness of the colony can vary greatly from species to species. For example, mouse and rat glial cells form compact colonies, but human glial cells do not. We have found that the best colonies for the study of cell differentiation are produced by glia from neopallia of C_3H/HeJ mice.

5. The frequency of occurrence of colonies of various morphologies is related to the age of the donor embryo. For example, cells from mouse embryos at E16–E18 produce colonies in which the centers are formed by epithelial-type immature cells (glioblasts) and toward the periphery various stages of astroglial differentiation can be identified, i.e., proastroblasts, which are vimentin-positive and glial fibrillary acidic protein (GFAP) negative; astroblasts, which are vimentin-positive and GFAP-positive; and small stellate astroglia, which are vimentin-positive and GFAP positive and contain very little actin (Fedoroff et al., 1990).

6. Colony cultures initiated from perinatal mouse or rat brain tissue are very plastic and cell fate can be affected to an extent by the composition of the culture medium. In regular medium containing 10–15% serum, astroglial cell colonies will predominate (e.g., Fedoroff and Doering, 1980). When colony stimulating factor-1 (CSF-1) is added to this medium, the number of astroglia colonies decreases and the number of microglia colonies increases (Fedoroff et al., 1991). In serum-free medium, the number of oligodendroglia colonies will increase. The addition of platelet-derived growth factor (PDGF) to the serum-free medium will further increase the number of oligodendroglial colonies (e.g., Noble et al., 1988).

7. To obtain clearly defined colonies that do not overlap and a sufficient number of colonies per dish to permit quantification, it is advisable to use 100-mm tissue culture dishes. In 100-mm dishes, as many as 300–400 good-sized colonies can form without overlapping.

8. In our experience, approx 20–25% of colonies form from single cells. The other colonies form from more than one cell. Therefore, colony is not equivalent to clone, unless it is proven that the colony began from a single cell. To obtain clonal cultures, one colony must be picked up from the culture dish, the cells disaggregated, and these cells used to initiate another colony culture. If this procedure is then repeated several times, there is a high probability that the colonies that eventually form are real clones.

9. When colonies are to be grown on coverslips (*see* Section 6.4.) for immunocytochemical studies, it is advisable to use round coverslips placed in nontissue culture Petri dishes. These dishes have hydrophobic surfaces, thus ensuring that the growth of the cells will be limited to the coverslips.

10. In general, it is very difficult to grow single cells or a very small number of cells in culture vessels. To do this, a feeder layer is needed. A feeder layer consists of cells from a cell line that have been irradiated to arrest cell proliferation. Cells of the STO cell line (mouse embryonic fibroblasts) are commonly used as a feeder layer. Irradiated STO cells can be obtained from the American Type Culture Collection (Rockville, MD), catalog number CRL-1503. Another method, although less satisfactory, is the use of transwell cultures, in which a large population of cells is separated from a single cell compartment by a membrane with a pore size permeable to medium only. A disadvantage of this method is that cell-to-cell contact, which in many cases is important for cell differentiation, is lacking.

5. PLATING EFFICIENCY ASSAY

The plating efficiency of a given cell population provides a convenient way to estimate the number of viable cells present (colony number) and their proliferative potential (colony size) and is therefore an excellent assay for cytotoxic and growth factors.

Cells in graded dilutions are plated in dishes and cultured for a specific time, depending on the cell type and their population doubling time. The cells are plated in numbers small enough that viable cells can attach to the substratum as single cells and form discrete colonies. The colony cultures are stained at specified times and the colonies counted and sized manually or by using an automatic colony counter.

Plating efficiency is the percentage of individual cells from the inoculum, which gives rise to cell colonies when inoculated into culture vessels.

The total number of cells in the inoculum, type of culture vessel, and the environmental conditions (medium, temperature, closed or open system, carbon dioxide atmosphere, (and so on) used in the assay should always be stated, when reporting plating efficiency.

5.1. Determination of Plating Efficiency

1. Materials:

    Single cell suspension from neopallium of newborn mice (*see* Section 1.–3.2.)

    Tissue culture dishes, 60 mm, sterile

    Modified Eagle's Minimum Essential Medium (mMEM) supplemented with 5% horse serum

2. Procedure:

    a. Plate cells into five tissue culture dishes, one each of 0.5, 1, 2, 4, and 8×10^4 viable cells/60 mm dish.

    b. Incubate the cultures at 37°C in a highly humidified atmosphere of 5% carbon dioxide in air.

    c. After 2–3 d of incubation, wash cultures with prewarmed medium and replace medium. Thereafter, do not feed cultures.

    d. After 10–12 d of incubation, fix and stain cultures using Coomassie brilliant blue (*see* Section 5.2.).

    e. Count and size colonies using an automatic colony counter (*see* Section 5.5.). It is also possible to count colonies manually and size them by microscopic examination.

5.2. Fixation and Staining of Colony Cultures

1. Materials:

    Hanks' BSS

    Absolute methanol (–20°C)

    Distilled water

    0.25% Coomassie brilliant blue R-250 (C.I. 42660)

2. Fixation of Colony Cultures: Wash the cultures three times with Hanks' BSS and fix with absolute methanol at –20°C for 10 min. (Cells may be left overnight at this point at room temperature, with sufficient methanol to allow for evaporation without the cells becoming dry.)

3. Staining the cultures:

    a. Dilute the methanol in the culture dish with distilled water.

    b. Decant and add distilled water.

    c. Decant the water, add 0.25% Coomassie brilliant blue R-250, and stain for 1–2 min.

    d. Decant the stain and wash the cultures in tap water.

    e. Dry the cultures in air.

Note: If cultures are stained too dark they can be destained by washing with methyl alcohol. If the stain is not dark enough, the staining procedure can be repeated (repeat step 3).

5.3. Calculation of Plating Efficiency (PE)

$$PE\ (\%) = (number\ of\ colonies\ counted\ per\ culture)/$$
$$(number\ of\ viable\ cells\ plated\ per\ culture) \times 100 \qquad (1)$$

5.4. Comments

1. The plating efficiency for primary cultures and cell lines may be determined by the method given. The number of cells that attach and form discrete colonies is different for each cell type, and plating efficiency for different cell types may vary from nearly zero to nearly 100%. A cell type with a high plating efficiency will require plating of a lower concentration of cells to achieve discrete colonies than a cell type with a low plating efficiency. To determine the best concentrations for use for either colony cultures or plating efficiency assays, a wide range of concentrations of cells should be plated initially.

2. To determine the plating efficiency, it is important to plate a graded number of cells. Theoretically, the plating efficiency for each concentration of cells plated should be the same, as illustrated by the following example:

Number of viable cells plated $\times 10^{-4}$	Number of colonies formed	Plating efficiency
2.0	200	1%
1.0	100	1%
0.5	50	1%

However, if the concentration of cells is too low for the culture vessel, the cells may not exert their conditioning effect and an erroneously low plating efficiency may result. If the concentration of cells is too high for the culture vessel, colonies may overlap, which may also result in a low plating efficiency.

5.5. The Automatic Colony Counter

The automatic cell/colony counter (e.g., Artek, Imaging Products, Chantilly, VA) is a highly sensitive video scanning instrument that counts and sizes micro- and macrosize objects. In cell/colony counting, accuracy depends on the ability to see colonies distinctly, whether by eye or electronically. In both methods, it is advantageous to employ plating procedures that enhance the visibility of colonies, that is, a uniform distribution, distinct morphology, and good contrast. In manual colony counting, statistical reliability decreases with time and operator fatigue. These variables are overcome in automatic colony counting. In general, 50–200 colonies/60 mm plate is the most accurate range when comparing manual and automatic counts. The automatic counts tend to be slightly lower than the manual, however, because of masking of colonies around the periphery of the plate and overlapping or clustered colonies that are not fully counted. A single percentage calibration factor determined experimentally can provide machine counts that will correlate well with precise manual counts.

6. APPENDIX

6.1. Solutions

1. Medium: Eagle's minimum essential medium (MEM) is modified to contain a fourfold concentration of vitamins, a double concentration of amino acids except glutamine, and 7.5 mM glucose (Gibco 90-5175). Before using the modified MEM for culturing, 5.2 mL of 1M sodium bicarbonate and 2.5 mL of 200 mM glutamine are added to 200 mL mMEM and the pH adjusted to 7.2 by bubbling 5% carbon dioxide into the medium. The prepared modified MEM is supplemented with 5% HS.

2. High sucrose phosphate buffer: This maintenance medium is for freshly dissected parts of the brain. It contains physiological ion concentrations (Na$^+$ and K$^+$), some buffering action, and an energy source. Sucrose is the best compound for adjustment of osmolality, because it is neither taken up by the cells nor extracellularly degraded. It consists of:

NaCl	8.00 g/L
KCl	0.40 g/L
Na$_2$HPO$_4$	0.024 g/L
KH$_2$PO$_4$	0.03 g/L
Glucose	0.90 g/L
Sucrose	20.0 g/L

   a. Dissolve chemicals in 1 L of high quality distilled water.
   b. Sterilize by filtration through a 0.2-μm filter, aliquot, and store at 4°C.

3. Coomassie Brilliant Blue, 0.25%:

Coomassie Brilliant Blue R-250	1.1 g
Absolute methanol	200.0 mL
Glacial acetic acid	40.0 mL
Triple-distilled water	200.0 mL

   Filter the stain through Whatman paper into amber-colored bottles. Store tightly sealed at 4°C.

6.2. Nitex Mesh-Covered Beakers

See Chapter 8, Section 5.2. for suppliers of Nitex mesh and for the preparation of Nitex mesh-covered beakers.

6.3. Wax Dishes

See Chapter 9, Section 4.4., for preparation and sterilization of wax dissecting dishes.

6.4. Preparation of Coverslips

The composition of glass is important for the attachment of neural cells. Manufacturers may change the composition of glass without any notice. We have found that coverslips made from German glass are consistently satisfactory.

1. Metso (Sodium Metasilicate): Dissolve 40 g Calgon and 360 g Metso in 3785 mL distilled water. Let stand overnight. Filter.
2. Using forceps, place coverslips in staining rack (cradle) (Arthur H. Thomas, staining rack #8542-E40)
3. Add filled rack to a boiling mixture of 20 mL stock Metso/1000 mL highly purified water. Boil for 20 min.

Note: Glass boiling beads (marbles) should be added to the boiling mixture prior to adding the rack of coverslips.

4. Remove rack from the hot soapy solution. Immediately rinse it through two changes of tap water, two changes of distilled water, and two changes of highly purified water. Each change of water should contain 500–1000 mL.
5. Dry coverslips in a drying oven.
6. When completely dry, place coverslips in glass Petri dishes and sterilize in a preheated oven at 375°C for 3 hs.

FURTHER READING

Brunette, D. M., Melcher, A. H., and Moe, H. K. (1976), Culture and origin of epithelium-like and fibroblast-like cells from porcine peridontal ligament explants and cell suspensions. *Archiv. Oral Biol.* **21,** 393–400.

Cannow, T. B., Barbarese, E., and Carson, J. H. (1991), Diversification of glial lineages: a novel method to clone brain cells in vitro on nitrocellulose substratum. *Glia* **4,** 256–268.

Fedoroff, S. (1984), A method for the study of neural cell lineages based on colony culture and transplantation of cultured cells into the CNS, in *Developmental Neuroscience: Physiological, Pharmacological and Clinical Aspects*, Caciagle, F., Giacobini, E., Paoletti, R., eds., Elsevier, Amsterdam, pp. 373–376.

Fedoroff, S., Ahmed, I., and Wang, E. (1990), The relationship of expression of statin, the nuclear protein of nonproliferating cells, to the differentiation and cell cycle of astroglia in cultures and *in situ. J. Neurosci. Res.* **26,** 1–15.

Fedoroff, S. and Doering, L. C. (1980), Colony culture of neural cells as a method for the study of cell lineages in the developing CNS: the astrocyte cell lineage. *Curr. Topics Dev. Biol.* **16,** 283–304.

Ham, R. G. (1972), Cloning of mammalian cells. *Methods Cell Physiol.* **5,** 37–74.

Labourdette, G. and Sensenbrenner, M. (1995), Growth factors and their receptors in the central nervous system, in *Neuroglia*, Kettenman, H. and Ransom, B. R., eds., Oxford University Press, New York, pp. 441–459.

Loret, C. Sensenbrenner, M., and Labourdette, G. (1989), Differential phenotypic expression induced in cultured rat astroblasts by acidic fibroflast growth factor, epidermal growth factor and thrombin. *J. Biol. Chem.* **264,** 8319–8327.

Miller, R. H. and Szigeti, B. (1991), Clonal analysis of astrocyte diversity in neonatal rat spinal cord cultures. *Devel.* **113,**353–362.

Moore, S. C., McCormack, J. M., Armendariz, E., Gatewood, J., and Walker, W. S. (1992), Phenotypes and alloantigen-presenting activity of individual clones of microglia derived from the mouse brain. *J. Neuroimmunol.* **41,**203–214.

Noble, M., Murray, K., Schoobaut, P., Waterfield, M. D., and Riddle, P. (1988), Platelet-derived growth factor promotes division and motility and inhibits premature differentiation of the oligodendrocyte/type-2 astrocyte progenitor cell. *Nature* **333,** 560–562.

Puck, T. T., Marcus, P. I., and Cieciura, S. J. (1956), Clonal growth of mammalian cells *in vitro*: growth characteristics of colonies from single HeLa cells with and without a "feeder" layer. *J. Exp. Med.* **103,** 273–284.

Skoff, R. P. and Knapp, P. E. (1995), The origin and lineage of macroglial cells, in *Neuroglia*, Kettenmann, H. and Ransom, B. R., eds., Oxford University Press, New York, pp. 135–148.

Temple, S. (1989), Division and differentiation of isolated CNS blast cells in microculture. *Nature* **340,** 471–473.

Temple, S. and Raff, M. C. (1985), Differentiation of a bipotential glial progenitor cell in single cell microculture. *Nature* **313,** 223–225.

Temple, S. and Raff, M. C. (1986), Clonal analysis of oligodendrocyte development in culture: evidence for a developmental clock that counts cell divisions. *Cell* **44,** 773–779.

Chapter Thirteen

Herpes Simplex Virus Vectors for Gene Therapy of the Nervous System

Angela P. Dyer and Frank Tufaro

1. INTRODUCTION

The basic idea of gene transfer arose in the late 1950s, after the discovery that viruses have an intrinsic capability to transfer their genetic material into infected cells. By this mechanism, some viruses, such as retroviruses, are able to establish life-long expression of a foreign gene in cells of diverse origins. Unfortunately, it is not possible to infect nondividing cells with retroviruses. This has led to the development of nontoxic mutants of other viruses, such as adenovirus and herpesvirus, to infect other cell types, such as neurons, which are refractory to infection by retroviruses.

Two general strategies are used to construct HSV vectors. In the first, the gene of interest is inserted into the genome of the vector, either wild-type virus or, more often, virus with deletions in genes either essential or nonessential for viral replication and growth. The second strategy uses HSV helper virus to package an HSV amplicon. An amplicon is a plasmid that contains the gene of interest, the HSV replication origin and the HSV packaging signal ("a" sequence). Amplicon DNA is transfected into animal cells followed by infection with helper virus (Protocol A). Alternatively, helper virus and amplicon DNA can be cotransfected into cells (Protocol B). Helper virus directs the replication of amplicon and the packaging of amplicon

Protocols for Neural Cell Culture, 2nd Ed. • Eds.: S. Fedoroff and A. Richardson • Humana Press, Inc., Totowa, NJ

concatemers into viral capsids. Helper virus particles are also generated. To reduce toxicity associated with helper virus, helper virus is typically replication-defective and, accordingly, transfections and infections are conducted using a cell line that expresses a viral gene product that complements the defect in the virus. A limitation of this strategy is that amplicon stocks may contain a high ratio of helper to amplicon virus. Passaging packaged stocks on fresh cells can, however, improve the yield of packaged amplicon particles (Wu et al., 1995). It is our experience that two passages of the original amplicon stock can increase infectious amplicon titer.

Procedures for working with herpes simplex viruses are described below. Remember that **HSV is a human pathogen. Exercise care at all times.**

2. GENERATION OF INFECTIOUS HSV AMPLICON PARTICLES

There are several different protocols for transfecting DNA into animal cells, including DEAE-dextran, calcium phosphate, cationic liposomes, and electroporation. The efficiency of transfection, using any one of these methods, will vary for different cell types. Our laboratory routinely uses Lipofectin® Reagent (Gibco-BRL [Gaithersburg, MD], 18292-011) for DNA transfections.

2.1. Protocol A: Transfection of Amplicon DNA

1. Materials:
   Lipofectin reagent.
   Tissue culture dishes, 100 mm round.
   Dulbecco Modified Eagle Medium (DMEM, Gibco-BRL 12800), serum free, antibiotic-free.
   Host cells: mouse L cells, BHK, COS, Vero, or any transfectable cell line can be used HSV-1 helper virus stock.
   Pipets, sterile: 1, 5, 10 mL.
   Fetal bovine serum (FBS).
   Tubes, sterile, plastic, capped.
2. Method:
   a. Seed host cells into 100-mm dishes 1 d prior to experiment (use DMEM with 10% FBS). Cells should be about 70–80% confluent after 24 h.
   b. The following solutions are prepared in separate tubes:
   Solution A: 5–50 µg amplicon DNA in 600 µL serum-free, antibiotic-free DMEM.
   Solution B: 65 µL Lipofectin Reagent in 600 µL serum-free, antibiotic-free DMEM.
   Note: Adjust reagent volumes accordingly if different-sized cell culture dishes are to be used.

c. Mix equal volumes of solution A and B and let sit for 15–45 min at room temperature. This is the DNA-Lipofectin® mix.

d. Rinse cell monolayer with 5 mL serum-free, antibiotic-free DMEM. Repeat once.

e. Remove serum-free, antibiotic-free DMEM from cell monolayer. Add 4.8 mL serum-free, antibiotic-free DMEM to the DNA-Lipofectin mix. Mix gently and add this solution to the cell monolayer.

f. Incubate for 6 h at 37°C.

g. After 6 h, add 6 mL antibiotic-free DMEM containing 10% FBS.

h. After 24 h, examine cells. If cells are losing adherence to the dish, replace media with fresh DMEM containing 10% FBS.

i. 48 h posttransfection, infect cells with HSV-1 helper virus stock at a multiplicity of infection (MOI) of 0.1 (MOI = 0.1 PFU/cell) (*see* Section 6.).

j. Let infection proceed for 2 d and then harvest the virus (*see* Section 3.).

2.2. Protocol B: Packaging Amplicons by Transfection of Viral and Amplicon DNA

This protocol is modified so that HSV DNA is transfected into the cells along with the amplicon plasmid DNA. This ensures that only those cells containing amplicons will package virus, and reduces the amount of unwanted helper virus particles produced.

1. Materials:
   Flasks, 175 cm², sterile for tissue culture.
   Tissue culture dishes, 60 mm, sterile.
   Host cell line: mouse L cells, BHK cells, COS cells, Vero cells, or other transfectable cell line.
   HSV-1 helper virus stock.
   Proteinase K (Gibco-BRL 25530-031).
   Cell scraper or rubber policeman.
   Flame-sealed Pasteur pipet.
   Lipofectin reagent.
   Phosphate-buffered saline (PBS).
   Lysis buffer (15 mL).
   Lysis buffer with proteinase K and sodium dodecyl sulfate (SDS) (Lysis K-SDS) (15 mL).
   Phenol:chloroform:isoamyl alcohol (50:48:2) (60 mL).
   Chloroform (45 mL).
   Isopropanol, ice-cold (30 mL).
   Tris EDTA buffer, pH 7.4.

2. Isolation of HSV DNA from infected cells:
   a. Seed 800 mL T-flasks with cells 24 h prior to infection. Grow cells in DMEM, 10% FBS, to approx 80% confluence.

b. Infect cells with helper virus stock at MOI = 3, so that each cell is infected with three infectious virus particles.

c. When the majority of cells are round (24–48 h), scrape cells into the growth medium using a rubber policeman or disposable, plastic cell scraper.

d. Centrifuge cells at $1500g$ for 10 min at 4°C to pellet infected cells. Discard supernatant into bleach.

e. Rinse cells once with PBS. Centrifuge as before to pellet cells. Discard supernatant.

f. Rinse cells once with lysis buffer.

g. Lyse cells by addition of 15 mL Lysis K-SDS buffer. Gently rock tube for 5 min. Incubate in 37–50° waterbath for at least 2–4 h or overnight.

h. **Gently** extract the lysate three times with phenol:chloroform:isoamyl alcohol (50:48:2). To do this, add an equal volume of phenol:chloroform:isoamyl alcohol, shake gently for a minute or so, and centrifuge at >10,000g for 5 min. Remove the aqueous phase (upper phase) to a new tube. After three extractions, there should be no remaining interphase between the upper aqueous and lower organic phase. If an interphase persists, continue extractions.

i. Gently extract the aqueous phase three times with an equal volume of chloroform. Remove the aqueous phase to a new tube each time.

j. Precipitate DNA by adding 2 vol of ice-cold isopropanol to the aqueous solution containing the DNA. Spool the precipitated DNA out of solution using a flame-sealed Pasteur pipet and allow to dry. Resuspend the DNA in Tris EDTA buffer, pH 7.4. DNA isolated in this manner is infectious, i.e., it will direct the synthesis of new HSV particles after the DNA is transfected into suitable host cells.

3. Cotransfection of HSV and amplicon DNA:

a. Seed cells to be transfected into a 60-mm dish 24 h prior to transfection (use DMEM with 10% FBS). Grow to 70–80% confluence.

b. Place 5 µg DNA (4 µg viral HSV DNA obtained from Section 2.2., step 2, 1 µg amplicon DNA in 50 µL or less) into a plastic tube. If a 100 mm dish is used, reagents are increased by threefold; if 35-mm dishes are used, reagents are decreased by threefold.

c. Add an equal volume of chloroform to the DNA. Shake the mixture gently and centrifuge the chloroform to the bottom of the tube. Remove the aqueous phase containing the DNA to a new tube. This procedure sterilizes the DNA prior to transfection.

d. Prepare the following two solutions:
Sterile DNA in 300 µL of serum-free, antibiotic-free DMEM.
10 µL Lipofectin reagent in 300 µL serum-free, antibiotic-free DMEM.

e. Mix the two solutions and incubate at room temperature for 10–15 min. This is the DNA/Lipofectin mix.

f. Rinse the cell monolayer to be transfected with 5 mL serum-free, antibiotic-free DMEM. Remove the medium from the cells.

g. Add 2.4 mL serum-free, antibiotic-free DMEM to the DNA/Lipofectin solution. Mix gently and add the entire volume to cell monolayer.

h. Incubate cells for 18 h at 37°C.

i. Replace media with DMEM containing 10% FBS.

j. Small plaques, or zones of dead cells, should appear in 2–3 d. When most of the cells round up, but before they detach from the dish, the viral stock should be harvested as described below.

3. HARVESTING VIRUS STOCK

3.1. Materials

1–2 mL freezing vials.
Cell scraper or rubber policeman.
PBS and disposable plastic centrifuge tubes.

3.2. Procedure for the Harvest and Storage of Virus Stock

At 48 h postinfection with HSV, most cells will be round in appearance. At this point the viral stock can be harvested as follows.

1. Scrape cells off the dish with a rubber policeman or a disposable cell scraper. Collect growth medium and cells in one disposable centrifuge tube.

2. Freeze cells at –70°C and thaw at 37°C. Repeat once. This will allow for the release of cell-associated virus into the growth medium.

3. Centrifuge cells at about 1500g for 10 min to pellet cell debris. Collect supernatant. This is your virus stock. Virus should be stored at –70°C or below in 1 mL aliquots in cryovials or other suitable containers. When needed, thaw by placing the vial in a waterbath at 37°C. The virus is stable at 37°C for several hours.

4. PRODUCING VIRAL STOCKS/PASSAGING PACKAGED AMPLICON STOCK

4.1. Materials

Host cell line: mouse L cells, COS cells, Vero cells.
Tissue culture dishes, 100 mm, sterile.
DMEM, 10% FBS.
Viral stock.

4.2. Procedure for Generating Viral Stocks

1. Distribute cells into 100-mm dishes 24 h prior to infection. They should be approx 80–90% confluent by the next day.
2. The next day, remove the growth medium from the cell monolayer to be infected.
3. Infect cells by adding 100 μL viral stock onto the monolayer. Incubate the cells for 1 h at 37°C, rocking the dish every 5–10 min to prevent the cells from drying.
4. Harvest new stock as described previously by scraping the cells into the medium, followed by freeze-thaw cycles and centrifugation. Store virus stocks in 1 mL aliquots at −70°C or colder.

5. PREPARATION OF PURIFIED VIRUS

This procedure allows for the purification and concentration of virus stocks. This may be required to ensure the delivery of adequate amounts of virus to infect tissues.

5.1. Materials

Sucrose.
Phosphate-buffered saline (PBS).
Disposable centrifuge tubes.
Tris buffer.
NaCl.

5.2. Preparation of Virus Stocks

1. Prepare a 30% (w/w) sucrose solution in PBS or a low-molarity (<50 mM) Tris buffer, pH 7.8, containing 50 mM NaCl. Chill on ice.
2. Chill virus stock on ice.
3. Gently layer the virus stock onto a 1.5 mL cushion of 30% sucrose in an ultracentrifuge tube. Centrifuge for 2–3 h at 134,000g, 4°C (SW 41 rotor). Following centrifugation, remove the supernatant, while being careful not to lose the virus pellet at the bottom of the tube.
4. Add 100 μL cold PBS or a low molarity Tris buffer, pH 7.8, containing 50 mM NaCl to the tube to cover the pellet. Do not attempt to resuspend the pellet at this time.
5. Store virus overnight at 4°C. Gently mix to dissolve pellet and transfer to cryotubes for storage at −70°C. If additional purity is desired, the virus suspension can be layered over a 30 mL continuous gradient of 5–45% sucrose in the same buffer and centrifuged (134,000g) for 1 h. Virus will appear as a white band in the gradient.

6. DETERMINATION OF VIRUS TITER

Using this method, it is possible to determine the number of infectious particles in a virus stock. Virus stocks always contain a mixture of infectious and noninfectious particles, and the ratio of the two types of particles may alter the usefulness of the virus stock. The ratio of total particles to the number of infectious particles (PFU = plaque forming unit) is called the particle/PFU ratio. Although it is rarely necessary to do so, the number of particles can be determined by counting negatively stained particles in the electron microscope. The number of PFU/mL (the titer) is a more important determinant of the usefulness of a virus stock.

The virus titer is determined by infecting monolayers of host cells with diluted virus, so that relatively few cells are infected. Infected cells are detected by allowing virus to spread to adjacent cells to form a plaque. A plaque is usually a clear zone or a zone of dead cells amid the monolayer of healthy cells. To prevent virus from forming satellite plaques in the monolayer, the monolayer is normally overlayered with 0.8% agarose (2X agarose is combined with 2X DMEM/FBS, which is then used to overlay the culture).

A good alternative when working with herpes simplex virus is to overlay the cultures with 0.1% pooled human IgG. Pooled human IgG contains anti-HSV antibodies, that inactivate virus particles as soon as they are released from infected cells. Plaques can still form because most viruses, including HSV, can spread to adjacent cells by direct cell-to-cell contact. This type of spread is not inhibited by antibodies.

6.1. MATERIALS

Host cell monolayers in 6-well tissue culture dishes or in flasks.
Snap-cap tubes, disposable, sterile (15 mL).
DMEM/FBS growth medium (10% FBS).
PBS.
DMEM with 4% FBS and 0.1% pooled human IgG (ICN Biomedicals, 823102) plaquing medium.
Virus stock to be tested.
Pasteur pipets.
1-mL sterile plastic pipets.
10-mL sterile plastic pipets.
Bleach container.
Ethanol, 70%.
Latex gloves.
5% Methylene blue in 70% methanol.

6.2. Preparation of Virus Inoculum

1. Put on latex gloves. Rinse work area in hood with 70% ethanol.

2. Immerse virus stock in a 37°C bath to quickly thaw the virus.
3. Remove the vial from the bath and rinse with 70% ethanol.
4. Open the vial in the hood and remove 1 mL to a 15-mL Snap-Cap tube. Label this tube A. Discard the virus stock vial in the bleach container.
5. Put 900 μL of DMEM into each of two sterile tubes. Label the tubes B and C.
6. Transfer 100 μL virus from tube A into tube B to make a 10-fold dilution.
7. Transfer 100 μL virus from tube B into tube C. Continue making serial dilutions in the same manner. Because the titer of HSV-1 rarely exceeds 10^9 PFU/mL, six serial 10-fold dilutions are usually adequate to obtain an accurate titer measurement.
8. Using a Pasteur pipet, remove the growth medium from each well.
9. Using a 1-mL pipet, transfer 100 μL of virus from each dilution tube into an individual cell monolayer growing in a flask or 6-well dish. Repeat this procedure for each virus dilution. Discard the pipets into the bleach container.
10. Rock the dishes every 10 min to redistribute the virus onto the monolayers. Do not let any part of the monolayer dry during this period.
11. After 60 min, remove the liquid from each well using a Pasteur pipet. Discard the pipette and liquid into bleach.
12. Rinse each well with 3 mL PBS or growth medium. Discard pipet.
13. Add DMEM/FBS/IgG plaquing medium to each well and place in a CO_2 incubator at 37°C for 3–4 d, by which time plaques will be visible.
14. After plaques develop, remove medium from the monolayers. Wash the monolayers once with PBS and cover cells with approx 2 mL methylene blue in 70% methanol. This will inactivate the virus.
Note: Sterile technique is no longer required.
15. Incubate at room temperature for 15–30 min. Pour off methylene blue stain and wash cells under tap water to remove excess stain.
Note: Wash with enough force to remove loosely adherent cells, so that they leave white spots among the uninfected blue cells. Some cell types are less adherent than others, so do not wash too hard.
16. Allow the dishes to dry. Count the plaques and determine the titer as follows:

$$\text{Titer} = \text{PFU/mL} = (\# \text{ plaques})/[\text{aliquot size } (100 \text{ μL})] \times 1000 \times \text{reciprocal of dilution factor} \qquad (1)$$

7. DETECTION OF VIRUS INFECTION

Many vector constructs contain the bacteriophage *lacZ* gene, which encodes β-galactosidase. β-galactosidase can be detected directly using a substrate or by immunohistochemical detection using an antibody. The substrate method is described below.

7.1. β-Galactosidase Assay

1. Materials:

    X-Gal (final concentration) in X-gal buffer (0.1%).

    PBS.

    Formaldehyde or paraformaldehyde in PBS (4%).

    PBS containing 1% bovine serum albumin (BSA) (fraction V; Sigma [St. Louis, MO] A3311).

    Disposable pipets (10 mL).

    Pasteur pipets.

2. Detection of β-gal activity:

    a. Remove medium from an infected cell monolayer and rinse cell monolayers with PBS.

    b. Add 4% formaldehyde in PBS to each well, so that the cells are covered. Incubate at room temperature for 5–10 min to fix cells. Sterile technique is no longer needed, because this procedure inactivates virus.

    c. Remove fixative and rinse once with PBS containing 1% BSA.

    d. Add 0.1% X-gal solution to cover the monolayer. Incubate monolayers at 37°C until blue cells appear. This can take up to 24 h, but can be visible within 1 h. Count the number of blue cells and determine the titer of blue cells/mL virus stock.

8. IMMUNOHISTOCHEMISTRY

For immunohistochemistry, following fixation, cells should be permeabilized by incubating the cell monolayers with 0.02% Triton X-100 for 3 min at room temperature. The monolayers should be rinsed with copious amounts of PBS containing 1% BSA to completely remove the Triton X-100 solution. Cells can then be incubated with antibodies diluted in PBS containing 1% BSA. Antibody detection using a secondary antibody conjugated to alkaline phosphatase or horseradish peroxidase can then be performed according to the manufacturer's instructions.

9. APPENDIX

9.1. Solutions

1. Phosphate-buffered saline (PBS) 10× solution:

$Na_2HPO_4 \cdot H_2O$	14.2 g
NaCl	80 g
KCl	2 g
KH_2PO_4	2 g

    Make up to 1 L of H_2O. Dilute before use.

2. Lysis buffer: 10 mM Tris, pH 8.0, 10 mM EDTA.
3. Lysis buffer with proteinase K and SDS (Lysis K-SDS): Add 0.25 mg/mL protein-ase K (Gibco-BRL #25530-031) and 0.6% sodium dodecyl sulfate to lysis buffer.
4. Tris-EDTA buffer:
   a. 1M Tris buffer, pH 7.4: Dissolve 121.1 g Tris base in 800 mL H$_2$O. Adjust the pH to 7.4 by adding 70 mL of concentrated HCl and sterilize by auto-claving.
   b. 0.5M EDTA: Add 186.1 g of disodium ethylenediamine tetra-acetate · 2H$_2$O to 800 mL of H$_2$O. Adjust the pH to 8.0 with NaOH and sterilize.
   c. Tris-EDTA buffer: Mix 0.5 mL 1M Tris-HCl, pH 7.4, with 0.1 mL 0.5M EDTA. Bring the volume to 50 mL with distilled water. Final concentra-tion is 10 mM Tris, 1 mM EDTA.
5. X-gal buffer:
   Potassium ferrocyanide   10 mM
   Potassium ferricyanide   10 mM
   MgCl$_2$ 2 mM
   Dissolve in PBS.

9.2. Safe Handling of Virus

All viruses used for gene therapy, including adenovirus, herpesvirus, and retroviruses, are potentially dangerous human pathogens. Although they have been debilitated in many instances, they are capable of replicating under certain condi-tions. The following guidelines should be followed carefully to reduce the risk of acci-dental exposure.

1. Syringes with needles should be used with viruses only when absolutely nec-essary. In general, syringes should not be used in the routine transfer of virus except when animals are to be infected. Thick gloves should be worn to reduce the risk of stabs.
2. Latex gloves should be worn at all times when handling virus. Double gloves are useful so that the first pair can be removed without touching them with bare hands.
3. Bleach inactivates most enveloped viruses quickly. The bleach should be rela-tively fresh, however, and pipets and tubes containing virus should be fully immersed to inactivate all traces of virus prior to discard. Pipets can be safely removed from bleach after a day or so and discarded in biohazardous waste containers.
4. Always place a sign in the work area to indicate that human pathogens are being used.

5. If you accidentally contaminate yourself by getting liquid containing herpes-virus on your skin, wash immediately with copious amounts of warm, soapy water. This will rapidly inactivate the virus.

FURTHER READING

Friedmann, T. (1994), Gene therapy for neurological disorders. *Trends Genet.* **10,** 210–214.

Glorioso, J. C., DeLuca, N. A., and Fink, D. J. (1995), Development and application of herpes simplex virus vectors for human gene therapy. *Annu. Rev. Microbiol.* **49,** 675–710.

Chapter Fourteen

Immunostaining and Identification of Antigens

Colin J. Barnstable

1. INTRODUCTION

Tissue culture provides an opportunity to study the function of the nervous system under strictly controlled conditions. A major variable in neural tissue cultures, however, is the heterogeneity of the tissue used for the culture. Without knowing the relative proportions of neurons and glia, or the relative proportions of different subclasses of neurons, it can be difficult to interpret experimental results. Antibodies provide by far the most useful way of characterizing cells in culture. Using appropriate antibodies it is possible to determine the number of cells of a particular type in a culture, whether all of these cells have the same morphology or level of expression of antigen, and whether there is any preferential association between particular cell types. Because antibodies can be used in combination, it is possible to obtain an even more precise definition of cell type of developmental status. Although some of these measurements can be made using other methods, such as transmitter uptake, antibodies have two other important advantages. First, some antibodies can be used to compare cells in culture with those in intact tissue. Second, antibodies can frequently be used both to label cells in culture and to aid in biochemical isolation of the antigen.

A large battery of antibodies recognizing several antigens has been produced and many of these are now readily available from standard commercial sources. In

Protocols for Neural Cell Culture, 2nd Ed. • Eds.: S. Fedoroff and A. Richardson • Humana Press, Inc., Totowa, NJ

addition, the methods for producing antibodies against any cell type of interest have now become almost routine. Although the specificity and sensitivity of antibodies are ideally suited for studies of neural cells in culture, it is important to remember that:

1. Antibodies and their antigen targets are biological materials, and are very susceptible to experimental manipulations, such as temperature and fixation;
2. Antibodies have extremely specific binding sites, and the efficiency of binding can easily be perturbed by changes in conformation or posttranslational modifications, such as acetylation or phosphorylation; and
3. An antibody binds to a small structure (of the order of half dozen sugar residues or amino acids).

Thus, binding of an antibody provides information only about the availability of that particular epitope. Many potential binding sites may be masked giving less reactivity, and conversely, very similar epitopes may be shared by different molecules, which will give more widespread reactivity.

2. PREPARATION OF CULTURES FOR IMMUNOSTAINING

2.1. Materials

Wash buffer: Dulbecco's phosphate buffered saline (DPBS) (50 mL).
Fixative: 1% paraformaldehyde in DPBS (3 mL).
Blocking buffer: 5% normal goat serum in DPBS (3 mL).
Aspirator.
Pipets (5 mL).
Pasteur pipets.

2.2. Procedure

1. Gently aspirate growth medium from the culture dish by tilting the Petri dish and aspirating the medium from the edge of the plate. Gently add about 3 mL DPBS by slowly pipeting the DPBS against the side of the Petri dish.
Note: It is essential to take care at this step, because vigorous treatment will break fine neuronal processes and may even remove many cells.
2. Gently aspirate DPBS from the culture dish and gently add an additional 3 mL DPBS.
Note: It is important to remove serum proteins as much as possible.
3. Aspirate DPBS from the culture dish and add 3 mL fixative. Incubate at room temperature for 30 min.
4. Gently remove the fixative and wash three times with 3 mL DPBS.

5. Remove the DPBS and add 3 mL blocking buffer. Incubate at room temperature for 10 min.

Note: This step will inactivate any free aldehyde groups that could potentially interact nonspecifically with the antibody.

3. IMMUNOSTAINING

3.1. Materials

Primary antibody: Polyclonal antisera generally need to be diluted at least 1:100 to reduce background staining. Good antisera should work at dilutions of 1:10,000 or greater. Monoclonal antibodies can be diluted at least 1:10 if used as culture supernatant or at least 1:1000 is used as undiluted ascites fluid. All of these numbers are, of course, only very approximate and the exact dilution necessary for staining should be determined for each antibody by using a range of dilutions.

Antibody diluent: 5% normal goat serum in DPBS.

Wash buffer: DPBS.

Secondary antibody: A commercially available peroxidase conjugated antibody is used; test dilutions of the secondary antibodies should be carried out to determine the optimal concentration for use.

3,3'-Diaminobenzidine (DAB) wash buffer: 50 mM Tris-HCl, pH 7.4.

DAB solution: 0.5 mg/mL DAB in 50 mM Tris-HCl, pH 7.4.

Hydrogen peroxide: 1% solution in distilled water.

Microliter pipets.

Disposable tips.

Pipets (1 mL).

3.2. Procedure

1. Remove blocking buffer and add 0.5 mL of primary antibody at the correct dilution/35-mm Petri dish.
2. Incubate 1 h at room temperature.
3. Remove antibody and wash three times with 3 mL DPBS.
4. Remove the final wash and add 0.5 mL of secondary antibody diluted to the optimum concentration.
5. Incubate 1 h at room temperature.
6. Remove antibody and wash two times with 3 mL DPBS.
7. Wash once with DAB wash buffer.
8. Remove and add 1 mL DAB solution to which 20 µL of 1% hydrogen peroxide has been added.
9. Incubate for appropriate length of time (10–30 min) until staining is apparent, but background staining is low.

10. Remove DAB and wash once in DAB wash buffer.
11. Examine the culture under a microscope.

4. IMMUNOBLOTTING

4.1. Materials

Culture wash buffer: DPBS.

Cell lysis buffer: 0.5% (w/v) Nonidet P-40™ in distilled water.

Gel sample buffer (4X): Tris-HCl (2.5M), pH 6.8; sodium dodecyl sulfate (SDS) (8%); glycerol (40%); 2-mercaptoethanol (20%); bromophenol blue (0.01%).

Laemmli gel consisting of:
1. Resolving gel; acrylamide (10%) (from 29.2% acrylamide/0.8% *bis*-acrylamide stock); Tris-HCl (0.375M), pH 8.8; and SDS (0.1%).
2. Stacking gel; acrylamide (3%); and Tris-HCl (0.125M), pH 6.8.

Note: Acrylamide is neurotoxic and should be handled with care.

Gel running buffer: Tris-HCl (0.025M), pH 8.3; glycine (0.192M); and SDS (0.1%).

Gel stain: 0.1% Coomassie brilliant blue in methanol:water:glacial acetic acid 42:51:7 by volume.

Gel destain: methanol:water:glacial acetic acid 42:51:7 by volume.

Transfer buffer: 4 parts (0.025M Tris-HCl, pH 8.3, 0.192M glycine) plus 1 part methanol.

Blocking buffer: 5% normal goat serum in DPBS.

Immunoblot wash buffer: DPBS.

Primary antibody: as for immunostaining.

Secondary antibody: as for immunostaining.

DAB wash buffer: 50 mM Tris-HCl, pH 7.4.

DAB solution: 0.5 mg/mL DAB in 50 mM Tris-HCl, pH 7.4.

Hydrogen peroxide: 1% solution in water.

Boiling water bath.

Sponge pad.

Plastic bag sealer.

Plastic bags.

3MM filter paper (Whatman, Hillsboro, OR).

Nitrocellulose paper (HAWP-304-FO; Millipore, Bedford, MA).

4.2. Materials for SDS Polyacrylamide Gel Electrophoresis (Laemmli, 1970)

Volumes are sufficient for one gel.

1. Resolving gel: Make up one of the mixtures given in Table 1 to give the appropriate acrylamide concentration, cool on ice, degas for 5 min, add 20 μL TEMED, mix, and pour to appropriate height.

Table 1
Mixtures to Generate Resolving Gels of Different Acrylamide Percentages

	Percentage final acrylamide				
	5.0	7.5	10.0	12.5	15.0
29.2% (w/v) acrylamide/0.8% (w/v) *bis* stock	5.00	7.50	10.00	12.50	15.00
Tris-HCl (0.75M), pH 8.8	15.00	15.00	15.00	15.00	15.00
SDS (10%, w/v)	0.30	0.30	0.30	0.30	0.30
Distilled water	9.55	7.05	4.55	2.05	0
Ammonium persulfate (10%, w/v)	0.15	0.15	0.15	0.15	0.15
Total	30.00	30.00	30.00	30.00	30.45

2. Stacking gel

	mL
29.2% acryl/0.8% bis	0.80
Tris-HCl (1M) (pH 6.8)	1.00
SDS (10%)	0.08
Distilled water	6.08
Ammonium persulfate (10%)	0.04
Total	8.00

3. Cool, degas, add 12.5 µL TEMED, mix, and pour.

4.3. Procedure

1. Wash cultures several times with culture wash buffer to remove serum proteins.
2. Cultures can now be either:
   a. Scraped up into approx 150 µL cell lysis buffer, centrifuged for 2 min in a microfuge, and the supernatant taken into a fresh tube containing 50 µL 4X gel sample buffer; or
   b. Directly extracted in 160 µL gel sample buffer. Once in the buffer containing SDS, the sample can be frozen or used immediately.
3. Use a 10% acrylamide gel with a 3% stacking gel. Boil the samples and apply to the lanes of the gel, which are mounted on the gel tank with running buffer added.
4. Run the gels at constant voltage (about 45 V) overnight or at 25–40 mA constant current for about 4 h.
5. When the bromophenol blue marker is about 1 cm from the bottom of the gel, switch off the current and disassemble the gel sandwich.
6. Open the blot holder and place a sponge pad, prewetted to remove air bubbles, on one side. Place wet filter paper on top of the pad. Place the gel on filter

paper. Place prewetted nitrocellulose paper (cut to the size of the gel) on the gel. Complete the sandwich by placing another sheet of prewetted filter paper on top of the nitrocellulose filter and a sponge pad on top. Assemble the blot holder in the tank with the gel toward the cathode and the nitrocellulose paper toward the anode. The blotting can be carried out for either about 4 h at 60 V (approx 0.17 A) or at higher field strength of approx 0.75 A for 1–2 h.

7. At the end of the run, take the blot sandwich apart. Wash the nitrocellulose filter in DPBS for 5 min to remove methanol and place the gel in the stain to ensure that all the proteins have been electrophoresed onto the nitrocellulose.

8. Place the nitrocellulose in blocking buffer for 15 min to eliminate all nonspecific binding sites.

9. Cut nitrocellulose into strips as appropriate. Place strips in plastic bags with primary antibody, seal, and incubate at room temperature for 1 h.

10. Cut open the bags, take the filter strips, and wash three times in 500 mL DPBS for 5 min each.

11. Place strips in fresh bags, add secondary antibody, and seal bags. Incubate 1–2 h at room temperature.

12. Cut open the bags, take the filter strips, and wash three times in 500 mL DPBS for 5 min each.

13. Wash once in DAB wash buffer.

14. Add strip to 50 mL of DAB solution to which 1 mL of 1% hydrogen peroxide has been added.

15. Incubate until bands are clearly visible.

16. Rinse in DAB wash buffer.

17. Dry strips in air.

18. Deactivate DAB with hypochlorite solution made with commercial bleach.

5. APPENDIX

5.1. Solutions

1. Paraformaldehyde (1%): Heat paraformaldehyde in DPBS with stirring until dissolved. Cool and filter to remove the undissolved material found in almost all batches of fixative. Store at 4°C.
   Note: This procedure must be performed in a fume hood.

2. Dulbecco's phosphate-buffered saline (Dulbecco and Vogt, 1954):

$CaCl_2$	0.10 g
KCl	0.20 g
KH_2PO	0.20 g
$MgCl_2\ 6H_2O$	0.10 g
NaCl	8.00 g
$Na_2HPO_4\ 7H_2O$	2.16 g

Dissolve in 1 L distilled water.

5.2. Comments

1. Fixation: Immunostaining for cell-surface antigens can be carried out on unfixed cultures. The problem with this is that it requires very gentle handling of the cells, so that fine processes are not broken and cell bodies do not detach from the dish. One important feature for many cell types is to keep calcium in the buffers. In calcium-free media, many cell types will rapidly detach. We have successfully used 0.5 and 1% paraformaldehyde as fairly gentle fixatives for this type of staining. Higher concentrations of paraformaldehyde: Other classes of fixatives can be used such as acetone or methanol/acetic acid but these tend to give poorer preservation of cell morphology. Such fixatives are, however, good for preservation and staining of cytoskeletal antigens.

2. Detergents: For internal antigens, it is advisable to include detergents in the antibody solutions. Detergent can also be added to blocking buffers and wash buffers, but this is not essential. Various detergents can be used, but 0.05% Triton X-100 is a reasonable first choice.

3. Blocking buffers: Blocking buffers come in many variations. Because we routinely use a goat secondary antibody, we tend to prefer normal goat serum as a blocking reagent. We have used other normal sera and even bovine serum albumin with equal success. Use of buffers containing glycine is also effective at mopping up aldehyde groups from the fixative.

4. Secondary antibodies and chromogens: The procedure described uses an enzyme-coupled secondary antibody. This method has the potential advantage that the enzyme can provide an intensification step and should be more sensitive than, for example, using fluorescently conjugated secondary antibodies. In practice, this gain in sensitivity is minimal. Fluorescence should have a greatly reduced background signal because all nonabsorbed excitation light is blocked by filters, whereas the light used to detect enzyme products all passes through the sample. In addition, fluorescence methods allow the integration of signal over time. With the increasing use of confocal microscopy to detect stained cells in culture, immunofluorescence is, once again, becoming more popular. The methods used are identical to those for enzyme-coupled secondary antibodies except that the sample can be viewed directly after washing to remove unbound antibody.

   Peroxidase-conjugated secondary antibodies remain one of the easiest enzyme-coupled secondary antibodies to use because of low background and ease of generating an insoluble reaction product. The other common enzyme used in these procedures is alkaline phosphatase, which can be used with a number of commercially available substrates. For staining of cultures with peroxidase-coupled antibodies we prefer DAB because of the density of the insoluble reaction product.

Note: DAB is a possible carcinogen. Minimize contact by using gloves and mask.

5. Gel systems: For the immunoblots, I have outlined our routine lab method. Other gel systems are possible, but the Laemmli discontinuous gel system gives very good resolution. A 10% gel will give detection of protein bands of mol wt 25,000–400,000. To obtain the best resolution of particular bands, it may be necessary to adjust the acrylamide concentration between 5–15% or to use gradient gels. For large extracellular molecules, such as proteoglycans, special gel mixtures and running conditions are necessary (*see*, for example, Zaremba et al., 1990). The times and currents used to run the gels can be varied to suit the experiment. We often run the gels overnight, so that we have the next day to carry out the blotting and antibody staining. A variety of dry or semidry transfer systems are now available. These have the advantage of using much less buffer and can shorten the transfer times.

6. Immunostaining: We use a transfer buffer that consists of gel running buffer without SDS and with 20% methanol. This gives good protein transfer and effectively removes the SDS.

   Once in an aqueous buffer, immunostaining of the nitrocellulose strips is the same as staining cultures or tissue. It is necessary to provide a blocking step and adequate washes between antibodies. As well as normal sera, effective blocking can be achieved by the use of low concentrations of Tween-40 detergent (0.1%) or a 10% solution of nonfat dried milk.

   If a strong primary antibody is being used, it is essential to keep it away from other strips. We frequently use a tubulin antibody as a positive control and, without care, can find tubulin bands appearing on all the strips. When the possibility of this type of crosscontamination arises, it can be avoided by carrying out all washes of each strip in separate containers.

   Staining immunoblots with peroxidase-conjugated secondary antibodies is robust and reproducible. As well as DAB, 4-chloronaphthol can be used to give a blue stain. More sensitivity can often be obtained by using alkaline phosphatase-conjugated secondary antibodies. Recently, a number of kits have come onto the market for chemiluminescent labeling. A peroxidase secondary antibody is used, and reaction of the substrate solution with the enzyme on the bound antibody gives out light. The light emission is stable for long enough to carry out several exposures of autoradiography film. Detection of bands is at least an order of magnitude more sensitive than the colorimetric enzyme reactions.

FURTHER READING

Akagawa, K. and Barnstable, C. J. (1986), Identification and characterization of cell types in monolayer cultures of rat retina using monoclonal antibodies. *Brain Res.* **383**, 110–120.

Andrews, A. T. (1986), *Electrophoresis. Theory, Techniques, and Biochemical and Clinical Applications.* 2nd ed., Oxford University Press.

Arimatsu, U., Naegele, J. R., and Barnstable, C. J. (1987), Molecular markers of neuronal subpopulations in layers, 4, 5, and 6 of cat primary visual cortex. *J. Neurosci.* **7,** 1250–1263.

Barnstable, C. J. (1985), Monoclonal antibodies as molecular probes of the nervous system, in *Hybridoma Technology in the Biosciences and Medicine*, Springer, T., ed., Plenum, New York, pp. 269–289.

Barnstable, C. J. (1987), Immunological studies of the diversity and development of the mammalian visual system. *Immunol. Reviews* **100,** 47–78.

Childs, G. V. (1986), *Immunocytochemical Technology.* Liss, New York.

Constantine-Paton, M., Blum, A. S., Mendez-Otero, R., and Barnstable, C. J. (1986), A cell surface molecule distributed in a dorsoventral gradient in the perinatal rat retina. *Nature* **324,** 459–462.

Dulbecco, R. and Vogt, M. (1954), Plaque formation and isolation of pure lines with poliomyelitis virus. *J. Exp. Med.* **99,** 167–182.

Harlow, E. and Lane, D. (1988), *Antibodies. A Laboratory Manual.* Cold Spring Harbor Laboratory, Cold Spring Harbor, NY.

Laemmli, U. K. (1970), Cleavage of structural proteins during the assembly of the head of bacteriophage T4. *Nature* **227,** 680–685.

Towbin, H., Staehelin, T., and Gordon, J. (1979) Electrophoretic transfer of proteins from polyacrylamide gels to nitrocellulose sheets. *Proc. Natl. Acad. Sci. USA* **76,** 4350–4354.

Zaremba, S., Naegele, J. R., Barnstable, C. J., and Hockfield, S. (1990), Neuronal subsets express multiple high-molecular-weight cell-surface glycoconjugates defined by monoclonal antibodies Cat-301 and VC 1.1. *J. Neurosci.* **10,** 2985–2995.

Chapter Fifteen

Elimination of Cell Types from Mixed Neural Cell Cultures

Richard M. Devon

1. INTRODUCTION

There are primarily three strategies that can be used to isolate cells directly from body tissues and establish highly enriched neural cells in cultures of specific cell type. The first strategy involves using differential gradients to separate and purify cellular populations through centrifugal force. This procedure is well-described by Pretlow and Pretlow (1983), as well as Yong and Antel in Chapter 11. The second strategy utilizes the presence of specific cell surface antigens and established cell markers to further purify and enrich populations of neural cells, through the application of fluorescent cell sorting techniques. Use of such approaches will not be discussed further in this chapter. The third strategy employs the addition of compounds or substitution of specific nutrients to the growth media for the elimination of certain cell types from mixed cell cultures.

Although simple in principle, the elimination of different cell types is compounded by the fact that the fetal nervous system contains a plethora of different cell types, including many classes of both developing and differentiated neurons, developing neuroglia (Schwann cells, astroglia, and oligodendrocytes), ependymal cells, meningeal cells, fibroblasts, and microglia, as well as endothelial cells. The following sections highlight those procedures that produce purified cell populations initiated from pri-

Protocols for Neural Cell Culture, 2nd Ed. • Eds.: S. Fedoroff and A. Richardson • Humana Press, Inc., Totowa, NJ

mary disaggregated mixed cell cultures, along with some of the pitfalls of utilizing these techniques. It should be noted that there are several different media available, including chemically defined media, that preferentially support the growth of one cell type over another.

2. CULTURES OF NEURONS

The age at which specific populations of neurons may be available for selection for culture depends on the timing of their differentiation. It is customary to use embryonic material at a stage when neurons have differentiated and stopped their proliferation (approx E15–E16 in mouse cerebrum). However, some populations of neurons, such as cerebellar granule neurons, are still dividing postnatally. An understanding of the developmental timing of these cells is critical, therefore, in order to select the appropriate population of postmitotic differentiated cells. In establishing these cultures, there are many other cell types, as listed above, that are continuing to divide and proliferate; the task is to maintain and purify the postmitotic cells, while reducing the population of dividing cells.

2.1. Use of Antimitotics

1. A procedure that appears well-suited for selection of a neuronal cell type from a mixed culture of either peripheral nervous system (PNS) or central nervous system (CNS) material is the use of antimitotics in the culture medium. Fluorodeoxyuridine (FUdR; or cytosine arabinoside) at concentrations of 10–50 μM is toxic to those cells that are still capable of DNA synthesis, interfering with their proliferation and subsequently killing them.

2. Coupled with low-density plating (7×10^4 cells/cm^2) of cells onto appropriate adhesion substrates (see below) and maintenance with glial-conditioned media to stimulate cell proliferation, this procedure yields cleaned neuronal cultures within 2 wk. It should be recognized, however, that these antimitotics may also be toxic to some populations of neurons. Cytosine arabinoside, for instance, has been shown to be toxic to cerebellar granule neurons (Seil et al., 1992) and to parasympathetic neurons (Banker and Goslin, 1992) at concentrations as low as $10^{-8}M$, and to those neurons that are still mitotically active during the first 5 d in aggregate cultures, such as GABA-ergic neurons (Honneger and Werfflei, 1988).

3. Purity of neuronal populations can be assessed by use of antibodies to cell surface markers, such as anti-Thy 1.1 (anti-Thy 1.2 for BalbC and C57 mice), or antibodies to intracellular proteins such as anti-MAP, anti-τ, anti-neurofilament protein, or anti-neuron specific enolase, on fixed coverslip samples of the culture.

Note:

a. Once the glial cells have been eliminated by the antimitotic agent, the neurons may die unless appropriate trophic support is provided. Glial-conditioned media is often used as a source for these trophic factors.

b. This problem of lack of support leading to neuronal death is further compounded by the fact that neurons will begin to detach from the surface of tissue culture plastic (and also die), unless an appropriate substrate, such as collagen for PNS neurons or polyornithine or poly-L-lysine for CNS neurons, is provided. Polymers of the D-isomer form of these amino acids are preferred by some, since these are not subject to breakdown by proteases, which cultured cells often release. Poly-L-lysine may be toxic to certain developing neuronal populations, i.e., fetal DRG neurons.

c. Anti-Thy 1.1 also labels fibroblasts, but these can be recognized, as compared to neurons, by their spindle-shaped morphology.

2.2. Protection of Neurons

1. The use of fluorodeoxyuridine in combination with uridine results in the elimination of most nonneuronal cells within a 2 wk period. The presence of uridine in the culture medium prevents the inhibition of RNA synthesis in the nondividing neurons.

2. To achieve this, a 2 d incubation in the antimitotic-containing medium is followed by a 2 d return to regular growth medium. This routine may be repeated several times over the 2 wk period to purify the neurons of any contaminating glia or fibroblasts.

3. Nonneuronal cell proliferation may be enhanced by the introduction of conditioned media or specific growth factors (such as FGF) or serum, to produce high rates of DNA synthesis during the incubation in the antimitotic-containing medium, thereby increasing the incorporation of the antimitotic agent.

2.3. Photo-Induced Killing of Dividing Cells

In those instances in which a population of slowly dividing nonneuronal cells remains, it may be necessary to employ a photo-induced killing procedure to remove contaminating glial cells (Shine, 1989).

1. Incubation of dividing cells for 24 h in the thymidine analog 5-bromo-deoxyuridine (5-BUdR) at a concentration of $10^{-5}M$ leads to its incorporation into the DNA of the cell.

2. A second incubation of these cells, with 5-BUdR substituted DNA in their nucleus, for 2–3 h in the presence of the fluorescent dye Hoechst 33258 (at a concentration of 2.5 µg/mL), renders the cells uniquely sensitive to light.

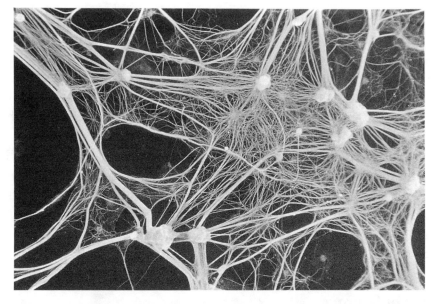

Fig. 1. Fluorescent light micrograph showing extent of neuritic growth and fasciculation between neurites in a 2-wk-old DRG neuronal culture that was purified by using photo-induced killing of dividing cells. Neurites stained with anti-neurofilament protein.

3. Exposure of the culture cells to bright or fluorescent light for 45 min, while incubating in 5% CO_2/95% air, increases the effectiveness of the method as well as the selectivity of the cells that are killed.

4. During the subsequent feeding and maintenance schedule of the purification procedure, neurons will begin to establish an elaborate and extensive network of neurites on the culture substrate (Fig. 1).

Note:

a. This technique, although rapid, should be used with caution, since 5-BUdR may also be toxic to certain neurons. The reader is encouraged to determine the appropriate conditions of photo-killing in their particular culture setup.

b. Neuronal cultures are maintained by either incomplete media changes or fed less regularly to enable the neurons to condition their culture medium and promote cell survival.

c. Care should be used in exposing the cells to the light source, to ensure that the temperature of the cultures does not exceed 37°C.

3. CULTURES OF ASTROGLIA

Complications in studying pure astroglial cultures that are derived from mixed dissociated cell cultures are that neurons, fibroblasts, oligodendrocytes, and microglia, as described in the opening paragraph, may contaminate these cultures. Astroglia, however, can proliferate both perinatally as well as postnatally in serum-containing media. These astroglia grow to confluency and can be subsequently purified through the elimination of the other contaminating cells.

3.1. Elimination of Fibroblasts

When older CNS material is trypsinized as starting material, or when the meninges are not entirely removed from the brain surface prior to disaggregation of the tissue, fibroblasts contaminate astroglial cultures (Bottenstein and Michler-Stuke, 1989).

1. Contaminating fibroblasts are best eradicated by avoiding the use of trypsin, by careful preparation of the starting material, and by plating the cells at high density.
2. Complement-mediated cell lysis employing the use of anti-Thy 1.1 antibody can also be used to specifically destroy fibroblasts, since astroglia do not exhibit the Thy 1.1 antigen recognition site on their membranes.
3. Fibroblasts can also be eradicated by the substitution of D-valine for L-valine in the culture medium (Estin and Vernadakis, 1989), since it has been demonstrated that the addition of D-valine kills fibroblasts (fibroblasts lack D-valine acid oxidase and are unable to convert D-valine into L-valine; Cholewinski et al., 1989).

Note: If the culture medium includes serum, then this must be dialyzed to remove all traces of L-valine, otherwise, fibroblasts can survive.

3.2. Elimination of Microglia

Contamination by microglial cells may present a problem in long-term astroglial cultures and becomes readily apparent when astroglial cultures are not fed regularly. Microglial cells and microglial precursor cells subsequently appear as a contaminating cell type after several weeks of growth.

1. Purification of astroglia cultures can be obtained by the addition of L-leucine methyl ester to preferentially kill the microglia (Theile and Lipsky, 1985).
2. Astroglia cultures are incubated in media containing low concentrations of L-leucine methyl ester (1, 5, 10 mM). The majority of microglia commence the formation of large vacuoles within 15–30 min of incubation and subsequently die following rupture of the cell membrane. Most microglia are killed by this procedure.
3. Reduction of microglial cell numbers can also be accomplished by inhibiting the proliferation of microglial precursor cells. These precursors require the presence of colony-stimulating factor-1 (CSF-1) in the medium. Astroglia are known to produce and secrete CSF-1 in culture (Hao et al., 1990). Therefore,

reducing CSF-1 by regular feeding of cultures (i.e., every second day) effectively limits the proliferation of microglia (*see* Chapter 9).

4. Complement-mediated cell lysis, employing the use of antibodies directed against the CR3 surface membrane receptor on microglial cells, will also remove microglial cell contamination, but not microglial progenitor cells.

5. When complement-mediated cell lysis is used to eliminate microglia, it is recommended that the procedure be done while cells are in suspension, because microglia can hide underneath the astroglia, thereby being unavailable to the antibody.

Note: Caution should be used when L-leucine methyl ester is used, since astrocyte viability and growth can also be affected at higher doses of L-leucine methyl ester (>10 m*M*).

3.3. Elimination of Oligodendrocytes and Neurons

The final possible contaminating cells for astrocyte cultures to be considered here are neurons and the other macroglial cell, the oligodendrocytes. Neurons (a minor contaminating population) and oligodendroglia are readily distinguished from astroglia in vitro, since they grow as small rounded cells supported by the underlying astroglia.

1. Many laboratories use the preferential adhesion of astroglia to tissue culture plastic to assist as an initial step in purification on initiating the cultures to limit the presence of neurons and oligodendrocytes.

2. Cells that remain attached to the astroglial layer may be easily removed from the mixed cultures by using the shaking method of McCarthy and de Vellis (1980).

3. Oligodendrocytes that remain after the shaking technique has been performed may be preferentially eliminated from these mixed cultures by growth in medium containing increased concentrations of serum.

4. If any oligodendrocytes remain, then complement-mediate cell lysis (utilizing an antibody directed against galactocerebroside in combination with exposure to complement) may be employed to selectively destroy this contaminating cell population.

3.4. Selective Media for Astroglial Purification

Astroglia do not require glucose or ketone bodies for respiration, since they possess appropriate enzymes for oxidizing fatty acids (i.e., glycogen phosphorylase, aldose reductase, and sorbitol dehydrogenase). It is possible, therefore, to selectively destroy the populations of oligodendrocytes, neurons, and microglia by growing astroglia in a glucose-free media containing both sorbitol and serum (Wiesinger et al., 1991).

1. Astroglial-rich cultures can be established by adding 25 mM sorbitol to a mixed glial culture that has previously been grown in glucose-containing media prior to switching to glucose-free media.

2. Alteration to this glucose-free media containing sorbitol can be performed 2–7 d after the mixed glial cultures are established on normal glucose-containing media.

3. Feeding the cultures for 14 d on the sorbitol-containing medium results in the establishment of an apparently homogeneous GFAP-positive population of astroglia (Wiesinger et al., 1991).

Note:

a. Cells cultured immediately in glucose-free media containing sorbitol, however, will not attach to the substratum and will die.

b. It should be stressed that even in these pure cultures, several subpopulations of astroglia may exist (for review, *see* Levison and McCarthy, 1989), depending on the age of the animal, the region chosen for obtention of the starting material, and the cell-plating density.

c. Astroglial cells that are prepared from immature brain do not mature in culture to the degree that occurs in vivo. As well, those astroglia prepared from mature brain cultures probably represent more immature forms of the adult cell type.

4. CULTURES OF OLIGODENDROCYTES

Disaggregated mixed glial cell cultures that are used as the starting material for purified oligodendrocytes cultures contain the same type of contaminating cells as listed above. In establishing purified oligodendrocytes cultures, astroglia are eliminated because of their preferential adhesion characteristics in shaking cultures, as outlined in the previous section. The cells that shake off the attached astroglia in the mixed cultures are collected and include bipotential glial progenitor cells, oligodendrocytes, neurons, and microglia cells.

4.1. Elimination of Microglia

If microglia survive in these cultures, a preadherence step can be used in the initial setting up of the cultures to facilitate the attachment of suspended microglia prior to establishing the oligodendrocyte cultures.

1. Microglia are very adhesive cells and will generally adhere to tissue culture substrata within a half hour, leaving oligodendrocytes suspended in the medium. The preadherence step will remove the majority of microglia; however, it is not always 100% effective.

2. The reduction of CSF-1 by frequent feeding of the cultures, as previously outlined in the section on astroglia, will control the proliferation of any remaining microglia and their progenitor cells; the use of anti-CR3 antibody in complement-mediated cytolysis (preferably in cell suspension) will eliminate microglia.

4.2. Selective Media for Oligodendrocyte Purification

1. In studying oligodendrogliogenesis, it has become obvious that serum is to be avoided in culturing these cells, since serum contains both inducers and repressors of oligodendrocyte differentiation (Bologa et al., 1988). Also, by excluding serum from the medium, neurons and other cell populations (such as astroglia and microglia) do not survive, leaving cultures that are highly enriched with these developing oligodendroglia.

2. Bottenstein et al. (1988) have demonstrated that the addition of B104 cell-conditioned medium into serum-free media selects a population of bipotential glial progenitor cells whose progeny proliferate in this culture.

3. The bipotential glial progenitor cells, which respond dose-dependently to the B104 cell-conditioned media, generate a progeny of cells that can be identified with specific immunological markers, and that represent various developmental stages of oligodendrocytes.

4. Serum-free media have also been formulated for the selection and maintenance of mature oligodendrocytes in long-term (3–4 wk) cultures (Espinosa de los Monteros et al., 1988). The medium is a combination of equal parts of Dulbecco's Modified Eagles medium (DMEM) and Ham's F12 medium, containing supplements of insulin, sodium selenite, putrescine, and D+-galactose. It should be noted, however, that contamination by a small number (<2%) of astroglia is still evident using this selection procedure.

Note:

a. B104 cell-conditioned medium appears to inhibit the proliferation of astroglia, but may induce a more morphologically differentiated astroglial cell under these growth conditions (Alosi et al., 1988).

b. In the presence of fetal bovine serum, bipotential glial progenitor cells differentiate in culture into a GFAP-expressing process bearing astroglia.

c. Neuronal contamination is seldom a problem in these cultures, but where it does occur, care should be taken to remove these cells. When tetanus toxin alone, or when anti-tetanus toxin antibody and complement is used for this purpose, special care must be taken, because immature oligodendrocyte cells contain several gangliosides (e.g., GM_1 and GC) that can readily bind cholera toxin, leading to their subsequent demise (Fields, 1985).

d. It is possible to select a population of pro-oligodendroblasts that differentiate into antigenically identifiable oligodendrocyte progenitors and mature oligodendrocytes (Hardy and Reynolds, 1991). Recently, it has been demonstrated that these cultures of pro-oligodendroblasts can also be purified by substituting lactate for glucose in the medium (*see* Chapter 10). Growth of cells in this medium, after establishing the cultures in glucose-containing medium, results in a purified population of maturing oligodendrocytes that grow to confluency. Switching to a differentiation medium results in the oligodendrocytes expressing MBP, GalC, and other oligodendrocytic markers, characteristic to mature oligodendrocytes, within 1 wk.

5. CULTURES OF MICROGLIA

As stated above, the starting population of mixed cells contains many different cell types that need to be eradicated to obtain purified cultures of microglia. This can be achieved by utilizing the protocols to remove astroglia, oligodendrocytes, and neurons as previously outlined in this chapter.

1. Purification of microglia is accomplished by exploiting the adhesiveness of this cell type in the shaking model previously outlined. In the initial preadherence step, following removal of surface cells from the underlying astroglial cells, the microglia preferentially adhere to the tissue culture plastic within the first half hour of culture.

2. Astroglia that contaminate microglial cultures can be effectively eradicated by reduced feeding of the cultures, thereby reducing the amounts of nutrients (*see* Chapter 9). The majority of astroglial cells die because of the lack of these nutrients. At this stage, recombinant CSF-1, or medium conditioned by CSF-1-producing cells, is added to the culture medium to facilitate microglial proliferation.

Note: Tumor necrosis factor and LPS (endotoxin) inhibit microglial responsiveness to CSF-1 (Fedoroff et al., 1993).

FURTHER READING

Alosi, F., Agresti, C., D'Urso, D., and Levi, G. (1988), Differentiation of bipotential glial precursors into oligodendrocytes is promoted by the interaction with type-1 astrocytes in cerebellar cultures. *Proc. Natl. Acad. Sci. USA* **85,** 6167–6171.

Banker, G. and Goslin, K. (1992), Primary dissociated cell cultures of neural tissues, in *Culturing Nerve Cells*, Banker, G. and Goslin, K., eds., MIT, Cambridge, MA, pp. 41–74.

Bhat, S. and Silberberg, D. H. (1989), Isolation and culture of rat and mouse brain oligodendrocytes, in *A Dissection and Tissue Culture Manual of the Nervous System*, Shahar, A., de Vellis, J., Vernadakis, A., and Haber, B., eds., Liss, New York, pp. 145–147.

Bologa, L., Cole, R., Chiapelli, F., Saneto, R. P., and de Vellis, J. (1988), Serum contains both inducers and repressors of oligodendrocyte differentiation. *J. Neurosci. Res.* **20,** 182–188.

Bottenstein, J. E. and Michler-Stuke, A. (1989), Serum-free culture of dissociated neonatal rat cortical cultures, in *A Dissection and Tissue Culture Manual of the Nervous System*, Shahar, A., de Vellis, J., Vernadakis, A., and Haber, B., eds., Liss, New York, pp. 109–111.

Bottenstein, J. E., Hunter, S. F., and Seidel, M. (1988), CNS neuronal cell-line-derived factors regulate gliogenesis in neonatal rat brain cultures. *J. Neurosci. Res.* **20,** 291–303.

Cholewinski, A. J., Reid, J. C., McDermott, A. M., and Wilkin, G. P. (1989), Purification of astroglial-cell cultures from rat spinal cord: the use of D-valine to inhibit fibroblast growth. *Neurochem. Int.* **15,** 365–369.

Espinosa de los Monteros, A., Roussel, G., Neskovic, N. M., and Nussbaum, J. L. (1988), A chemically defined medium for the culture of mature oligodendrocytes. *J. Neurosci. Res.* **19,** 202–211.

Estin, C. and Vernadakis, A. (1989), Purification of glial cell cultures: medium chemical conditions for the culture of astrocytes, in *A Dissection and Tissue Culture Manual of the Nervous System*, Shahar, A., de Vellis, J., Vernadakis, A., and Haber, B., eds., Liss, New York, pp. 112–114.

Fedoroff, S., Hao, C., Ahmed, I., and Guilbert, L. J. (1993), Paracrine and autocrine signalling in regulation of microglia survival, in *Biology and Pathology of Astrocyte-Neuron Interactions*, Fedoroff, S., Juurlink, B. H. J., and Doucette, R., eds., Plenum, New York, pp. 247–261.

Fields, K. (1985), Neuronal and glial surface antigens on cells in culture, in *Cell Culture in the Neurosciences*, Bottenstein, J. E. and Sato, G., eds., Plenum, New York, pp. 45–93.

Giullian, D. and Baker, T. J. (1986), Characterization of amoeboid microglia isolated from developing mammalian brain. *J. Neurosci.* **6,** 2163–2178.

Hao, C., Richardson, A., and Fedoroff, S. (1990), Production of Colony-Stimulating Factor-1 (CSF-1) by mouse astroglia in vitro. *J. Neurosci. Res.* **27,** 314–323.

Hardy, R. and Reynolds, R., (1991), Proliferation and differentiation potential of rat forebrain oligodendroglial progenitors both in vitro and in vivo. *Development* **111,**1061–1080.

Honneger, P. and Werfflei, P. (1988), Use of aggregating cell cultures for toxicological studies. *Experientia* **44,** 817–822.

Levison, S. W. and McCarthy, K. D. (1989), Astroglia in culture, in *Culturing Nerve Cells*, Banker, G. and Goslin, K., eds., MIT Press, Cambridge, MA, pp. 309–336.

McCarthy, K. D. and de Vellis, J. (1980), Preparation of separate astroglial and oligodendroglial cell cultures from rat cerebral tissue. *J. Cell Biol.* **85,** 890–902.

Meistrich, M. L. (1983), Separation by centrifugal elutriation, in *Cell Separation: Methods and Selected Applications*, vol. II, Pretlow, T. G. II and Pretlow, T. P., eds., Academic, New York, pp. 33–62.

Owen, C. S. (1983), Magnetic cell sorting, in *Cell Separation: Methods and Selected Applications*, vol. II, Pretlow, T. G. II and Pretlow, T. P., eds., Academic, New York, pp. 127–143.

Pretlow, T. G. and Pretlow, T. P. (1983), *Cell Separation: Methods and Selected Applications*, vol. II, Academic, London.

Seil, F. J., Drake-Baumann, R., Herndon, R. M., and Leiman, A. L. (1992), Cytosine arabinoside effects in mouse cerebellar cultures in the presence of astrocytes. *Neuroscience* **51,** 149–158.

Shine, H. D. (1989), Efficient photo-induced killing of dividing cells in neural cultures with 5-bromodeoxyuridine and Hoechst dye 33258, in *A Dissection and Tissue Culture Manual of the Nervous System*, Shahar, A., de Vellis, J., Vernadakis, A., and Haber, B., eds., Liss, New York, pp. 169–171.

Thiele, D. L. and Lipsky, P. E. (1985), Modulation of human natural killer cell function by L-leucine methyl ester: monocyte-dependent depletion from human peripheral blood mononuclear cells. *J. Immunol.* **134,** 786–793.

Wiesinger, H., Schuricht, B., and Hamprecht, B. (1991), Replacement of glucose by sorbitol in growth medium causes selection of astroglial cells from heterogeneous primary cultures derived from newborn mouse brain. *Brain Res.* **550,** 69–76.

Chapter Sixteen

Quantification of Cells in Culture

Arleen Richardson and Sergey Fedoroff

1. HEMOCYTOMETRY AND DETERMINATION OF NUMBER OF VIABLE CELLS BY DYE EXCLUSION

Cell enumeration using the hemocytometer is applicable when determining the number of cells in a suspension and when the number of samples to be analyzed is relatively small. Hemocytometry is also useful for determining the proportion of singly dispersed cells in a suspension and an estimation of the frequency of viable cells.

The average error in counting cells using the hemocytometer approaches 15–20% although it may be kept as low as 5–8%. Many of the errors inherent in cell enumeration by this method caused by incorrect sampling caused by improper mixing, chambers not properly filled, cells not evenly distributed, presence of clumps of cells, or too few or too many cells in the initial sample. The optimal number of cells to be counted is 1×10^5 cells/mL.

1.1. Determination of Cell Number

1. Materials:
    Hemocytometer and coverglass.
    Test tube, capillary or Pasteur pipet.
    Serological pipets, sterile, 1 mL.
    Ethanol, 95%.
    Soft lint-free gauze or tissue.
2. Preparation for counting cells:

Protocols for Neural Cell Culture, 2nd Ed. • Eds.: S. Fedoroff and A. Richardson • Humana Press, Inc., Totowa, NJ

a. Cleaning the hemocytometer:
    i. Using a lint-free gauze or tissue, clean the surfaces of the counting chamber of the hemocytometer and the coverglass with water. Do not scratch the counting surfaces.
    ii. Repeat the cleaning using 95% ethanol. Completely dry surfaces and coverglass.
    iii. Mount the coverglass over the ruled areas of the two chambers.

b. Sample preparation and filling the hemocytometer:
    i. Mix the cell suspension thoroughly by trituration and immediately fill a capillary pipet or tip of a Pasteur pipet.
    ii. Fill the counting chambers: Place the tip of the pipet on the edge of the hemocytometer chamber, being careful not to move the coverglass, and allow the cell suspension to fill the chamber by capillary action. The rate of flow can be regulated by placing a finger over the top of the pipet A micropipet can also be used to fill the chamber. (Approximately 20 µL cell suspension is necessary to fill one chamber).
    Note: This step should be done quickly to avoid settling of the cells in the pipet, which would cause uneven distribution of cells in the hemocytometer.
    Then fill the second chamber.
    Note: Be careful not to overfill the chambers since this will cause counting errors. If the chamber is filled improperly, clean the hemocytometer and coverglass and repeat the procedure.

3. Determining the cell number (Fig. 1):
a. Using the microscope, count all cells in the four large corner squares in both counting chambers (total of eight large corner squares). In counting the cells, count those that touch the left and upper lines (if the chamber has triple outside lines, count the cells that touch the middle of the three outside lines on these two sides) and disregard those touching the right and lower lines.
b. If the counts in the two chambers differ by more than 20% of the mean, clean and refill the chamber and repeat the counts.
c. Remove the coverglass and place both the coverglass and the hemocytometer into a container of distilled water. Clean and dry the hemocytometer and coverglass.

1.2. Determination of Number of Viable Cells by Dye Exclusion

Any cell suspension will contain both live and dead cells. To prepare cell suspensions for planting cells in cultures, it is important to base dilutions on the number of viable cells in suspension rather than on the total cell number. The number of viable

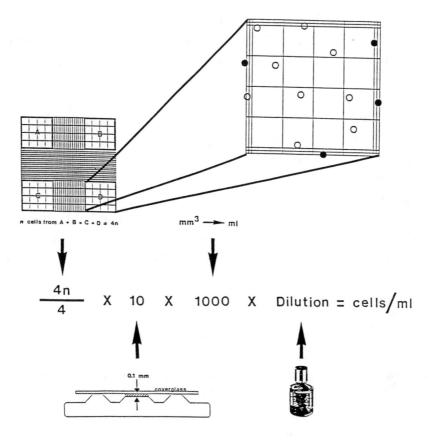

Fig. 1. Calculation of cell number by using the hemocytometer and the dye exclusion method. One large corner square of the hemocytometer is enlarged to illustrate the counting of cells. Count all cells within the area bounded by the triple lines and in addition, count the cells that touch the middle of the outer triple boundary lines on the top and on the left side (open circles). Do not count cells that touch the middle outer boundary lines on the bottom and right side of the square nor any on the other sides that do not touch the middle outer boundary line (filled circles).

cells varies depending on the age and species of the animal from which the cells were obtained, the type of tissue, and the procedure of cell disaggregation. The number of viable cells in cell suspensions prepared from cultures depends on whether the cells in the culture were in the logarithmic or stationary phase of growth.

1. Preparation for counting viable cells:
    a. In addition to the materials listed in Section 1.1., item 1, a dye, such as 0.4% trypan blue or 0.3% nigrosin, is required.
    b. Clean the hemocytometer as described in Section 1.1., item 2a.
    c. Prepare an aliquot of the cell sample for counting cells.

    i. Add 0.2 mL nigrosin followed by 0.8 mL cell suspension to a test tube. (Smaller amounts can be used but the proportion of nigrosin to cell suspension must be maintained).

    ii. Mix the contents of the tube by gentle agitation by hand. Allow to stand for a few minutes but not longer than 10 min.

      Note: If the cells remain in the dye solution too long, the cells may settle out or may be injured. Such suspensions will give wrong estimates of viable cell numbers.

    iii. Gently mix the cell suspension with the pipet and immediately fill a capillary pipet or tip of a Pasteur pipet.

    iv. Fill the counting chambers as described in Section 1.1., item 2b.

2. Using the microscope, count all unstained cells (viable cells) and all stained cells (nonviable cells) in the four large corner squares in both counting chambers (*see* Section 1.1., item 3b).

3. General comments:

    a. The determination of the number of viable cells by dye exclusion is based on the principle that living cells exclude dyes, such as trypan blue, eosin, erythrosin B or nigrosin, in colloidal suspension. When cell membranes are injured, dyes in colloidal suspension can enter the cell and bind to the proteins of the cytoplasm, thus staining the cell. Cells that stain with the dyes may, therefore, be considered dead (or of low viability).

      Not all unstained cells, however, are viable cells. If the cells have been injured severely enough so that the cytoplasmic protein leaks out of the cell (cell lysis), the cells will not stain with the dye even though they are "dead". This is especially true when cells are killed because of immunocytolytic reactions.

    b. The dye exclusion method includes as viable cells, cells that are still in the cell cycle, as well as cells that have exited from the cell cycle, i.e., nondividing but still viable cells.

    c. Another method for determining the number of viable cells in a suspension is to determine the plating efficiency of the cells. This method determines the number of cells in a suspension that can attach to a substratum and proliferate. This assay excludes viable but nondividing cells. For details of this method *see* Chapter 12.

1.3. Calculation of Cell Number

1. For each cell count (total or viable), add up the number of cells in eight large squares and divide by eight to obtain the mean number of cells in one large corner square.

2. Multiply by 10 because the mean number of cells for one large corner square (0.1 mm^3) was determined in step 1.
3. Multiply by 1000 to convert from 1 mm^3 to 1 mL.
4. Finally, multiply by the factor of cell dilution used to prepare the cell suspension (e.g., in the procedure described, the dilution factor is 10/8).
5. Equation for calculating cells/mL:

$$\textbf{Number of cells in 8 squares/8} \times \textbf{10} \times \textbf{1000} \times \textbf{10/8} = \textbf{cells/mL} \qquad (1)$$

1.4. Calculation of Frequency of Viable Cells

1. The percentage of viable cells in suspension is a good indicator of variability in the procedures used and can be compared from experiment to experiment.
2. Equation for calculating frequency of viable cells:

$$\textbf{\% of viable cells = (viable cells counted)/(total cells counted)} \times \textbf{100} \qquad (2)$$

2. ELECTRONIC CELL COUNTER

The electronic cell counter is particularly useful when a large number of samples must be counted. The procedure is fast, the counts are reproducible, and when operated properly, yield single counts with an error of no more than 10% and multiple counts with an error as low as 1–2%. In addition, some counters are capable of providing information about the size of cells. For accurate cell enumeration using the electronic cell counter, optimum instrument settings should be determined for each cell type, the aperture should be examined for blockage, the cell suspension should be examined for cell debris and cell aggregates that may be indiscriminately counted, and sampling errors resulting from improper mixing should be eliminated. The electronic cell counter cannot distinguish between viable and nonviable cells and therefore an estimate of these parameters is best done using the dye exclusion technique and hemocytometry.

2.1. Materials

Counting solution.
Palo dispensing flask.
Counting cuvet and lid.
Cell suspension.

2.2. Preparation of the Sample

1. Dispense 24.5 mL of counting solution into a clean counting cuvet using the Palo dispensing flask.

2. Mix cell suspension to be counted and immediately add 0.5 mL of the cell suspension to the cuvet containing the counting solution. Rinse the pipet three times using the counting solution in the cuvet. Place lid on the cuvet.
3. Immediately prior to counting, mix the cell suspension by inverting the cuvet several times.

Note: Avoid mixing the cell suspension too vigorously. This may cause erroneous counts because of air bubbles in the cell suspension or ruptured cells.

2.3. Operation of Counter

See operating manual supplied for the model available.

2.4. Electronic Cell Counting: General Comments

1. Principle: An aperture is placed between two platinum electrodes. An electric current flows between the electrodes and through the aperture. By applying a vacuum, cells are drawn through the aperture, which changes the resistance between the two electrodes causing a voltage pulse with a magnitude proportional to the size of the particles. These impulses are amplified and recorded on a counter. A mercury manometer, with appropriately placed electric leads, permits a sample of exactly 0.5 mL to pass through the aperture. Voltage pulses resulting from cell passage through the aperture show continuously on an oscilloscope. Interpretation of oscilloscope patterns can be of valuable assistance in determining aperture current and amplification settings, blockage of the aperture, and distribution of the cells in the sample.
2. Threshold settings:
   a. Some electronic cell counters are equipped with both an upper and a lower threshold. No particles smaller than the lower threshold settings are counted and no particles larger than the upper threshold setting are counted. This ability to count the number of particles in a certain range or window makes it possible to count the cells in several different windows and consequently, a size distribution curve can be obtained.
   b. The threshold can be determined by performing a series of electronic counts on a cell sample. Begin determinations with the aperture current switch set at 2 or 3. The series can be repeated using different aperture current settings if an increased width of plateau is required. The threshold selector should be moved by increments beginning at zero until a plateau is reached. The optimum threshold is equivalent to the center of the plateau.
3. Aperture current: The aperture current switch controls the amount of current flowing in the aperture and produces the pulses when the particles enter.

The pulses produced in the aperture are amplified according to the amplification setting. It is desirable to have the least amount of aperture current that is allowed for the particular particle being counted, and this minimum is reached when the most desirable oscilloscope pattern is seen. The pulses seen on the oscilloscope should be such that they average approximately one-half of the screen in height.

4. Counting solution: Commercially available counting solutions, such as Isoton by Coulter (Hialeah, FL), are available from many suppliers. It has been found that 0.85% saline was less adequate in counting human cells than a diluting fluid that contained a dispersing agent. However, for many cells or particles, normal saline is suitable.

3. COUNTING CELL NUCLEI IN CULTURES

Two visual methods that utilize nuclear stains to count cells in culture are described: the Feulgen stain for use with light microscopy and the Hoechst 33258 stain for use with fluorescent microscopy. The advantage of these methods is that all cell nuclei are visible and easy to count, regardless of the density of the cultures. The Hoechst stain is more cumbersome because fluorescence microscopy must be used. Its advantage, however, is that the cells can be double- or triple-immunostained in addition to the Hoechst staining, thus allowing determination of the frequency of different cell types in the culture. If the cultures are densely populated, it is possible to count only predetermined areas in the culture and then to extrapolate the number obtained to the whole culture.

3.1. Feulgen DNA Method

The Feulgen method, when used properly, is specific for DNA. The reactive aldehyde groups liberated by acid hydrolysis of the purine deoxyribose bond (but not the purine ribose bond) are stained with Schiff's reagent, resulting in DNA-containing structures being stained magenta or a red-purple color.

The specificity of the reaction may be checked by incubating sections with deoxyribonuclease. The presence of free aldehydes (which would give false-positive staining and may be blocked by treatment with sodium borohydride) may be detected by omitting the acid hydrolysis.

Two important aspects of the method are the hydrolysis time and the method of fixation. The optimal hydrolysis time, which produces the most darkly stained nuclei, should be determined, since too long a hydrolysis may completely depolymerize and extract the DNA, producing a negative result. The hydrolysis time is dependent on the fixative used on the cells. In addition, some fixatives such as glutaraldehyde may contain free unsaturated aldehyde groups and others, such as Bouin's fixative, may cause overoxidation of the nucleic acid.

The following procedure for confluent layer cell cultures uses Carnoy A as a fixative. Since this fixative contains acid, the hydrolysis time is shortened to about 90 min.

1. Materials:
   Hanks' balanced salt solution (BSS).
   Carnoy A fixative.
   5N HCl.
   Schiff reagent.
   Fast green.
   Ethanol (50%).
   Ethanol (70%).
   Ethanol (95%).
   Ethanol (100%).

2. Procedure:
   a. Wash cultures three times with Hanks' BSS. It is very important to wash cells gently, since at this time they are not fixed.
   b. Remove the last wash from the culture and incubate the culture in Carnoy A fixative for a minimum of 5 min at room temperature.
   c. Rinse in two changes of absolute ethanol, allowing 1 min in each rinse.
   d. Hydrate as follows, allowing 2 min in each solution:
      i. Ethanol (95%).
      ii. Ethanol (70%).
      iii. Ethanol (50%).
      iv. Distilled water.
   e. Hydrolyze in 5N HCl for 90 min at room temperature.
   f. Wash well in three changes of tap water, allowing 2 min in each change.
   g. Rinse for 2 min in distilled water.
   h. Stain in Schiff reagent (prewarmed to room temperature) for approx 15 min or until the nuclei are well stained.
   i. Wash well in three changes of tap water, allowing 2 min in each change.
   j. Rinse for 2 min in distilled water.
   k. Dehydrate as follows, allowing 1 min in each solution:
      i. Ethanol (70%).
      ii. Ethanol (95%).
   l. Counterstain, if desired, with fast green prepared in 95% ethanol.
   m. Remove excess fast green by rinsing with 95% ethanol.
   n. Complete dehydration by rinsing with two changes of 100% ethanol, allowing 1 min in each solution.

o. If the cells are grown on coverslips, clear in xylene and mount. If the cells are grown on plastic, air-dry the cultures and use paraffin oil to mount the coverslips.

3. Solutions:
   a. Fixative: Carnoy A: 20 mL glacial acetic acid, 60 mL absolute ethanol.
   b. 5N hydrochloric acid: Add 429.5 mL concentrated hydrochloric acid to 570.5 mL high-quality distilled water to make a total of 1000 mL.
   c. Schiff reagent:
      i. Dissolve 1 g basic fuchsin (C.I. 42510) in 200 mL boiling distilled water in a 1-L flask.
      ii. Stopper and shake for 5 min.
      iii. Cool to 50°C, filter, add 30 mL of 1N hydrochloric acid to the filtrate.
      iv. Cool to 25°C and add 3 g potassium metabisulfite.
      v. Store in the dark for 24 h. After 24 h, while shaking the solution, add small amounts of activated charcoal until the solution becomes colorless (0.1 g/200 mL).
      vi. Filter to remove the charcoal. Wrap the container of solution in aluminum foil and store in the dark at 0–4°C.

   Note: A good solution is almost colorless and any pink coloration is an indication that it has lost some of its potency, at which time it should be discarded. Schiff's reagent is stable for about 6 mo. A chemical fume hood should be used during its preparation.

   d. Fast green: 0.5 g fast green FCF (C.I. 42053), 100.0 mL ethanol (95%).

3.2. Hoechst 33258

Hoechst 33258 (Aldrich Chemical Co., Milwaukee, WI), a benzimidazole derivative, is a DNA-binding fluorochrome. The dye is readily distinguishable from fluorescein and rhodamine, and therefore, can be used in conjunction with immunocytochemistry. Hoechst 33258 exhibits fluorescent excitation at 350–365 nm and emission over 450 nm. The dye is generally nontoxic to cells, except in the presence of light when the cells have incorporated 5-bromodeoxyuridine.

1. Materials:
   Hoechst working solution of 1 µg/mL.
   Dulbecco's phosphate buffered saline (Dulbecco's PBS).
2. Method:
   a. Staining with Hoechst 33258 dye can be done by itself or in conjunction with other immunocytochemical procedures that use probes labeled with fluorescein, rhodamine, or Texas red. When used in conjunction with other procedures, use Hoechst staining as the last step.

   b. Stain cells using the Hoechst 33258 dye for 5 min at room temperature.
   c. Wash cells with PBS for 5 min. Repeat this wash twice more.
   d. Mount and observe using the fluorescent microscope with excitation filter 350–365 nm and emission filter 450 nm.
3. Solutions:
   a. Hoechst 33258 stock solution:
      i. Dissolve 1 mg Hoechst 33258 in 10 mL PBS. This stock solution of 100 µg/mL is 100 times more concentrated than the working solution.
      ii. The bottle of stock solution should be wrapped in aluminum foil and stored in the dark at 0–5°C. The solution is stable for approx 2 wk under these conditions. The stock solution may also be frozen in aliquots at −20°C. At this temperature, the stock may be stored indefinitely.
   b. Hoechst 33258 working solution: Dilute 0.1 mL Hoechst 33258 stock with 9.9 mL PBS. This gives a working solution of 1 µg/mL.

4. FLUORESCENT ASSAYS FOR DETECTION OF LIVE AND DEAD CELLS IN CULTURES

Several fluorescent probes are available for assessing frequency of live and/or dead cells in cultures. These methods are reproducible and can be used for quantification of live and dead cells together or separately.

One method to identify live cells utilizes a fluorogenic esterase substrate, calcein AM, that passively crosses the cell membrane in a near neutral form and in live cells is then converted to a membrane-impermeable green fluorescent product by intracellular esterases. There are many other esterase specific dyes, e.g., *bis*-carboxymethylcarboxyfluorescein (BCECF), fluorescein diacetate, and so forth, that vary in pH sensitivity, retention time, and wavelength. Other live cell stains are dependent on peroxidase substrates (e.g., dihydrorhodamine) and membrane potential (e.g., rhodamine 123).

Dead cells can be stained with DNA-specific fluorescent probes. In living cells, such probes are impermeable to cell membranes. When cells are injured and the membranes are disrupted, then probes can enter the cell. Commonly used DNA-specific probes are ethidium bromide and propidium iodide. Various kits for determination of live and dead cells in culture are available commercially (LIVE/DEAD® EukoLight™ Viability/Cytotoxicity Kit, Molecular Probes, Inc. Eugene, OR).

5. GROWTH ASSAYS

The following growth assays are rapid, sensitive, reproducible, avoid the use of enzymes, and make possible the processing of large numbers of cultures. A known number of cells (as a single cell suspension) are plated in multiwell culture dishes and the agent to be tested is added in progressive dilutions. The effects on growth or cytotoxicity effects can be evaluated by direct determinations in cell cultures and values obtained are read from standard curves. Precautions should be taken to avoid increased evaporation in edge wells in multiwell plates during incubation.

5.1. [³H]-Thymidine Incorporation Assay

Tritiated thymidine is incorporated into cells that are synthesizing DNA during the S-phase of the cell cycle. This assay therefore measures the degree of DNA synthesis that has occurred during the time the cells have been incubated with tritiated thymidine. The assay does not determine the number of cells present in the culture at the end of the experiment.

1. Materials:
    [³H]-thymidine solution.
    96-well plate containing cells at a suitable stage of growth.
    Cell harvester.
    Scintillation solution.
    Scintillation vials.
    Multichannel pipet.
    Absorbent glass-filter paper.
2. Procedure:
    a. Add 20 μL [³H]-thymidine solution to each well of the multiwell plate using a multichannel pipet.
    b. Incubate the multiwell plate at 37°C for 4 h.
    c. Harvesting of cells
        i. Nonadherent cells: Nonadherent cells may be harvested directly onto absorbent glass-filter paper using a cell harvester.
        ii. Adherent cells: Add 100 μL of 0.1% Triton X-100 to each well of the culture plate, gently agitate the multiwell plate for 2 min, and harvest onto absorbent glass-filter paper using a cell harvester.
    d. Dry the absorbent glass-filter paper containing the cells for 30 min in a drying oven (or air dry overnight).
    e. Cut circles containing the cells from the glass-filter paper. Place each circle of glass-filter paper into a scintillation vial.
    f. Add 1 mL liquid scintillation solution.
    g. Measure the radioactivity of each sample by using a scintillation counter.
3. [³H]-Thymidine solution:
    a. Stock solution: 1 μCi of [³H]-thymidine (New England Nuclear, Boston, MA) with a specific activity of 20 Ci/mmol.

    b. Dilute stock solution 1:19 in culture medium for use.

Note: It may be necessary to increase the amount of [³H]-thymidine when using medium that contains thymidine as a nutrient.

5.2. Neutral Red Assay

The use of neutral red is based on the principle that neutral red passes through the intact plasma membrane and becomes concentrated in the lysosomes of viable cells. The cells are then lysed and the neutral red is measured spectrophotometrically at 540 nm. The total neutral red uptake by the cells is proportional to the number of viable cells in the culture.

1. Materials:
   96-well plate containing culture to quantitate.
   Multichannel pipet reservoirs (3).
   Tips with holder.
   Multichannel pipet.
   Calcium-formaldehyde solution (25 mL).
   Acid alcohol solution (25 mL).
   Microplate reader.
2. Addition of Neutral red:
   a. Keep the 96-well plates at an angle of approx 45° and gently aspirate the medium from the cells without actually touching the bottom of the wells.

   Note: Do not remove medium from rows that serve as blank controls.

   b. Add 200 µL neutral red to each sample well.
   c. Incubate in a 37°C incubator containing a humidified atmosphere of 5% CO_2-95% air for 3 h.
3. Fixation and quantification:
   a. After the 3 h incubation, gently remove the neutral red solution from all wells. Keep the plates at an angle of approx 45° when aspirating medium.

   Note: Do not touch the bottom of the wells with the pipet when aspirating. The cells that have taken up the neutral red are very fragile.

   b. Add 200 µL of the calcium-formaldehyde solution to each well. Fix cells no longer than 2 min.

   Note: Fixation damages the lysosomes, which will result in extraction of the dye; therefore, fixation time should be kept to a minimum.

   c. Gently aspirate the fixative and add 200 µL of the acid alcohol solution to each well.

   Note: Variations in the amount of acid alcohol added will contribute to the experimental variation.

d. Mix the contents of each well by pipeting up and down using the multi-channel pipet.

e. Using a microplate reader equipped with a 540-nm filter, read the plate.

Note: A conventional spectrophotometer at a 540-nm wavelength can also be used for this assay by using larger culture dishes or by pooling the extracted supernatant.

4. Solutions for neutral red assay:

a. Neutral red (C.I. 50040):

   i. Stock Solution (0.4%): neutral red 0.4 g/100 mL ultrapure water; filter stock through a 0.2-μm filter and shield stock solution from light by covering the bottle with foil. Store at 4°C.

   ii. Working solution: Prepare a fresh dilution for each use. Make a 1:80 dilution of the neutral red stock using culture medium so that the final concentration of dye is 50 μg/mL. Incubate the diluted solution at 37°C for 8–12 h prior to use to allow fine precipitates of dye crystals to develop. Centrifuge for 5 min at 1500g or filter through a 0.2-μm filter to remove dye crystals.

b. Calcium-formaldehyde solution (1% formalin, 1% calcium chloride):

40% Formaldehyde	10 mL
10% Anhydrous calcium chloride	10 mL
Distilled water	80 mL

c. Acid alcohol solution:

Glacial acetic acid	1 mL
50% Ethanol	100 mL

Note: Acid should be added into water, **not** water into acid.

6. COLORIMETRIC ASSAYS

6.1. MTT

The MTT (3-[4,5-dimethylthiazol-2-yl]-2,5-diphenyltetrazolium bromide) colorimetric assay is based on the reduction by mitochondria of the soluble yellow tetrazolium salt to a blue insoluble formazan product. The formazan product can be measured spectrophotometrically and is directly proportional to the number of metabolically active cells in the culture. *See* Chapter 6 for the detailed procedure.

6.2. XTT

The XTT (sodium 3'-[1-[(phenylamino)-carbonyl]-3,4-tetrazolium]-*bis*(4-methoxy-6-nitro) benzene-sulfonic acid hydrate) assay is similar to the MTT assay. Both MTT and XTT are cleaved by mitochondrial dehydrogenase to produce a colored formazan derivative, that can be measured spectrophotometrically and the sensitivities of the assays are equivalent. However, the formazan derivative produced by XTT is water soluble, whereas the product produced by MTT is insoluble and requires additional steps to solubilize the formazan derivative. An XTT assay kit (Sigma [St. Louis, MO], Tox-2) and an MTS assay kit (Promega Corp., CellTiter 96™ AQueous), which is similar to XTT, are available commercially.

FURTHER READING

Bainbridge, D. R. and Macey, M. M. (1983), Hoechst 33258: a fluorescent nuclear counterstain suitable for double-labelling immunofluorescence. *J. Immunol. Methods* **62,** 193–195.

Baserga, R. (1989), Measuring parameters of growth, in *Cell Growth and Division,* Baserga, R., ed., IRL, New York.

Borenfreund, E. and Puerner, J. A. (1985a), A simple quantitative procedure using monolayer cultures for cytotoxicity assays (HTD/NR-90). *J. Tissue Culture Methods* **9,** 7–9.

Borenfreund, E., Puerner, J. A. (1985), Toxicity determined *in vitro* by morphological alterations and neutral red absorption. *Toxicol. Lett.* **24,** 119–124.

Borenfreund, E., Babich, H., Martin-Alguacil, N. (1988), Comparisons of two *in vitro* cytotoxicity assays—the neutral red (NR) and tetrazolium MTT tests. *Toxicol. In Vitro* **2,** 1–6.

Branch, D. R. and Guilbert, L. J. (1986), Practical *in vitro* assay systems for the measurement of hematopoietic growth factors. *J. Tissue Culture Methods* **10,** 101–108.

Clark, G. (1981), *Staining Procedures* 4th ed., Williams and Wilkins, Baltimore, MD.

Demalsy, P. and Callebaut, M. (1967), Plain water as a rinsing agent preferable to sulfurous acid after the Feulgen nuclear reaction. *Stain Technol.* **42,** 133–136.

De Tomasi, J. A. (1936), Improving the technic of the Feulgen stain. *Stain Technol.* **11,** 137–144.

Dulbecco, R. and Vogt, M. (1954), Plaque formation and isolation of pure cell lines with poliomyelitis viruses. *J. Exp. Med.* **99,** 167–182.

Elias, J. M., Conkling, K., and Makar, M (1972), Cold feulgen hydrolysis: its effect on displacement of tritiated thymidine. *Acta Histochem. Cytochem.* **5,** 125–131.

Hamilton, L. H. (1956), Errors in blood cell counting. 1. Technical errors. 2. Statistical errors. *Can. J. Med. Tech.* **18,** 8–14.

Hanks, J. H. and Wallace, R. E. (1958), Determination of cell viability. *Proc. Soc. Exper. Biol. Med.* **98,** 188–192.

Harris, M. (1959), Growth measurements on monolayer cultures with an electronic cell counter. *Can. Res.* **19,** 1020–1024.

Hilwig, I. and Gropp, A. (1972), Staining of constitutive heterochromatin in mammalian chromosomes with a new fluorochrome. *Exp. Cell Res.* **75,** 122–126.

Jones, K. H. and Senft, J. A. (1985), An improved method to determine cell viability by simultaneous staining with fluorescein diacetate propidium iodide. *J. Hist. Cytol.* **33,** 77–79.

Kaltenbach, J. P., Kaltenbach, M. H., and Lyons, W. B. (1958), Nigrosin as a dye for differentiating live and dead ascites cells. *Exp. Cell Res.* **15,** 112–117.

Kjellstrand, P. T. T. (1977), Temperature and acid concentration in the search for optimum Feulgen hydrolysis conditions. *J. Histochem. Cytochem.* **25,** 129–134.

Kolber, M. A., Quinones, R. R., Gress, R. E., and Henkart, P. A. (1988), Measurement of cytotoxicity by target release of the fluorescent dye bis-carboxymethyl-carbosyfluorescein (BCECF). *J. Immunol. Meth.* **108,** 225–264.

Latt, S. A. and Stetten, G. (1976), Spectral studies on 33258 Hoechst and related bisbenzimidazole dyes useful for fluorescent detection of deoxyribonucleic acid synthesis. *J. Histochem. Cytochem.* **24,** 24–33.

McLimans, W. F., Davis, E. V., Glover, F. L., and Rake, G. W. (1957), The submerged culture of mammalian cells: the spinner culture. *J. Immunol.* **79,** 428–433.

Moore, P. L., MacCoubrey, I. C., and Haugland, R. P. (1990), A rapid, pH insensitive, two color fluorescence viability (cytotoxicity) assay. *J. Cell Biol.* **111,**304 (abstract).

Mullbacher, A., Parish, C. R., and Mundy, J. P. (1984), An improved colorimetric assay for T cell cytotoxicity in vitro. *J. Immun. Methods* **68,** 205–215.

Parish, C. R., Mullbacher, A. (1983), Automated colorimetric assay for T cell cytotoxicity. *J. Immun. Methods* **58,** 225–237.

Pevzner, L. Z. (1979), *Functional Biochemistry of the Neuroglia.* Consultants Bureau, New York.

Phillips, H. J. and Andrews, R. V. (1959), Some protective solutions for tissue-cultured cells. *Exper. Cell Res.* **16,**678–682.

Phillips, H. J. and Terryberry, J. E. (1957), Counting actively metabolizing tissue cultured cells. *Exper. Cell Res.* **13,**341–347.

Roehm, N. W., Rodgers, G. H., Hatfield, S. M., and Glasebrook, A. L. (1991), An improved colorimetric assay for cell proliferation and viability utilizing the tetrazolium salt XTT. *J. Immunol. Methods* **142,**257–265.

Sanford, K. K., Earle, W. R., Evans, V. J., Walts, H. K., and Shannon, J. E. (1951), The measurement of proliferation in tissue culture by enumeration of cell nuclei. *J. Nat. Canc. Inst.* **11,**733–795.

Schrek, R. (1944), Studies *in vitro* on the physiology of normal and of cancerous cells. II. The survival and the glycolysis of cells under anaerobic conditions. *Arch. Path.* **37,** 319–327.

Thornthwaite, J. T. and Leif, R. C. (1978), A permanent cell viability assay using Alcian blue. *Stain Technology* **53,** 199–204.

Waymouth, C. (1956), A rapid quantitative hematocrit method for measuring increase in cell population of strain L (Earle) cells cultivated in serum-free nutrient solutions. *J. Nat. Canc. Inst.* **17,**305–313.

Yip, D. K. and Auersperg, N. (1972), The dye exclusion test for cell viability: persistence of differential staining following fixation. *In Vitro* **7,** 323–329.

Chapter Seventeen

Procedures for Subculturing Cells

Arleen Richardson and Sergey Fedoroff

1. INTRODUCTION

Cells attach to the culture substratum with varying degrees of adherence. Some types of cells do not adhere at all and grow as cell suspensions in the medium. Such cells are referred to as nonadhering cells (nonanchorage-dependent cells). Cells that have to attach to the substratum to proliferate are referred to as adhering cells (anchorage-dependent cells).

When cells proliferate in culture, they eventually populate the culture vessel and then must be transplanted. This process is referred to as subculturing (passaging). Sometimes it is desirable to keep cells growing logarithmically. To achieve this, it is important to know how many cells must be subcultured to a fresh culture vessel. In practice, this is referred to as "splitting," and indicates the number of new flasks of cultures that can be initiated from a culture that has become confluent. Slow-growing cell cultures are split twice, i.e., cells from one confluent culture are passed to two new cultures. Rapidly growing cell cultures may require splitting as many as six or eight times. It is convenient to arrange cell subculturing for every 7–10 d and to feed cultures every 3–4 d.

There are situations in which cells are extremely sensitive to subculturing. To propagate cells of such a line and to adapt them for subculturing may require that several flasks of cultures be combined rather than split. This will ensure that the new culture will be started with a sufficient number of cells to make it viable.

It is easy to subculture cells of nonadhering cell types, since they grow in suspension. An aliquot containing a defined number of cells may simply be used to inoculate fresh flasks filled with medium.

Protocols for Neural Cell Culture, 2nd Ed. • Eds.: S. Fedoroff and A. Richardson • Humana Press, Inc., Totowa, NJ

Subculture of adherent cells requires a number of strategies to remove the cells from the substratum with the least damage and to prepare a cell suspension for subculturing into fresh culture vessels. Two basic approaches are used: mechanical separation or chemical separation from the substratum.

2. MECHANICAL PROCEDURES

Mechanical procedures are used for lightly adherent cells and for cells that may not tolerate chemical treatment. Mechanical procedures are also used in experiments that dictate avoidance of chemical treatment.

2.1. Shaking

When the culture contains only loosely adherent cells, a portion of the medium is removed and the cells in the small volume of remaining medium are dislodged from the substratum by sharply rapping the culture vessel against the hand or by using a mechanical shaker. Creation of air bubbles or frothing of the medium should be avoided.

2.2. Washing

When the cells are not firmly attached to the substratum, they may be removed by repeated washing of the culture with medium flushed from a Pasteur pipet. Begin washing at the top of the flask and proceed toward the base, holding the flask at a slant. Avoid creating air bubbles or frothing of the medium.

2.3. Scraping

1. A soft rubber policeman may be used to remove the cells by gentle scraping. The most efficient type of rubber policeman has the end sealed flat and cut on an angle. The wing type rubber policeman will also work, but is difficult to insert in the neck of a small flask. A rubber policemen inserted onto a 45° short bend of a glass rod is particularly useful for scraping flasks and can be made to any length.
2. A number of disposable cell scrapers and lifters are available commercially. Cell scrapers usually have blades that swivel and the variable length handles are angled for easy access into flasks (Falcon, Corning-Costar). The lifters are designed to be used on cells grown in dishes (Corning-Costar).

3. CHEMICAL PROCEDURES

3.1. Versene

The disodium salt of ethylenediaminetetra-acetate (versene), in a calcium- and magnesium-free medium, may be used to chelate the calcium ions and disaggregate cells. This procedure is often used in conjunction with enzymatic digestion. It should not be used with enzymes that require calcium for activation.

Versene in the transfer solution will be quickly neutralized by the high concentration of inorganic ions present in the growth medium. Always use the lowest effective concentration of versene.

3.2. Proteolytic Enzymes

Enzymes may be used to digest the extracellular matrix proteins responsible for cell adhesion to the substratum. The enzyme most commonly used for this purpose is trypsin, since it can be easily inactivated. Crude trypsin preparations have been found to be more effective than crystalline trypsin; this has been attributed to the presence of other enzymes in the crude trypsin preparations. Crystalline trypsin, however, has been found to be less toxic and less variable from batch to batch. Crude trypsin is commonly used at concentrations of 0.025–0.05 (w/v) and crystalline trypsin at concentrations of 0.01–0.05 (w/v). The concentration of the enzyme used will depend on the characteristics of the cell, but should always be kept as low as possible. In general, the smallest possible volume and the shortest possible exposure time should be used. Temperature is also important. When possible, trypsinization should be done at 4°C. At that temperature, trypsin does not enter the cell.

Some cells are not easily dislodged from the substratum or are more sensitive to damage by trypsin. Other enzymes, such as pronase, dispase, and collagenase, or a combination of the two, may be used. These enzymes require the activation of calcium and are not, or are only partially, neutralized by serum. Therefore, these enzymes should be removed by centrifugation. Other more specific enzymes, such as elastase, hyaluronidase, and DNase, are used in specific situations.

3.3. Neutralization of Enzyme Activity

When enzymes are used, it is essential to neutralize their activity after the cells have become detached from the substratum. Unless neutralization is complete, the subcultured cells will not adhere properly to the new flask or flatten out in the normal fashion, but will remain rounded, with a considerable number floating freely in the culture medium.

1. Serum contains natural trypsin-inhibiting factors that neutralize trypsin and facilitate the cells to adhere to the flask. An equal volume of medium containing 5–10% serum is added to the cell-trypsin solution to inactivate the trypsin.
2. If serum-free medium, or medium low in serum, is used, the cells may be centrifuged out of the enzyme solution, washed with Hanks' balanced salt

solution (HBSS) and resuspended in medium for plating into another culture vessel. This procedure involves some risk of damaging the cells during the centrifugation.

3. In serum-free medium and medium low in serum, soybean trypsin inhibitor (1 mg/mL) may be added to the medium to neutralize the trypsin. Excess of the antitryptic agent should be avoided, since it is somewhat inhibitory to cell growth. Crude trypsin contains a variety of enzymes and the soybean trypsin inhibitor does not neutralize all the enzymes. Therefore, either crystalline trypsin should be used in this procedure, or, after trypsinization with crude trypsin, the cells should be centrifuged, washed, and resuspended for culturing.

4. COMMENTS

1. Cells grown in a serum-containing medium that are to be detached from the substratum by use of proteolytic enzymes should first be rinsed with a BSS to remove all traces of serum before the addition of the enzyme. A calcium- and magnesium-free BSS, such as Puck's, is used for this step when trypsin is used. Other enzymes, such as collagenase, dispase, and pronase, require the presence of calcium for their activity, and should be rinsed with a BSS containing calcium and magnesium, e.g., Hanks' BSS.

2. The pH of the enzyme solution is important for enzyme activity. Trypsin, for example, is nearly inactive below pH 7.0. Raising the pH above 8.0 may damage the cells. It is recommended that trypsin be used at a pH of about 7.5.

3. The crude trypsin may contain viruses, mycoplasma, and various bacteria. Therefore, careful filtration of crude trypsin is necessary and special attention must be paid that the final 0.2 μm filter is intact. Even though the trypsin may be sterile, it may contain variable amounts of endotoxins, which is a good reason for using crystalline trypsin.

4. To avoid crosscontamination between cell lines or primary cultures during subculturing, each cell line or primary culture should be handled separately, including separate bottle of media, BSS, trypsin, and other solutions for each cell line or primary culture. No two cell lines should share a solution from a common bottle.

5. Any method of subculturing cells, mechanical or chemical, causes some damage to the cells. The procedure should be carried out as rapidly as possible, to minimize this damage. The method of subculturing should be appropriate for a given cell line. Procedures effective with one cell line are not necessarily suitable for use with a different cell line.

5. APPENDIX

5.1. Trypsin-Versene Method for Removing Cells from the Substratum

1. Remove the medium and add calcium- and magnesium-free Puck's BSS.
2. Wash cells and remove Puck's BSS.
3. Add just enough 0.025% trypsin and 0.01% versene mixture to cover the cells and incubate at room temperature, until cells round up and begin to come off the tissue culture vessel (observe under the microscope). Disperse the cells by pipeting gently several times.
4. When the cells are dispersed, add growth medium containing 5% serum and triturate the cells to disperse them in the medium. Avoid the creation of air bubbles.
5. Count well-suspended cells immediately in hemocytometer, if required. Make a suitable cell dilution in medium for subculturing.
6. Add the cell suspension to the new culture vessel and incubate.

5.2. Preparation of Solutions

1. 1% Trypsin:
   a. Add 2.5g 1:250 trypsin (Gibco-BRL, 27250) to approx 200 mL Puck's BSS. Stir until totally dissolved and make up to 250 mL with Puck's BSS.
   b. Filter through stacked filters of 5.0, 1.2, 0.45 μm, and 0.2 μm pore size.
   c. Aliquot and store at −20°C.
2. 0.02% Disodium ethylenediaminetetra-acetate (EDTA or versene):
   a. Dissolve 0.2 g EDTA (disodium salt) in 1000 mL Puck's BSS.
   b. Dispense in convenient amounts and sterilize by autoclaving.
3. Trypsin-Versene solution for disaggregation of cells for subculturing: 1 part 0.05% trypsin in Puck's BSS and 1 part 0.02% Versene (EDTA).
4. Puck's BSS, magnesium- and calcium-free (Puck's BSS):

NaCl	80.0 g
KCl	4.0 g
$Na_2HPO_4 7H_2O$	0.9 g
KH_2PO_4	0.6 g
Glucose	10.0 g

   Dissolve the above quantities in 1000 mL high quality water. Sterilize by filtration through a 0.2-μm filter.

   Note: 0.02 g phenol red solution may also be added (if desired) before sterilization of the stock solution.

FURTHER READING

Bottenstein, J. , Hayashi, I., Hutchings, S., Masui, J., Mather, J., McClure, D. B., Ohasa, S., Rizzino, A., Sato, G., Serrero, G., Wolfe, R., and Wu, R. (1979), The growth of cells in serum-free hormone-supplemented media, in *Methods in Enzymology Cell Culture*, Jakoby, W. B. and Pastan, I. H., eds., Academic, New York, pp. 94–109.

Melnick, J. L. and Wallis, C. (1977), Problems related to the use of serum and trypsin in the growth of monkey kidney cells, in *Developments in Biological Standardization*, Perkins, F. T. and Regamey, R. H., eds., S. Karger, Basel, pp. 77–82.

McKeehan, W. L. (1977), The effect of temperature during trypsin treatment on viability and multiplication of single normal human and chicken fibroblasts. *Cell Biol. Int. Reports* **1**, 335–343.

Waymouth, C. (1982), Methods for obtaining cells in suspension from animal tissues, in *Cell Separation Methods and Selected Applications,* vol. 1, Pretlow, T. G. and Pretlow, T. P., eds., Academic, New York, **1,** 1–29.

Waymouth, C. (1993), *Tissue Dissociation Guide*, Worthington Biochemical Corporation, Freehold, NJ, pp. 1–78.

Chapter Eighteen

Preparation of Tissue-Cultured Material for Electron Microscopical Observation

Richard M. Devon

1. INTRODUCTION

Electron microscopy is an invaluable tool that has enabled investigators to visualize, at high resolution, the fine structure of cells. Many steps are required in preparing tissue for electron microscopy; these include fixation, dehydration, embedding (infiltration and polymerization), mounting, and sectioning, as well as collection and staining of the sections. At each step, it is possible to introduce artifacts that affect the end results. Therefore, an understanding of the rationale for performing each step (i.e., rates of penetration for various types of fixatives, buffer combinations, infiltration rates, and temperatures used) will assist the investigator in preventing, or at least reducing, the number of possible artifacts that can cause the deterioration of the final image obtained by the electron microscope.

Many of the variables outlined above are less problematic when using electron microscopy as a tool to investigate cells in culture. Cells are more readily available to the fixatives because of the reduced distances that fixatives have to penetrate and the increased surface area for the action of the fixative. There is also the advantage that once fixed, cells or tissues in culture can be embedded directly within the tissue culture chambers, thus preserving natural cellular structure and cellular relationships. Fine structural details of cells in culture can be correlated with light or phase

Protocols for Neural Cell Culture, 2nd Ed. • Eds.: S. Fedoroff and A. Richardson • Humana Press, Inc., Totowa, NJ

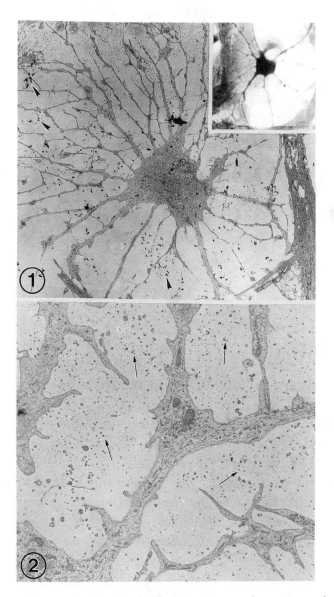

Fig. 1. Low power electron micrograph showing an en face view of a cultured glial cell exhibiting numerous processes. Arrowheads denote osmium blacks precipitate attached to both the culture substratum and the cell processes. Inset, light micrograph of the same cell in culture, embedded and stained with toluidine blue prior to sectioning for electron microscopy.

Fig. 2. Electron micrograph of a culture that was not washed free of serum proteins prior to fixation. These serum proteins precipitate and can be seen attached to the culture substratum as well as to the glial cell processes, giving the appearance of a dirty or gritty background.

contrast images (Fig. 1). The following method has been developed to optimize the fixation of cells in cultures, but may be also applied to thin explant, slice, or aggregate cultures by increasing the fixation, dehydration, and infiltration times (*see*

Section 2.). It should also be emphasized that extreme caution should be exercised in using most of the solutions for electron microscopy (i.e., cacodylate buffer, osmium tetroxide, glutaraldehyde, formaldehyde, potassium ferricyanate, Araldite) because of their carcinogenic or toxic qualities.

2. PREPARATION OF CULTURES FOR ELECTRON MICROSCOPY

2.1. Materials

Cells grown on Aclar or Thermanox coverslips or on plastic tissue culture substrate.
Hanks' balanced salt solution (BSS).
Formaldehyde (2%).
Glutaraldehyde (25%).
Osmium tetroxide (4%).
Stock solutions of 0.08, 0.1, and $0.11M$ sodium cacodylate.
Potassium ferricyanide (2.5%).
Epon 812.
Dodecenyl succinic anhydride hardener/964 (DDSA).
Araldite 502.
2,4,6-tri(dimethyl amino methyl)phenol (DMP) 30.
Stock solutions of 50, 70, 90, 95, and 100% ethanol.
Electron microscope grids.
Formvar (0.5%).
Toluidine blue (1%).
Uranyl acetate (4%).
Lead citrate.

2.2. Procedure

2.2.1. FIXATION

1. Rinse cultures twice in Puck's or Hanks' BSS prewarmed to 37°C to remove any serum proteins.
2. Remove the rinse with a Pasteur pipet.
3. Carefully add primary fixative, preheated to 35–37°C, to the culture dish or onto the coverslip. Fix for a minimum of 15 min.
4. Replace with preheated fresh fixative; continue fixing for an additional 15 min.
5. Rinse the cultured cells twice in $0.08M$ cacodylate buffer (at room temperature) for 5 min each rinse. Remove the rinse completely with a Pasteur pipet.
6. Gently add the secondary fixative to the cells by filtering the osmium blacks solution through a 10 mL syringe, with a 0.2 μm filter attached, and postfixing the cells for a minimum of 40 min.

7. Remove the spent fixative and repeat the postfixation by adding fresh osmium blacks for another 30 min.
8. Rinse with two 5-min rinses in 0.08M cacodylate buffer.

Note:
a. If the serum proteins are not removed from the cultured cells, they will precipitate out of the growth medium on fixation and attach to the culture substrate or cell processes, giving the cultured cells a gritty appearance (Fig. 2, arrows) under the electron microscope.
b. The secondary fixative is freshly prepared by adding the osmium tetroxide to 2.5% potassium ferricyanide to form osmium blacks (NB: Osmium blacks are more reactive than straight osmium tetroxide, rapidly crosslinking membrane phospholipids and proteins and thereby better preserving the fine structure of membranes. This mixture is recommended for revealing the fine structure of myelin membranes). The osmium blacks solution must be filtered through a 0.2-μm filter, otherwise large precipitates of osmium will remain attached to the culture substrate and interfere with visualization of the cells (Fig. 1, arrowheads).

2.2.2. DEHYDRATION

1. After the buffer rinses, dehydrate the cells by immersion through two 5-min changes of cold 50, 70, 90, and 95% ethanol.
2. Complete the dehydration stage by immersing the cells in three changes of 100% ethanol for 10 min each. The final change in 100% ethanol is allowed to come to room temperature.

Note:
a. The ethanol is stored in a refrigerator to keep it at 4°C at all times. Cold dehydration minimizes cellular distortion and limits the formation of shrinkage artifacts.
b. If block staining is required, this should be performed at the 70% ethanol dehydration stage; tissue should be brought to room temperature and the block stained and dehydrated at room temperature (*see* Section 3. for solutions).

2.2.3. EMBEDDING—INFILTRATION AND POLYMERIZATION

1. Prepare increasing concentrations of 25, 50, 75, and 100% Epon/Araldite and pipet them, in turn, onto the cultured cells (at room temperature) for 1 h intervals each. During this infiltration process, wear disposable gloves and take care to ensure that the cells are always covered.
2. Infiltrate the cells overnight in pure Epon/Araldite and change with fresh Epon/Araldite to a depth of 2–3 mm the next day.

3. Polymerize the Epon/Araldite by placing the cells in a vacuum oven at 55°C for 24–36 h. Once polymerized, remove the embedded material from its surrounding tissue culture plastic while still warm.

Note:

a. Infiltration of the embedding material is generally assisted by using propylene oxide as the penetrating medium. However, use of this medium rapidly destroys any type of tissue culture plasticware. To circumvent this problem, we prefer to use ethanolized Epon/Araldite as the penetrant for the embedding material (Unicryl may also be used). This must be prepared well in advance, since ethanol and Epon/Araldite do not readily mix.

b. If cells are grown on Aclar® or Thermanox® coverslips, the coverslips may be left on or stripped off, depending on the plane of sectioning, since this will not affect sectioning perpendicular to the culture surface. It is important to ensure that the polymerization temperature is not allowed to rise above 55°C, since it becomes more difficult to separate the embedded material from its attached and surrounding tissue culture plastic. The surface of the embedded material should resemble a polished surface when the separation occurs properly.

2.2.4. STAINING AND MOUNTING

1. Stain the embedded cells by floating the polymerized Epon/Araldite for 1–2 h on a weak solution of toluidine blue (*see* Section 3.) that has been preheated to 50°C.
2. Select an appropriate or representative area of cells and cut these areas out of the embedded material with a small coping saw (or remove with a leather punch apparatus).
3. Mount cells to be cut en face (i.e., in the same plane as the growth substrate) on aluminium stud mounts with fast-setting epoxy resin.
4. Trim appropriate areas for ultramicrotomy.

Note:

a. Cells can be stained with a weak solution of toluidine blue (Humason, 1979; after Trump et al., 1961), since they are in close proximity to the external surface of the polymerized embedded material. Cells that take up the stain can be visualized through a light or dissecting microscope (Fig. 1, inset).

b. Material that is to be transversely sectioned (i.e., sections cut perpendicular to the growth substrate) can be mounted directly onto an ultramicrotome for light and electron microscopy sectioning.

2.2.5. SECTIONING

1. Cut silver to gray thin sections using a diamond knife on the ultramicrotome.

2. Collect the sections on the surface of the water bath.
3. Immerse a cotton tip into 100% chloroform.
4. Chemically stretch the sections with chloroform vapor by holding the cotton tip close to the sections.
5. Mount the sections on 2-mm 100 meshcopper grids and store in a grid holder.

Note:

a. Section thickness is monitored by visualizing the reflective coloring of the sections. The following table lists the sequence of colors correlated with the approximate thicknesses of sections:

Dark gray	<40 nm
Gray	40–50 nm
Silver	50–70 nm
Gold	70–90 nm
Purple	>90 nm

It is generally accepted that the thinner the section, the better the resolution and final appearance on the electron micrograph. The optimum section thickness for general electron microscopy work using regular staining techniques is between silver and gray.

b. Sections are chemically stretched to minimize drift when they are placed under the electron beam.

c. When large areas of section are to be photographed, it is easier to mount the sections on Formvar (or carbon) coated 2-mm slot grids. This gives the sections the support they require to withstand the electron beam and allows visualization of larger areas of cultured tissue, including complete aggregates. The Formvar coating will slightly reduce the contrast of the image, however.

2.2.6. STAINING FOR ELECTRON MICROSCOPY

1. Prepare a large drop of uranyl acetate for each grid by adding one drop of 100% ethanol to each.
2. Stain the sections in uranyl acetate by picking up the grid with fine jeweler's forceps, wetting the section on the grid with double-distilled water, and placing the grid section-side down onto the drop for 12 min.
3. Rinse the grids by repeated immersion (30×) in a beaker containing 50% ethanol.
4. Rinse further in a gentle stream of double-distilled water for 30 s.
5. Dry the grid by placing filter paper between the tines of the forceps to absorb excess water.
6. Stain the section in lead citrate by placing the grid section-side down on a fresh drop of lead citrate (*see* Section 3.) for 15 min.

7. Rinse the sections in a gentle stream of double-distilled water for 30 s.
8. Dry the grid by again placing the filter paper between the tines of the forceps to absorb excess water.
9. Store the grids in a numbered grid box.
10. Examine under the electron microscope.

Note:

   a. Staining of cytoplasmic proteins is achieved by initial staining in uranyl acetate. Magnesium uranyl acetate (4%) is stored in a 10-mL syringe kept in the cold at 4°C and is filtered through 0.2 μm filter just prior to use.

   b. Grids must be held parallel to the flow of the stream of water to minimize section destruction.

   c. Staining of membranous structures is achieved by secondary staining in Reynold's lead citrate.

   d. Although there are many modifications that can be made to these methods, a high degree of reproducibility in forming good electron microscopic images (Fig. 3) can be achieved by following this schedule.

2.2.7. COMMENTS

1. To optimize fixation, there must be rapid penetration within the cell or tissue, so that cessation of biochemical processes rapidly occurs and the integrity of ultrastructural organelles is preserved. If the cell is not killed rapidly by the fixative, artifacts may be produced, and therefore the fine structural compartments of the cell may not be readily identified under the electron microscope, leading to problems in analysis and quantification. Certain fixatives, such as osmium tetroxide, may cause certain artifacts, such as gross swelling, as well as hardening of the tissue during fixation. Shrinkage often occurs in the dehydration stage. Tissues can also swell during infiltration by embedding resins (Hayat, 1981).

2. Regular fixation protocols do not suit all aspects of electron microscopy. If immuno-electron microscopy is required, an appropriate choice of fixatives (such as periodate lysine or low concentration formaldehyde; Hayat, 1981) must be considered, since some fixatives render the antigenic binding sites on cell membranes inactive. In addition, infiltration and polymerization with embedding materials, such as water-soluble methacrylate or Unicryl®, must be employed, since the heat required for proper polymerization of many embedding materials will also destroy antigenic sites in the cells or tissues. Referring to an appropriate text on electron microscopy techniques, such as Meek (1973) or Hyatt (1981), will minimize the production of such problems.

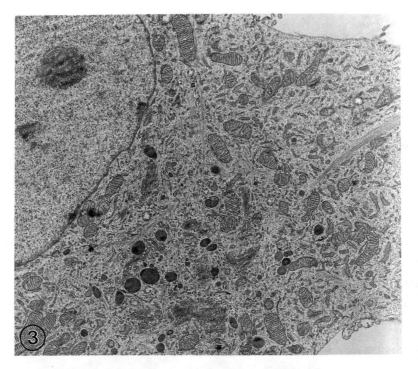

Fig. 3. Electron micrograph taken from a silver-gray section of a glial cell, showing excellent ultrastructural preservation and resolution of cellular organelles, as well as even staining of cytoplasmic components. Note the excellent preservation of membranous structures. There is very little artifactual precipitate.

3. APPENDIX

3.1. Solutions

1. Sodium cacodylate (BDH Chemicals, Poole, England)
   a. Make up a 0.2M sodium cacodylate stock: 21.403 g of sodium cacodylate in 500 mL of distilled water.
   b. Make up 0.11M sodium cacodylate (for potassium ferricyanide): Add 20 mL of distilled water to 25 mL of 0.2M sodium cacodylate.
   c. Make up 0.08M sodium cacodylate (for rinsing): Add 37 mL of distilled water to 25 mL of 0.2M sodium cacodylate.
2. 2% Formaldehyde (stored as stock solution at 4°C):
   a. Weigh out 0.4 g paraformaldehyde (BDH Chemicals, Toronto, Canada) and add to 10 mL distilled water.
   b. Heat while stirring in fume hood to 55°C (do not exceed 60°C).
   c. When temperature is reached, add 2 drops of 1M NaOH (BDH Chemicals) to clear.

    d. Filter while hot through Whatman #1 filter paper.

    e. Add 10 mL of this solution to 10 mL of 0.2M cacodylate buffer (final cacodylate concentration = 0.1M).

3. 2.5% Potassium ferricyanide (make fresh for each fixation) (J. T. Baker, Phillipsburg, NJ):

    a. Weigh out 0.5 g potassium ferricyanide.

    b. Add to 20 mL of 0.11 M sodium cacodylate.

    c. Stir on a magnetic stirrer until completely dissolved.

4. Primary fixative:

    a. Add 6.75 mL of 0.08M sodium cacodylate to 6.75 mL of stock 2% formaldehyde.

    b. While swirling, add 1.5 mL of 25% TAAB-EM grade glutaraldehyde (Marivac, Halifax, Nova Scotia, Canada).

    c. Now add 2 drops of 5% $CaCl_2$ (Fisher Scientific, Fair Lawn, NJ).

    d. Heat to 37°C just prior to fixing the cultured material (0.9% formaldehyde; 2.5% glutaraldehyde; 0.09M cacodylate; osmolarity = 320 mOsm).

5. Secondary fixative (after Russell and Burguet, 1977):

    a. In a fume hood, measure out 2 mL of 4% aqueous osmium tetroxide (Polysciences, Warrington, PA) into a 10-mL graduated cylinder.

    b. Add 6 mL of 2.5% potassium ferricyanide.

    c. Draw this solution up into a 10-mL syringe.

    d. Place 0.2 µm filter on the syringe and filter secondary fixative directly onto the cultures (1.88% potassium ferricyanide; 1% osmium tetroxide; 0.082M cacodylate).

    Note: Potassium ferrocyanide can also be used for excellent preservation of glucose and phospholipids in brain tissues (*see* de Bruijn and Den Breejen, 1975).

6. Epon/Araldite (Modification of Mollenhauer, 1964):

    a. Measure out in a disposable plastic graduated beaker the following: 50 mL of Epon 812 (Fisher Scientific); 40 mL of Araldite 502 (Polysciences); and 120 mL DDSA (J.B. EM Supplies, Dorval, Quebec).

    b. Mix these compounds using a magnetic stir bar for 90 min.

    c. Add 4.2 mL of DMP 30 (Ted Pella, Redding, CA).

    d. Mix this in thoroughly and rapidly.

    e. Stir for an additional 1 h.

    f. Store in 60-mL syringes in freezer until required.

    g. Use within 4 mo.

3.2. Stains

1. Toluidine blue (Fisher Scientific):
   a. Weigh out 1 g of toluidine blue.
   b. Add to 100 mL of 1% sodium tetraborate (Fisher Scientific, Nepean, ON).
   c. Boil solution and filter while hot through a Whatman #1 filter paper.
   d. For staining solution, add 10 mL of stock stain to 100 mL of distilled water.

   Note: Sections embedded in plastic will stain satisfactorily with basic dyes in alkaline solutions in the pH 11.0 range. Whole cells embedded in Epon/Araldite will stain when floated on a weak solution of toluidine blue (<1.0%) incubated at 60°C for 2 h (Fig. 1, inset). Areas of the culture can then be scanned and selected for sectioning.

2. Uranyl acetate (BDH Chemicals, England):
   a. Prepare an aqueous solution of 20% magnesium uranyl acetate.
   b. Weigh out 4 g of magnesium uranyl acetate.
   c. Add 100 mL of distilled water.
   d. Stir on magnetic stirrer until dissolved.
   e. Keep stock solution in air-tight syringe at 4°C.
   f. Filter through 0.2 μm filter prior to use.

3. Lead citrate (Modification of Reynolds, 1963): Stocks (all 1M):
   a. Dissolve 35.7 g of sodium citrate (Fisher Scientific, NJ) in 100 mL of double-distilled water.
   b. Dissolve 33.1 g of lead nitrate (Fisher Scientific) in 100 mL of double-distilled water.
   c. Dissolve 4 g of sodium hydroxide (BDH Chemicals, Canada) in 100 mL of double-distilled water.

   Technique:
   a. Measure out 16 mL of double distilled water into a clean graduated cylinder.
   b. Add 3 mL of 1M sodium citrate. Cover with Parafilm® (American National Can, Greenwich, CT) and shake.
   c. Add 2 mL of 1M lead nitrate. A white precipitate will form.
   d. Shake this precipitate until the solution becomes milky.
   e. Add 4 mL of 1M sodium hydroxide to obtain a clear solution. The solution will clear after the addition of 2 mL of sodium hydroxide, but 4 mL is necessary. Shake this solution to convert all precipitate. **If this solution does not clear, start again with clean glassware** or, if using old stocks, make up fresh stocks.
   f. Store in a clean glass container.

g. Pour paraffin oil on top of storage container to exclude air.

This solution will store at 4°C for several months.

3.3. Notes for Fixation of Tissue Slices or Aggregates

When using thicker tissues, such as aggregates, slices, or explants, the fixation, dehydration, and infiltration times are increased as follows:

1. Primary fixation: 1 to 2 hr with rotation stirring followed by fresh change overnight at 4°C.
2. Buffer rinses: 30 min minimum.
3. Secondary fixation.
   2-4 h with rotation stirring at room temperature.
4. Dehydration: 30 min minimum each change for 50% through to 95% ethanol; 1 h change for 100% ethanol.
5. Embedding: infiltration of 1–2 h with rotation stirring; final change into 100% Epon/Araldite, overnight at room temperature. Block out into fresh change of 100% Epon/Araldite prior to polymerization in a vacuum oven.

FURTHER READING

Buckley, I. K. (1971), A simple technique for comparative light and electron microscopy of designated living cultured cells. *Lab. Invest.* **25**, 295–301.

de Bruijn, W. C. and Den Breejen, P. (1975), Glycogen, its chemistry and morphologic appearance in the electron microscope. II. The complex formed in the selective contrast staining of glycogen. *Histochem. J.* **7**, 205.

Giammara, B. L. and Hanker, J. S. (1986), Epoxy-slide embedment of cytochemically stained tissues and cultured cells for light and electron microscopy. *Stain Technol.* **61**, 51–58.

Hayat, M. A., ed. (1981), *Fixation for Electron Microscopy*, Academic, New York.

Humason, G. L., ed. (1979), *Animal Tissue Techniques*, W. H. Freeman, San Francisco.

Meek, G. A., ed. (1973), *Practical Electron Microscopy for Biologists*, Wiley-Interscience, London.

Mollenhauer, H. H. (1964), Plastic embedding mixtures for use in electron microscopy. *Stain Technol.* **39**, 111–114.

Reynolds, E. S. (1963), Use of lead citrate at high pH as an electron-opaque stain in electron microscopy. *J. Cell Biol.* **17**, 208–212.

Russell, L. and Burguet, S. (1977), Ultrastructure of Leydig cells as revealed by secondary tissue treatment with a ferrocyanide-osmium mixture. *Tissue Cell* **9**, 751.

Trump, B. F., Smuckler, E. A. and Benditt, E. P. (1961), A method for staining epoxy sections for light microscopy. *J. Ultrastruct. Res.* **5**, 343–348.

Chapter Nineteen

Tips in Tissue Culture

Arleen Richardon and Sergey Fedoroff

1. BIOLOGICAL CONTAMINATION

1.1. Use of Antibiotics

Good aseptic technique is superior to the use of antibiotics in tissue culture. In certain cases, however, the prophylactic use of antibiotics is invaluable. Antibiotics should be used when the starting material for primary cultures is not sterile, e.g., tissue obtained from the abattoir, human tissue obtained during surgery or postmortem, and tissue from nasal passages, gastrointestinal and urogenital tract, and skin. In such cases, the tissue should be bathed in a solution containing a high concentration of antibiotics before initiating cultures. Antibiotics can also be used in the cultures, but for as short a period of time as possible, up to a maximum of 2 wk of culturing. Antibiotics can also be used prophylactically in experiments in which the cultures are terminated at the end of the experiment. In exceptional cases, antibiotics may be used to decontaminate irreplaceable cultures *(see below)*.

1.1. Bacterial Contamination

Bacterial infection in cultures is manifested by cell debris, a decrease in pH of the medium, and turbidity of the medium. Bacteria can be seen under the microscope at high power. A low level of bacterial contamination or slow growing bacteria may go undetected; however, the cells in the culture will exhibit slowed and uncharacteristic growth.

Protocols for Neural Cell Culture, 2nd Ed. • Eds.: S. Fedoroff and A. Richardson • Humana Press, Inc., Totowa, NJ

Cultures containing bacteria, as well as any reagents used with those cultures, must be autoclaved and discarded. In exceptional cases, an attempt can be made to save irreplaceable cultures by extensive washing, treatment with high concentrations of antibiotics, and subculturing the cells into as many cultures as possible to enhance the probability that some will be free of contamination. If the use of antibiotics is unacceptable, extensive washing (ten times or more) of the culture and subculturing into 96-well plates may produce some cultures free from bacterial contamination.

1. Procedure for decontamination:
   a. Prepare a solution of antibiotics in Hanks' balanced salt solution (HBSS). We use a high concentration penicillin and streptomycin solution, which has a broad bactericidal spectrum against gram-positive and gram-negative bacteria. The solution is made up at 50× the recommended working concentration *(see below)*.
   b. Wash the culture with Hanks' BSS at least five times, or more, if heavily infected.
   c. Treat with the antibiotic solution for 1–3 h. Examine the cultures about every 20 min. As soon as the morphology of the cells begins to change (round up), remove the antibiotic solution and replace with fresh medium.
   Note: The antibiotics at 50× the recommended concentration can be cytotoxic to cells; therefore, it is important to remove the solution as soon as the cells show any sign of change in normal morphology.
   d. Incubate cultures for 24 h at 37°C.
   e. After 24 h, examine the cultures for the presence of bacteria. If bacteria are present, the cultures may be washed, split into many small cultures using 96-well plates, or steps a–d may be repeated.
2. Solutions:
   a. Penicillin and streptomycin solution: The recommended concentrations of antibiotics for prophylactic use in cell culture are 100 U/mL penicillin G and 100 μg/mL streptomycin. However, the concentration of antibiotics tolerated by cells will vary for the cell type.

      The high concentrations of antibiotics in Hanks' BSS that we use for decontamination are: penicillin G 5000 U/mL; streptomycin 5000 μg/mL.
   b. Hanks' BSS:

NaCl	8.0 g/L
KCl	0.4 g/L
$Na_2HPO_4 2H_2O$	0.06 g/L
KH_2PO_4	0.06 g/L
$CaCl_2$	0.14 g/L
$MgSO_4 7H_2O$	0.2 g/L

NaHCO$_3$	0.35 g/L
Phenol red	0.02 g/L
Glucose	1.0 g/L

3. Comments:

    a. The sensitivity of cells to antibiotics can be determined by the neutral red, MTT or XTT assays (see Chapter 16), since the toxic effects of the antibiotic reduces the uptake of the dye. The combination of two or more antibiotics may lower the concentration at which cytotoxicity occurs for each of the individual antibiotics and, therefore, should be tested in the combination in which they will be used.

    b. Gentamicin sulfate is a broad spectrum antibiotic sometimes used in place of streptomycin. It is bactericidal in vitro and is effective against gram-negative and some gram-positive bacteria, some penicillin-resistant strains of bacteria, and some mycoplasmas. The effective prophylactic concentration is 50 μg/mL.

1.2. Fungal Contamination

Common fungi in cultures grow as single cells, such as yeast, or multicellular mycelium (molds). A change in pH and turbidity of the medium may indicate the presence of yeast. However, mold infections of cultures may be unnoticed until they have grown large enough to be readily apparent (many long intertwined branching filaments in one section of the culture dish). Yeast is usually noticed first when the culture is examined under the microscope. Yeast appears as refractile ovals in chains or branches, or showing evidence of budding, and is usually found throughout the culture. The common sources of fungal contamination in the tissue culture laboratory are humidified incubators, cardboard, and the tissue culture personnel.

Cultures containing fungi must be autoclaved and discarded. In addition, the incubators in which the cultures were grown must be thoroughly cleaned and disinfected, and all reagents used with the contaminated cultures discarded.

1. Antifungal agents commonly used in tissue culture include amphotericin B (Fungizone®) and nystatin (mycostatin®). The prophylactic concentration of amphotericin B is 2.5 μg/mL and that of nystatin is 50 μg/mL or 100 U/mL.

2. Amphotericin B, depending on the concentration used and the susceptibility of the fungal contamination, is either fungistatic or fungicidal. Nystatin is fungistatic. Therefore, if these antibiotics are used prophylactically, they should be used continuously throughout the experiment, since removal of the antibiotic may allow any fungi present to proliferate.

1.3. Other Biological Contaminants

1. Mycoplasma: Mycoplasmas have many effects on cell cultures, e.g., changes in growth rate and metabolism of cells, induction of chromosomal aberrations, depletion of arginine in culture medium, and so on, but are difficult to detect. The major sources of mycoplasma in the tissue culture laboratory are cross- contamination from infected cell cultures, serum and nonautoclavable medium additives, primary tissue (gastrointestinal and respiratory tract), and laboratory personnel.

   Since contamination of cell cultures by mycoplasma is difficult to detect, periodic screening of cultures is recommended. Although there are many screening methods available (see ATCC Quality Control Methods for Cell Lines, 1992) it is usually more accurate, less time consuming, and therefore cheaper to send samples to a laboratory that specializes in testing for mycoplasma contamination (ATCC, Rockville, MD; Bionique Testing, Saranac Lake, NY). **Note:** Mycoplasmas are not removed by conventional 0.2 μm filters.

   Cultures and cell lines infected with mycoplasmas and all reagents used with them must be autoclaved and discarded.

2. Endotoxins: Endotoxins (lipopolysaccharides) from the membranes of gram-negative bacteria are common contaminants in tissue culture. They have many and varied effects on cells, even when present in nanogram quantities. Endotoxins are released during the growth of bacteria, when the membranes are sloughed off or when the bacteria die and lyse. Bacterial contamination in the water purification system or during preparation of culture media will result in contamination with endotoxins, even if the bacteria are removed by filtration. Water is the major source of endotoxin contamination, but endotoxins are also present in sera and other biological materials, such as soybean trypsin inhibitor, bovine serum albumin, growth factors, and so on.

   a. The *Limulus* Amebocyte Lysate (LAL) test is recommended for the quantification of endotoxin in water and for monitoring levels in reagents and in tissue culture media and additives. Kinetic turbidimetric and gel clot method kits are available (Associates of Cape Cod, Inc., MA), both of which are quick and easy to use.

   b. Serum used in tissue culture medium should be selected for its low endotoxin level.

2. WATER

The importance of high quality water in cell culture cannot be overemphasized. High quality water is essential not only as a solvent for culture medium and reagents, but also as the final rinsing step used in the preparation of glassware for tissue culture. Water quality is especially critical when cells are grown in serum-free medium.

2.1. Water Purification

Water can be purified by distillation, ion exchange (deionization), carbon adsorption, microporous membrane filters, ultrafiltration, and reverse osmosis. Each of these procedures has certain advantages and disadvantages, but no one procedure by itself is satisfactory for obtaining water of a quality high enough for tissue culture purposes. The solution is to combine a number of the procedures in sequence. Systems are available that use a number of replaceable cartridges for carbon adsorption, ion exchange, ultrafiltration, and finally a 0.2-μm filter. Such a system can remove by ultrafiltration particles with a molecular weight of more than 10 kDa. Most endotoxins (lipopolysaccharides) are larger than 20 kDa and therefore are removed by ultrafiltration. A 0.2-μm final filter removes all particles and microorganisms larger than pore size. Sometimes it is necessary to prepurify the water before it is fed into the system, to extend the life of the cartridges.

Using equipment composed of several purification steps, it is possible to obtain large amounts of ultrapure, type I reagent grade water as defined by the College of American Pathologists (CAP), the American Society for Testing and Materials (ASTM), and the National Committee for Clinical Laboratory Standards (NCCLS). Water acceptable for tissue culture use must be free of endotoxins and organic contaminants, be essentially ion free, and have a resistivity close to 18 MΩ/cm at 25°C (resistivity of chemically pure water has been calculated to be 18.3 MΩ/cm).

The water content of inorganic and ionizable solids, organic contaminants, and particulate matter varies from one geographical region to another and, therefore, the requirements for purification of water may vary. The best way to determine the quality of the water is to send a sample of the water for analysis to Barnstead/ Thermolyne, IA, or to Millipore, MA, or to analyze the quality of the water by a resistivity monitor (purity meter) and by high performance liquid chromatography (HPLC). The water purification system to be used depends greatly on the amount of water required and the geographical location.

1. Ultrapure water should be used within a day of its production and should not be stored longer, since the highly purified water has the capability of leaching out impurities from the storage container (Pyrex™ or plastic). These contaminants then become part of the medium and tissue culture solutions or are deposited on glassware.
2. All water purification systems require monitoring, proper maintenance, and cleaning to ensure continued water quality. All tubing in contact with the

water purification system should be changed frequently to prevent microbial and algae growth. Bacterial growth can occur in resin beds, storage vessels, distillation apparatus, and so on, and therefore maintenance should be carried out on a regular basis.

3. STERILITY CONTROL

3.1. Autoclaving

Autoclaves are effective sterilizers only if materials to be autoclaved are properly wrapped and placed in such a way that the steam has access to them. The autoclave should not be overloaded. The autoclave must be operating properly, maintaining both temperature and pressure (121°C, 15 psi).

To ensure that sterilization has occurred, commercial indicators can be used. The best indicators of sterilization take into account the parameters of time, temperature, and steam penetration. Indicators such as Steriolmeter-plus® (ATI, Somerville, NJ) can be placed in the center of a pack, inside capped tubes, and so forth and only when the temperature is reached (121°C), and 12–16 min have elapsed, do the indicators change color. It should be noted that the endpoint for most indicators is variable and that the minimum autoclaving time is 15 min.

Autoclave tapes are available to attach to the outside of packs. They change color during autoclaving; most do not indicate that the product is sterilized, but simply indicate that items have been exposed to autoclaving.

Nontoxic materials should be used to wrap items to be autoclaved. There are many commercially available wrappers (Dualpeel® Tubing, Baxter Healthcare, IL; SteriLine® white paper bags, Thomas Scientific, Swedesboro, NJ) designed for use in autoclaves. In addition, unbleached cotton muslin may be used for bagging large glassware and envelopes of various sizes can be constructed from 27 lb uncoated vegetable parchment paper (available from restaurant supply companies).

Steam used for sterilization in autoclaves can contain many impurities, including the contaminants present in the feedwater and additives that prevent scale formation and corrosion. These contaminants are deposited on the sterilized material, which then can be dissolved in solutions used in cell culture. The addition of a steam filter (Balston, MA), placed as close to the steam inlet as possible, eliminates impurities in the steam before it enters the autoclave. The steam filters should be changed on a regular basis.

3.2. The Laboratory Environment

The tissue culture laboratory may be a single room designated for cell culture or may simply be space in a larger multipurpose room. It is usually defined by the presence of a laminar flow cabinet and an incubator. A laminar flow hood is advantageous for maintaining a sterile environment for preparation of cultures and provides personnel or product protection, or both. However, a laminar flow hood is not an absolute requirement for tissue culture. A desk top that is clean and in a dust-free environment can be used for tissue culture purposes if aseptic techniques are meticulously followed.

It is important to be familiar with the environment of the room in terms of air flow, traffic patterns, and possible sources of contamination. The placement of bacteriological plates throughout the room and at different times of day and night can aid in determining the changes needed to optimize the area for cell culture. The plates should be exposed for 30 min to 1 h and then incubated as usual. Bacterial (sheep blood agar, tryptic soy agar, and so on) and fungal (Saboraud dextrose agar and others) plates are placed in front of all air vents and around doors entering the room. Plates are also placed on and around major equipment in the room (centrifuges, refrigerators, ice machines, and the like), on and around the laminar flow hood and incubator, and areas of traffic (including the floor) that are near the working space. The growth of bacteria or fungi on the plates will pinpoint problem areas and appropriate steps can then be taken to eliminate or minimize the sources of contamination.

3.3. Medium and Other Cell Reagents

It is important to monitor the sterility of media and other cell reagents as an integral part of a quality control program. Media may be tested for bacteria and fungi by inoculating fluid thioglycolate broth, trypticase soy broth, Sabouraud dextrose broth, and blood agar plates. A bacteria and fungi detection kit may be purchased from ATCC.

To ensure sterility of large volumes of media, it is important that adequate sampling is done. In our laboratory, we remove a sample of the filtered medium at the beginning and end of filtration and in addition, a 25 mL sample is removed after filtering every liter of medium. All bottles of filtered medium and samples are numbered in sequence so that problems that occurred during filtration can be readily identified. These samples are incubated at room temperature until the entire batch of medium is used. Any samples that show signs of microbial contamination are matched to the numbers on medium bottles. Those bottles of medium are discarded.

Media are also tested for growth-promoting qualities on primary cultures or cell lines that are routinely used in the laboratory. In addition, media can also be tested using a plating efficiency assay (*see* Chapter 12).

3.4. Incubators

1. Carbon dioxide: For better control of pH during culturing, incubators in which the amount of carbon dioxide in the atmosphere can be controlled are used.

It is important for proper pH control that the carbon dioxide concentration in the incubator corresponds to the concentration of the bicarbonate buffer in the medium. Purchased media with specified concentrations of bicarbonate buffer require specified concentrations of carbon dioxide. For example, Eagle's Minimum Essential Medium (MEM) with Hanks' BSS does not require additional carbon dioxide in air. Such a medium is designed for a regular atmospheric environment. Eagle's MEM with Earle's salts requires an atmosphere of 5% carbon dioxide in air; Dulbecco's modified Eagle's medium requires an atmosphere containing 10% carbon dioxide.

The gas mixtures fed into the incubator from pressurized tanks may contain impurities that may be cytotoxic. Therefore, an in-line hydrophobic filter should always be inserted between the gas cylinder and the incubator.

2. Cleaning incubators: Incubators that have high humidity and operate at 37°C provide an excellent environment for growth of molds and yeasts. Therefore, incubators should be cleaned on a regular basis (every 2–3 mo), or at the first sign of mold or yeast contamination. We use the following method to clean our incubators:

   a. The incubator is turned off and unplugged.

   b. All removable parts (shelves, and so forth) are taken out, washed, rinsed with good quality water, and autoclaved.

   c. The incubator is dried with lint-free towels and carbon dioxide sensors are covered with plastic. The incubator is then sprayed with a good quality disinfectant (not bleach) (e.g., Super Bacterole, Magic White Western, SK.), paying particular attention to corners, seam lines, and so on. The incubator is closed and left for approx 2 h.

   d. The incubator is rinsed with distilled water until all traces of the disinfectant are removed. It is then dried with lint-free towels.

   e. The incubator is sprayed with 70% ethanol, again paying particular attention to corners and seam lines. A pan of 70% ethanol is placed in the incubator. The incubator is closed and left for approx 24 h.

   f. After 24 h, the 70% ethanol is removed, all surfaces are dried and the incubator is reassembled.

4. VISIBLE FLUORESCENT LIGHT

Visible fluorescent light is detrimental to media, sera, and cells in culture because of the generation of free radicals in the media. Light affects tryptophan and tyrosine, with riboflavin acting as a photosensitizer. Wavelengths up to 450 nm are responsible for the deleterious effects and to eliminate them certain precautions must be taken.

1. Fluorescent tubes in the light fixtures in the laminar flow hoods and in the tissue culture room can be replaced by yellow fluorescent tubes (Westinghouse 40 Watt, F 4OGO Gold; General Electric Gold). This will reduce the formation of free radicals in media.

2. Sera, especially fetal bovine and calf serum, which have low levels of catalase activity, should be stored in the dark and protected from light by the use of yellow plastic bags.

3. HEPES-containing media is particularly sensitive to the effects of visible fluorescent light. Bottles containing media with HEPES as a buffering agent should always be wrapped in aluminum foil.

4. As a rule, all media should be stored and cultures grown in the dark. Incubators with glass doors must have the glass covered to prevent any light from entering the incubator.

FURTHER READING

(1992), Testing for microbial contaminants, in *ATCC Quality Control Methods for Cell Lines*, Hay, R. J., Caputo, J., and Macy, M. L., eds., American Type Culture Collection, Rockville, MD, pp. 19–48.

Fogh, J., ed. (1973), *Contamination in Tissue Culture*. Academic, New York, pp. 1–288.

Gabler, R., Hegde, R., and Hughes, D. (1983), Degradation of high purity water on storage. *J. Liquid Chromatog.* **6,** 2565–2570.

Goule, M. C. (1984), Endotoxin in vertebrate cell culture: its measurement and significance, in *Uses and Standardization of Vertebrate Cell Cultures*, Tissue Culture Association, MD **5,** 125–136.

Mather, J., Kaczarowski, F., Gabler, R., and Wilkins, F. (1986), Effects of water purity and addition of common water contaminants on the growth of cells in serum-free media. *BioTechniques* **4,** 56–63.

Perkins, J. J. (1969), *Principles and Methods of Sterilization in Health Sciences*. Charles C, Thomas, Springfield, IL, pp. 1–549.

Perlman, D. (1979), Use of Antibiotics in cell culture media, in *Methods in Enzymology: Cell Culture,* vol. 58, Jacoby, W. B. and Pasten, I. H., eds., Academic, New York, pp. 110–116.

Rottem, S. and Barile, M. F. (1993), Beware of mycoplasmas. *Trends Biotechnol.* **11,** 143–150.

Ryan, J. A. (1994), Understanding and managing cell culture contamination. Corning, Inc. Technical Publication TC-CI-559, Corning, NY.

Taylor, W. G. (1984), Toxicity and hazards to successful culture: cellular responses to damage induced by light, oxygen or heavy metals, in *Uses and Standardization of Vertebrate Cell Cultures*, Patterson, M. K., ed., Tissue Culture Association, MD, 58–70.

Wang, R. J. and Nixon, T. (1978), Identification of hydrogen peroxide as a photoproduct toxic to human cells in tissue-culture medium irradiated with "daylight" fluorescent light *In Vitro* **14,** 715–722.

Zigler, J. S., Lepe-Zuniga, J. L., Vistica, B., and Gery, I. (1985), Analysis of the cytotoxic effects of light-exposed HEPES-containing culture medium. *In Vitro Cell. Devel. Biol.* **21,** 282–287.

Chapter Twenty

Use of Dissecting
Instruments in Tissue Culture

Arleen Richardson

1. INTRODUCTION

Dissecting instruments must be used to remove tissues from live animals. Surgical procedures that involve the cutting of the skin and removal of tissues usually require *medium-fine instruments. Fine instruments* are essential when the operational area is small and the operator has to work with the aid of a head loupe or dissecting microscope.

2. STERILIZATION OF DISSECTING INSTRUMENTS

Effective sterilization of instruments depends on how well the instrument has been cleaned prior to sterilization. Instruments in contact with tissue may retain dried material that resists penetration by the sterilizing agent. Therefore, the first step in sterilization is proper cleaning of the instrument.

2.1. Cleaning Dissecting Instruments

Immediately after use place the instrument in a tray containing distilled water and lined with a soft material. Never drop an instrument into a container, and be especially careful to avoid damaging the tips of fine instruments.

Protocols for Neural Cell Culture, 2nd Ed. • Eds.: S. Fedoroff and A. Richardson • Humana Press, Inc., Totowa, NJ

1. Manual cleaning: Soak the instruments for a short while, then remove them one at a time and clean carefully with gauze, clean cloth, or soft brush to remove any tissue remnants or blood. A very dilute nontoxic soap solution may be used for cleaning, but careful rinsing with hot tap water followed by distilled water is necessary. Dry the instruments thoroughly before storage or sterilization.
2. Ultrasonic cleaning:
    a. Follow the manufacturer's recommendations for the cycle time.
    b. Instruments should be in the open position and completely submerged. Instruments of similar metal content should be cleaned together.
    c. After ultrasonic cleaning, instruments should be rinsed carefully in warm tap water followed by distilled water to completely remove cleaning solution.

2.2. Sterilization and Disinfection by Alcohol

Alcohols leave no residues on surfaces and are effective agents for sterilization and disinfection. Methanol, ethanol, and isopropanol are used as bactericidal agents at concentrations of 70–80% alcohol in water.

1. Alcohol dip:
    a. Immerse instruments in 70% ethanol and allow to dry in air inside the laminar flow hood.
    b. Repeat this procedure three times.
2. Alcohol flaming:
    Note: All instruments that have been heated should be allowed to cool before use.
    a. Immerse instrument in 70% ethanol (in a heat-proof container with metal lid). Remove the instrument from the ethanol, replace the lid on the ethanol container, and pass the instrument through the flame of a gas burner. Repeat this three times for each instrument.
    Caution: Make sure the flame is completely out before reimmersing the instrument in the ethanol. If the ethanol does catch on fire, immediately replace the metal lid.
    b. General comments:
        i. Flame scissors in alcohol in the open position.
        ii. It is sufficient to flame the distal third of the instrument, since the handle of the instrument does not have to be sterile.
        iii. **Do not** carry too much alcohol with the instrument to be flamed!
        iv. **Do not** keep the instrument in the gas flame while the alcohol is burning.
        v. **Never** heat the instruments to red-hot heat.

Note: Instruments may be damaged by high heat, depending on the alloy used and the degree of hardness. Titanium alloy, for example, is heat resistant to temperatures up to 500°C.

2.3. Autoclaving Instruments

1. Instruments may be placed in an instrument box or wrapped individually, in the open position, for sterilization. Autoclave at 121°C for 30 min on a "wrapped" cycle. After autoclaving, run a dry cycle or place instruments in a drying oven.

Note: Sterilization of instruments by autoclaving is rapid and efficient; however, instruments that are not stainless steel will be damaged by rust unless they are completely dried.

2. Secure instruments firmly when using an instrument box, so that they do not move when the box is handled. Tips of forceps may be placed in glass tubes, so that the points do not reach the end of the tube, thus protecting them from damage. Gauze may be placed between layers of instruments.

2.4. Glass Bead Sterilizers (Inotech Biosystems International, Lansing, MI)

1. Fill the well of the sterilizer with glass beads.
2. Switch on the sterilizer approx 20 min before use.
3. After the temperature reaches 250°C, insert dry and clean instruments for at least 5–10 s, depending on their size.
4. Place instruments in a sterile glass Petri dish and allow them to cool before use.

3. PREPARATION OF STERILE INSTRUMENTS FOR USE

Keep the sterilized instruments in a sterile glass Petri dish in such a way that the handles of the instruments rest on the edge of the Petri dish and the tips are inside. Use the lid of the Petri dish to cover the tips of the instruments.

4. APPENDIX

4.1. Comments

1. An instrument should be used for the purpose for which it is designed. The most common mistake is to try to cut or handle larger or harder tissues than the particular instrument is able to do. Irreparable damage may result from these attempts and the instrument may become useless. Most fine instruments are manufactured from hardened stainless steel and some from titanium. The handling and care of fine instruments differs from the handling

and care of ordinary laboratory instruments. The price of the fine instrument is generally very high.

2. Fine instruments selected for a particular project should be regarded as personal items and never be made available for general use by many people in a laboratory.

3. The care of the instruments after use is important. The dealers usually recommend the use of fine oil for the lock screw of moving parts of the scissors, and so on. However, instruments for fine dissection purposes in the tissue culture laboratory are **not** to be oiled, since this may create problems with the oil mixing with the dissected tissues or becoming burned on the steel. Scissors with spring handles should be stored open to prevent tiring of the spring. Short lengths of flexible tubing may be used as tip protectors during storage. Every instrument should be examined before usage under a dissecting microscope. The ends of forceps and scissors should be of equal length, the tips should meet perfectly, and in addition, the shearing edges should be sharp.

4. Any repair of fine instruments should be done by a professional. Remember that the cutting parts of a pair of scissors can be easily overheated by the grinding process and ruined because of the change in the hardness of the steel.

Abbreviations and Definitions

acryl	acrylamide
anhyd	anhydrous
Ara-C	cytosine arabinoside
A/2	half the normal area
A2B5	monoclonal antibody that identifies common sialogang-liosides and sufatides in cell surface membranes of neurons, neuroendocrine, and goal cells
5-BUdR	5-bromodeoxyuridine
bis	bisacrylamide
BSA	bovine serum albumin
BSS	balanced salt solution
CD14	cluster of differentiation 14; anti-CD14, monoclonal antibody that identifies cell surface membrane glycoprotein in human microglia and monocytes
CD45	cluster of differentiation 45; anti-CD45, monoclonal antibody that identifies leukocyte common antigen
CD45^{hi}	leukocyte cell population having a high expression of common leukocyte antigen
cDNA	complementary DNA
C.I.	color index
CNS	central nervous system
CSF-1	colony stimulating factor-1, also known as macrophage colony stimulating factor (MCSF)
CUSA	Cavitron™ ultrasonic aspiration
DAB	3,3'-diaminobenzidine
DDSA	dodecenyl succinic anhydride
DlL-ac-LDL	1,1'-dioctadecyl-3,3,3',3'-tetramethyl-indocarbocyanate per chlorate, labels low density lipoproteins in lysosomes
DM5	chemically defined serum free medium
DME(M)	Dulbecco's modified Eagle's medium
DME(M)/F12	Dulbecco's modified Eagle's medium and Ham's nutrient mix ture F-12

DMP	2,4,6-tri(dimethylaminomethyl)phenol
DMSO	dimethyl sulfoxide
DNA	deoxyribonucleic acid
DNase	deoxyribonuclease
DPBS	Dulbecco's phosphate-buffered saline
DRG	dorsal root ganglion
DRGN	dorsal root ganglion neuron
E	embryonic age (e.g. E18 = 18-d-old embryo)
EBM	Eagle's basal medium
EDTA	ethylenediaminetetra-acetic acid (versene)
EGF	epidermal growth factor
ELISA	enzyme-linked immunosorbent assay
EM	electron microscope
EMEM	Eagle's minimum essential medium
F4/80	cell surface membrane antigen of unknown function, restricted to cells of mononuclear phagocyte system
FBS	fetal bovine serum
FUdR	5'-fluoro-2'-deoxyuridine
GalC, GalCer	galactocerebroside expressed on cell surface membrane in oligodendroglia
GBSS	Gey's balanced salt solution
GD3	a ganglioside, major glycolipid component of immature neuroectodermal cells and immature oligodendroglia
GFAP	glial fibrillary acidic protein, protein of intermediate filaments in astroglia
GHAP	glial hyaluronic acid protein
GQ1 c	a ganglioside expressed on cell surface membrane, used as marker for oligodendroglia precursor cells
GS	glutamine synthetase
Ham's F12	Ham's nutrient mixture F-12
H-Buffer	homogenization buffer
HEBM	Eagle's basal medium with supplements
HEPES	N-2-hydroxyethylpiperazine-N'-2-ethanesulfonic acid, used as buffer in media
HS	horse serum
IgG	immunoglobulin G
IL	interleukin, a cytokine, usually identified by number (e.g., IL-1)

L-15	Leibovitz's L-15 medium
Leu-M5	human monocyte, macrophage, and microglia antigen, a subunit of CD11c heterodimer
LPS	lipopolysaccharide (endotoxin)
Mac-1	monoclonal antibody that identifies complement 3 receptor (CR3), used as marker for microglia and macrophages
Mac-3	glycoprotein on mouse mononuclear phagocytes outside bone marrow
MAP2	microtubule-associated protein 2, present in neurons
MAP5	microtubule-associated protein 5, present in neurons
MBP	myelin basic protein
MEM	minimum essential medium
MEMg	minimum essential medium with glucose
MEMgi	minimum essential medium with glucose and insulin
MHC	major histocompatibility complex
μCi	microcurie
mMEM	modified Eagle's minimum essential medium
MOG	myelin oligodendrocyte glycoprotein
mRNA	messenger RNA
MTT	3-(4,5-dimethylthiazol-2-yl)-2,5-diphenyltetrazolium bromide
N1	defined culture medium supplement
N2	defined culture medium supplement
NF H	neurofilament (180–200 kDa)
NF L	neurofilament (60–70 kDa)
NF M	neurofilament (130–170 kDa)
ng	nanogram
NGF	nerve growth factor
nm	nanometer
nM	nanomolar
NMA	nadic methyl anhydride
NTF	neurotrophic factor
0-2A	oligodendrocyte progenitor cell
04	monoclonal antibody, recognizes sulfide, used as an oligodendroglia marker
OD	optical density
OPM	oligodendroglial precursor cell medium
OPM-G	oligodendroglial presursor cell medium with glucose
P0	postnatal d 0 (day of birth)

P7   postnatal d 7
PBS   phosphate-buffered saline
PE   plating efficiency
P/G (Pen/Glu)   penicillin/glutamine
PNS   peripheral nervous system
Puck's D-GS   Puck's salt solution D and gentamicin-sulfate
RIA   radioimmunoassay
RT97   antibody to neurofilament protein
SCG   superior cervical ganglion
SDS   sodium dodecyl sulfate
SM131   antibody to neurofilaments, phosphorylated M and H subunits
STO   mouse embryonic fibroblast cell line
SYN   synaptophysin
TEMED N,N,N',N'-tetramethylethylenediamine
Thy-1   cell surface membrane glycoprotein; in mice two acetic forms are expressed, thy-1.1 and thy-1.2
TNF   tumor necrosis factor
v/v   volume per volume
Vim   vimentin, protein of intermediate filaments

Index